# Socio-cultural Dimensions of Emerging Infectious Diseases in Africa

Godfrey B. Tangwa • Akin Abayomi
Samuel J. Ujewe • Nchangwi Syntia Munung
Editors

# Socio-cultural Dimensions of Emerging Infectious Diseases in Africa

## An Indigenous Response to Deadly Epidemics

Springer

*Editors*
Godfrey B. Tangwa
Department of Philosophy
University of Yaounde 1
Yaounde, Cameroon

Cameroon Bioethics Initiative (CAMBIN)
Yaounde, Cameroon

Global Emerging Pathogen Treatment
Consortium (GET) Consortium
Lagos, Nigeria

Samuel J. Ujewe
Global Emerging Pathogens Treatment
Consortium
Lagos, Nigeria

Canadian Institute for Genomics
and Society
Toronto, ON, Canada

Akin Abayomi
Global Emerging Pathogen Treatment
Consortium (GET) Consortium
Lagos, Nigeria

Nigerian Medical Research Institute
(NIMR)
Lagos, Nigeria

Faculty of Medicine and Health Sciences
University of Stellenbosch
Stellenbosch, South Africa

Nchangwi Syntia Munung
Department of Medicine
University of Cape Town
Cape Town, South Africa

Global Emerging Pathogen Treatment
Consortium (GET) Consortium
Lagos, Nigeria

ISBN 978-3-030-17473-6 ISBN 978-3-030-17474-3 (eBook)
https://doi.org/10.1007/978-3-030-17474-3



This Springer imprint is published by the registered company Springer Nature Switzerland AG.
The registered company address is: Gewerbestrasse 11, 6330 Cham, Switzerland

# Preface

Epidemics caused by emerging infectious diseases (EIDs) are fueled by a variety of complex drivers, and it becomes imperative that a strategic plan to prevent or manage epidemics or outbreaks of EIDs will have multiple facets.

The West African Ebola outbreak which commenced in December 2013 and was only recognized as Ebola in March or April 2014 is a perfect example of a multifaceted health problem. It soon became apparent that indigenous medical and cultural practices were the key catalysts of the rapid spread of the epidemic. The Global Emerging Pathogens Treatment Consortium (GET), was born at the height of the epidemic in August 2014. GET is a consortium made up of African indigenous experts drawn from all walks of life, with the required expertise to mount a holistic response to an EID outbreak. GET grew rapidly with the support of many international collaborators, and organized itself into work groups addressing issues related to: research ethics; clinical trials; blood product component therapy; community engagement; anthropological and social issues; biobanking; biocontainment; and logistics.

One of the major drivers of the rapid spread of the EVD outbreak in West Africa were social and cultural practices; thus, the Cultural, Anthropological, Social and Economic (CASE) work group was formed and became a leading player in the strategic response to the outbreak. Cultural practices that were driving the outbreak as well as those that were retarding response strategies were quickly targeted by the CASE work group with the aim of mitigating and adapting to the changing dynamic of the situation.

It could even be said that one of the interventions that helped to turn around the momentum of the outbreak were in the socio-cultural domain - interventions related to: sanitation, traditional burial practices, stigmatization and discrimination.

The CASE work group has grown from strength to strength. Led by its Chairperson, Professor Godfrey B Tangwa, the work group rapidly conceptualized a documentary of cultural, economic and anthropological issues on the micro and macro levels. It was clear that, as a global community, we often forget, during public health emergencies, to address socio-cultural issues that could engender global secuity risk.

The 2014 Ebola outbreak has taught us many things. It has taught us, most importantly, that during periods of a dangerous epidemic, it is easy for human rights to be abused and for cultural sensitivities to be sidelined. This is amplified when the epidemic has the potential of transforming into a pandemic.

This book is concieved as an inter-/intra-disciplinary publication with contributions from several knowledge domains. Some of its chapters are jointly authored by experts from different disciplinary perspectives. It would therefore have a broad appeal across disciplines including: medical sciences, research ethics, regulation and governance, health communication and the social sciences. It is our hope that this book will be an encouragement for all global health stakeholders, who are committed to improving basic health standards in Africa, a continent that has historically borne the heavy burden of enslavement, colonisation, exploitation, poverty and, disease, all in spite or perhaps because of its enormous resources and potentialities.

We are therefore happy to present this compilation that highlights many of the philosophical, scientific, social and anthropological issues experienced during the 2014 Ebola outbreak in West Africa. This by no means exhausts issues that need discussion. However, it is arguably the first comprehensive attempt by African scholars, researchers and their collaborators to address major socio-cultural concerns linked to the management of EIDs such as Ebola, Lassa Fever, Monkeypox and Zika for all global communities to deliberate upon because pandemics know no boundaries, and all communities are at risk and vulnerable.

We hope that you will enjoy this collection and that it would stimulate further reflection and preparedness on how to contain future epidemics of EIDs.

Lagos, Nigeria
Yaounde, Cameroon
Cape Town, South Africa
Toronto, Canada

Akin Abayomi
Godfrey B. Tangwa
Nchangwi Syntia Munung
Samuel J. Ujewe

February 2019

# Contents

# About the Editors

**Godfrey B. Tangwa** is emeritus professor of the University of Yaounde 1, Cameroon, where he was head of the Department of Philosophy from 2004 to 2009. He is a fellow of the Cameroon Academy of Sciences (CAS) and the African Academy of Sciences (AAS), vice chairperson of the Cameroon Bioethics Initiative (CAMBIN) which he founded in 2005, an executive committee member of the Pan-African Bioethics Initiative (PABIN) and chairperson of the Cultural, Anthropological, Social and Economic (CASE) work group of the Global Emerging Pathogens Treatment Consortium (GET). He has extensive teaching and research experience in the domains of philosophy and bioethics. He obtained a BA (1977) from the University of Nigeria, Nsukka; an MA (1979) from the University of Ife (now Obafemi Awolowo University), Ile Ife; and a PhD (1984) from the University of Ibadan, all in Nigeria. He has served on several expert advisory committees for the WHO, has been a member of the Scientific Ethics Advisory Group (SEAG) of Hoffmann La Roche since 2005 and is currently also an advisory board member of both ALERRT and SARETI. His publications' record shows about 10 books, 35 book chapters and 45 journal articles.

**Akin Abayomi** is professor of Medicine at the Nigerian Institute of Medical Research in Lagos, Nigeria. Prior to that, he was the chief pathologist and head of the Division of Haematology, Faculty of Medicine and Health Sciences, Stellenbosch University, Cape Town, South Africa. A specialist in internal medicine and haematology, environmental health and biosecurity, Professor Abayomi studied at the Royal Medical College of St Bartholomew's Hospital in the University of London where he attained his first graduate degree in Medicine. He has obtained fellowships from the Royal College of Medicine and Pathology in the United Kingdom and the College of Medicine of South Africa. He has worked in several countries around the world in both internal medicine and haematology and has been exposed to a variety of geographical variations and disease patterns within these areas. His focus has mainly been on the concept of emerging diseases like Ebola, HIV and TB and the development of laboratory and clinical capacity in Africa. He is the cofounder and principal investigator of the Global Emerging Pathogens Treatment Consortium (GET).

**Samuel J. Ujewe** is a scholar, researcher and analyst in Bioethics and Health Policy, especially health research ethics, healthcare ethics, mental health ethics, indigenous populations' health ethics and policy, global health ethics and policy, ethics of infectious disease management and international and cross-cultural bioethics. His research interests span through integrating major ethical theories with relevant indigenous principles and values to enhance just, responsible and actionable health policies and interventions, especially in African health systems. His research focuses on the intersection of ethics and policy, using a moral compass that aligns with indigenous contexts. He obtained a PhD in Bioethics and Health Policy from the University of Central Lancashire, UK; a Master of Health Sciences (MHealSc) in Bioethics from the University of Otago, New Zealand; and a First Class BA Hons in Philosophy from the University of Zimbabwe. He has since completed two Postdoctoral Fellowships at the University of Pretoria, South Africa, and McMaster University, Canada. He is currently an adjunct research fellow at the Canadian Institute for Genomics and Society, where he undertakes collaborative research on the ethical implications of genomic innovations for indigenous settings.

Dr. Ujewe is an associate fellow of the Higher Education Academy, UK; a member of the International Forum of Teachers of Ethics, Bioethics and Medical Law (IFT); and a fellow of the Global Emerging Pathogens Treatment Consortium (GET), working with the "Cultural, Anthropological, Social and Economic (CASE) Impact Work Group". He has also held Visiting Research Fellowships at the University of Central Lancashire in Cyprus and The Nathaniel Center, New Zealand.

**Nchangwi Syntia Munung** is based at the University of Cape Town (UCT), South Africa. She holds an MSc in Biochemistry and in Medicine. Her current research focus is on the governance of global health research, with a focus on justice and fairness in genomics research and biobanking in Africa. She also has an interest in science communication and public engagement with science.

# Chapter 1
# Editorial: African Perspectives and Approaches for African Healthcare Challenges

**Samuel J. Ujewe, Nchangwi Syntia Munung, Akin Abayomi, and Godfrey B. Tangwa**

## 1.1 Introduction

Sub-Saharan Africa is heavily endowed with natural and human resources. Yet, these same resources appear to be the bane of its poor development. "*Until the rotten tooth is pulled out, the mouth must chew with caution*", says a Nigerian proverb. Despite being surrounded by wealth, several existing challenges deter African populations from taking full advantage as others have in other regions of the globe. Crucial among these challenges is the health of the population and nature of healthcare accessible to them. African populations cannot enjoy the benefits of their great resource endowment until their health and wellbeing receive considerable attention. By 'Africa', we refer to countries south of the Sahara that largely represent the

S. J. Ujewe (✉)
Canadian Institute for Genomics and Society, Toronto, ON, Canada

Global Emerging Pathogens Treatment Consortium, Lagos, Nigeria

N. S. Munung
Department of Medicine, University of Cape Town, Cape Town, South Africa

Global Emerging Pathogen Treatment Consortium (GET) Consortium, Lagos, Nigeria

A. Abayomi
Global Emerging Pathogen Treatment Consortium (GET) Consortium, Lagos, Nigeria

Nigerian Medical Research Institute (NIMR), Lagos, Nigeria

Faculty of Medicine and Health Sciences, University of Stellenbosch, Stellenbosch, South Africa
e-mail: abayomi@sun.ac.za

G. B. Tangwa
Department of Philosophy, University of Yaounde 1, Yaounde, Cameroon

Cameroon Bioethics Initiative (CAMBIN), Yaounde, Cameroon

Global Emerging Pathogen Treatment Consortium (GET) Consortium, Lagos, Nigeria



G. B. Tangwa et al. (eds.), *Socio-cultural Dimensions of Emerging Infectious Diseases in Africa*, https://doi.org/10.1007/978-3-030-17474-3_1

World Health Organisation's Africa Region (World Health Organisation 2017). The Sub-Saharan Africa region consists of several independent states, with varying geographical landscapes and diverse social and cultural outlooks. Yet, there are underlying commonalities that cut across the region:

> There is a great variety and diversity between the different African ethnicities, but they are all united by commonalities that give them a remarkable family resemblance analogous to the family resemblance of groupings that are in some ways remarkably different from one another but all justifiably bracketed under the term "Western" (Tangwa 2017, 104).

Countries in the Sub-Saharan region have at least three things in common: cultural heritage, high burden of disease, and relatively low financial commitment to healthcare (Ujewe 2016). Among the several healthcare problems weighing on Africa's populations, the burden of infectious diseases, such as malaria, tuberculosis, dengue fever, yellow fever constitute over 60% of the disease burden in most African countries (World Health Organization 2014a). Among these, malaria, tuberculosis and HIV/AIDS have some of the highest contribution to mortality and morbidity in the region (Steenhuysen 2015; IHME and The World Bank 2013; WHO 2017). Most countries in the region are endemic with one or more of these diseases. Further to the challenge of the perennial epidemics of these infectious diseases is the frequent outbreak of emerging and re-emerging infectious diseases across the region. The 2013–2015 Ebola epidemic in West Africa brought economic and social life to a halt in Liberia, Sierra Leone and Guinea, and stirred up the social atmosphere in Nigeria and Ghana. These had varying consequences for the countries (UNDG 2015; Cha 2017). Another Ebola outbreak in the Democratic Republic of Congo in 2018 received immediate international attention, and measures were galvanised to contain the disease (WHO 2018; MSF 2018). The renewed effort to contain the DR Congo Ebola outbreak involved local experts, health workers and communities, as well as needed expertise from West Africa and the rest of the world. This partly shows that reliance on local knowledge, experience and understanding of the context can enhance the success of interventions.

Healthcare remains one of the most difficult challenges most African populations bear; yet many countries' annual budgetary allocation to healthcare is well below the 15% recommended by the WHO (World Health Organization 2014b). The challenge lies in the relatively high burden of health expenditure incurred by households in the region, averaging 62% of total country expenditure (World Health Organisation 2017). Additionally, recent reports show that the number of people living in poverty in the region is rising; and with 330 million poor in 2012, the region accounts for 36% of the world's poor (OPHI 2018; The World Bank 2016). With the number of people in poverty rising in the region and high out-of-pocket expenditure for healthcare, the burden of disease is even greater. By implication, this means that those who have money can buy the available healthcare and those without may have to trade off healthcare for other daily needs. Some countries, like South Africa, have advanced healthcare infrastructure and free public healthcare. However, as described in Chap. 19 there are serious questions around accessibility, as the private health facilities generally offer better care than the public facilities, and are not affordable to a large proportion of the population.

The lack of commitment by governments to address healthcare challenges around the region is highlighted by the number of African heads of states seeking medical treatment outside of Africa. In 2017, the President of Nigeria was on a medical vacation in the United Kingdom for over 100 days, following several of such trips previously (Searcey and Iyare 2017). This is similar to other countries in Africa like Angola, Cameroon, Republic of Benin, Gabon, Zambia and Zimbabwe where quite recently, there have been consistent media reports of government leaders leaving their countries to seek healthcare in countries outside of Africa (Zane 2017; Liedong 2017). It is alleged that Nigerians spends $1 billion annually on medical tourism (Nasir 2017), which if invested in the healthcare in Nigeria can make a significant impact, given the low national budgetary allocation to healthcare. Understandably, this figure also accounts for other citizens who seek medical treatment abroad using their own funds. In Uganda, it was alleged that money spent on treating government officials abroad annually is sufficient to build ten higher level hospitals (Ladu 2012). One logical conclusion from this trend is that government leaders in the region do not have confidence in the same health systems they govern. If they do not, who should? Africa's healthcare problems are thus not only of finance and infrastructure, but also of leadership, as noted by the WHO (Musvanhiri 2017).

Notwithstanding the disproportionate burden of disease on Africa, the low total health expenditure for many countries in the region indicates the need for a closer and continuous engagement with the issues. African scholars stand at a vantage position of local knowledge and experience to offer a valuable perspectives and ways forward. Perspectives and approaches motivated from within Africa or by African scholars, researchers, or policy makers may present a clearer outlook of problems and help to device better response strategies. We describe a virtual silence of African voices in the global discourse about healthcare problems affecting the region. While there is a recognisable volume of literature on the economic dimensions of infectious diseases, there is little to none on the socio-cultural implications and impact of emerging deadly infectious diseases, like Ebola and Lassa fever, among others. This is highlighted by the paucity of literature on local perspectives and approaches to the relevant issues. Understanding the socio-cultural underpinnings of emerging deadly infectious diseases in Africa is crucial towards establishing effective and sustainable strategies or frameworks to adequately address existing and future challenges. This will help to create context specific solutions that speak to the uniqueness of African settings in which these diseases occur.

## 1.2 The Virtual Absence of African Perspectives and Approaches

Godfrey Tangwa (2017) highlights the virtual absence of an African voice and perspective in the global discourses of medical research ethics. He notes the sustained dominance of Western ethical ideals, despite Africa being a hub of major infectious diseases and home to numerous medical research and trials. In furthering Tangwa's concern, we note that this observation extends beyond health research ethics to the management and control of infectious diseases in Africa. The envisioned approaches have potentials to better engage African healthcare contexts for better outcomes.

There are volumes of literature that speak to the infamous Ebola epidemic in Africa. In particular, the literature on the socio-economic drivers and impact of the epidemic has gained traction – to mention only a few (Elston et al. 2017; Pálsdóttir et al. 2016; Ordaz-Németh et al. 2017; Himelein and Kastelic 2015; Kastelic and Kastelic 2015; Himelein et al. 2015; Pellecchia et al. 2015; Ippolito et al. 2015; Parpia et al. 2016; Novelli et al. 2018; Maconachie and Hilson 2015; UNDG 2015). The literaturerepresents diverse perspectives about the crisis, providing various recommendations for such epidemics in future. There is also a plausible representation of African voices in this regard. For instance, one edited volume provides a comprehensive outlook of the political economy of the epidemic (Abdullah and Rashid 2017). And another dwells on the broad political underpinnings of the crisis, with a plausible African perspective (Hofman and Au 2017). However, not much attention has been given to the social-cultural and socio-ethical dimensions of the epidemic. In particular, there is a paucity of literature representing African voices in this regard. One edited volume, explores what transpired in the crisis and offers a cautious way-forward towards a future outbreak (Evans, Smith, and Majumder 2016). Yet, only one chapter highlights what may be regarded as presenting an African outlook and future considerations for future Ebola epidemics (Folayan and Haire 2016). The chapter emphasises an African perspective to the outbreak and offers relevant considerations for what a future response should entail. It highlights what the broad focus for managing and controlling infectious disease epidemics in Africa should look like.

Among the sparse presentation in the literature, effort has been made to present: a medical and socio-cultural aspects (Ikuomola 2015); socio-cultural factors associated with the epidemic generally, as well as for specific countries, like Liberia and Guinea (Whembolua et al. 2015; Ravi and Gauldin 2014; Carrión Martín et al. 2016). Of particular interest is the effort to include socio-cultural considerations in containing the Ebola outbreak in the DR Congo in 2018 (Bedford 2018). Giving the crucial place of social, cultural and ethical dimensions of successful interventions during medical emergencies, it is important to advance greater research to enhance the knowledge pool with African perspectives. This will ensure more adequate understanding of the underlying problems from the perspectives of affected populations. It will also engender outcomes that address local needs and aspirations of affected communities. A volume of socio-cultural dimensions of epidemics in Africa, representing African perspectives, is thus a crucial additional resource to broader search for viable solutions for future epidemics. By African response, we mean research, projects, or works that provide local perspectives and response to the challenges of infectious diseases among African populations.

The relevant volume on socio-cultural dimensions of deadly infectious disease epidemics should offer a broad outlook and extensive exploration of Africa-specific perspectives and approaches towards addressing present and future challenges of such crises on the continent. It should provide various local perspectives to local understanding and outlook of deadly infectious diseases in Africa. This would yield context-specific results where they may be urgently needed.

## 1.3 Significance of a Local Perspective and Approach

An objection may be raised regarding the significance of an African-specific outlook and response. Why insist on such approach since various strategies have already been proffered in existing literature? How different will an Africa-specific approach be from those that already exist, especially towards infectious disease management? Although various innovative approaches may already be proffered in existing literature, these largely underestimate the place of context. This is especially applicable to measures derived from universal global health approaches for application in African settings. Global health approaches have obvious benefits for African health systems. There are several examples of how such strategies have been used to alleviate desperate health challenges around the continent.

One example is the "3 by 5" program of the World Health Organisation that aimed to make HIV/AIDS treatments accessible to three million people, especially in Africa, by 2005 (Macklin 2004; World Health Organization 2005). The main strategy of the program hinged on an ethical framework called "accountability for reasonableness" (Daniels 2000, 2007). It is a practical ethical tool that offers guidance towards fairness in healthcare decision-making. It is underpinned by four conditions: (i) *publicity condition,* requiring transparency about the reasons for a decision; (ii) *relevance condition,* specifying what reasons are acceptable; (iii) *appeal/revision,* providing opportunity to review decisions to incorporate new evidence or views; and (iv) *regulative condition,* providing a mechanism to check the implementation of policy decisions. The framework was instrumental in the delivery of the 3-by-5 project. Yet, more could have been achieved, as the anticipated targets were not met. Part of the challenge was that the framework was developed as a universal tool, and little to no attention was paid to the contextual differences in global health (Ujewe 2016). Recognising and understanding the underpinning differences and subtleties in different healthcare contexts is crucial to the success of innovative interventions.

A more comprehensive global health strategy that was extensively applied to African health systems was the Structural Adjustment Programs (SAPs) formulated for use in developing countries and invariably imposed on African countries in the 1980s (Logie and Woodroffe 1993). It was an economic initiative to alleviate poverty in poor countries across the globe. The initiative included trade liberalisation, currency devaluation, removal of government subsidies and price control, and cost recovery in healthcare and education. African countries, being among the poorest in the world, were obliged to enlist for these programs in order to access loans (Logie and Woodroffe 1993). The strategic formulations of the SAPs suggested that their use in Africa would achieve great benefits for its populations. Yet, the outcomes were opposed to the projections, as the failure of the program had adverse effects on African countries that adopted them. For instance, there was a marked depression in health status, marked by increased food insecurity and malnutrition, rising prevalence of ill health, and a decrease in access to healthcare in two-thirds of the African countries that adopted SAPs (Ujewe 2016).

Nevertheless, in the same period, Cuba adopted a locally developed healthcare approach that broadly conflicted with the SAPs strategies, as the blueprint for its healthcare revolution (Brouwer 2011). The Cuban approach has been effective in sustaining greater health and wellbeing for its populations, as Cuba's overall health outcomes in terms of mortality now compares well with, and in some cases better than, those of the United States (Ujewe 2016). Yet, in 2017, the World Health Statistics comparing various health outcomes puts those of most African countries well below those of the United States (World Health Organisation 2017). The points is that a universally endorsed approach does not always or necessarily apply to a variety of local contexts, and that locally conceptualised approaches may be more viable for healthcare contexts in Africa (Ujewe 2016).

Considering the success of Cuba in employing a context-specific healthcare strategy, it is reasonable to proffer similar progress in Africa's healthcare if the strategies employed bear on local outlooks of the relevant health problems, especially those relating to deadly infectious diseases. Cuba's experience becomes a point of reference for health system reforms in Africa. The reforms should draw substantively from the kind of perspectives that present local outlooks to the varied challenges, as well as context-specific responses/approaches towards addressing Africa-specific healthcare challenges. It is thus crucial to present foundational explorations of African local perspectives and response to Africa's healthcare challenges, especially the socio-cultural dimensions.

## 1.4 Contents and Potential Value of an African Perspective and/or Approach

What should constitute relevant perspectives and approaches to population health and healthcare in Africa? It is easy to assume that since population health is a global concern, universal strategies, as developed or promoted by global agencies, like the WHO and World Bank, should suffice for healthcare development or reforms in African contexts. Yet, past events show otherwise, and prompt us to consider different approaches towards healthcare reforms around Africa. For instance, in the early stages of the program to eliminate Onchocerciasis in Africa, led by the WHO and World Bank, a "community-based strategy" (Katabarwa et al. 2000) was adopted as the gold-standard. The idea was to invoke community participation and to appoint and train community-based distributors to distribute Ivermectin, which is the most effective Onchocerciasis drug to date, in their communities.

However, the program and training personnel overlooked the social structure of local communities, and training was only provided in terms defined by 'modern' or 'Western' health-delivery systems (Foster 1987). This led to a failure of the program: for although 'community-based', it involved only a mere request for 'community tolerance' and 'community compliance' (Katabarwa et al. 2000). As an alternative, a "Community-Directed Treatment with Ivermectin (CDTI)" was proposed, tried, and presented towards the ultimate success of the Onchocerciasis control program in Africa. The CDTI approach invites community members collectively to: (a) discuss a relevant health or developmental challenge, and to determine possible interventions; (b) design an approach to implement the intervention within their community; (c) identify the kind of resources needed to accomplish the intervention; and (d) plan how, when, where and by whom it should be implemented (Katabarwa et al. 2005).

The new approach has seen greater success for the Onchocerciasis control program in Africa over the past two decades (Katabarwa et al. 2015). The key to the success was that the CDTI approach incorporated significant social aspects and cultural values of the communities where the program was implemented. It sufficiently engaged local contexts and initiated a co-ownership of the project with relevant communities. In short, it took seriously the African outlook and understanding of the problem, and adopted strategies evolving from the context-specific outlook to address the problem.

Going forward with the broader context of infectious diseases, population health, and healthcare in Africa, the relevant perspectives and effective strategies should be those that similarly recognise the uniqueness of African contexts. African contexts are not unilateral across the board; yet, they have inherent underlying commonalities that form the basis for common action. The context-specific approaches may thus be adapted in varying proportions in different parts of the continent. Also, adopting these approaches should not imply express dismissal of strategies developed and proposed from elsewhere. Externally developed strategies should be subjected to critical scrutiny in the light of African social contexts and the specific understanding of the health care problems from an African outlook. Although Africa is geographically vast and culturally diverse, there are established shared socio-cultural values and moral outlooks (Tangwa 2017), the healthcare problems experienced in much of the of continent are similar, as statistical evidence shows (World Health Organisation 2017). The relevant healthcare intervention approaches must account for African socio-cultural contexts, as these invariably define specific health problems in different parts. They must aim to reflect what affected African communities consider important to their healthcare; not simply what the "world" thinks is important for Africa.

## 1.5 Conclusion: Overview of Book Sections

What is the potential value of African perspectives or approaches to its varied health problems? Or what difference would these make to what is already being achieved through global contributions? The example from the Onchocerciasis control program in Africa may suffice for a response. It is also important to note that the developmental challenges of African countries that bear on healthcare do not translate to limitedness in local context-specific perspectives and/or approaches, and hence of local capacities to address them. The Onchocerciasis case shows, for instance, that local African communities' outlook of their own health problems was overlooked in the effort to provide them with needed health intervention. Presenting African perspectives and adopting African approaches to healthcare will offer a better chance at addressing the varied healthcare challenges.

As part of the effort to advance African perspectives and approaches, the chapters in this book explore various dimensions of emerging and re-emerging deadly infectious diseases. They aim to present the challenges in the light of the socio-cultural dimensions of healthcare and diseases in Africa. The book is divided into four broad sections: Emerging deadly pathogens and clinical practice; Social determinants of EIDs; Global health and governance; Ethics and Policy in the context of EIDs; and Narratives from the field. The first section on Emerging deadly pathogens and clinical practice presents a historical and contemporary overview of emerging infectious diseases in Africa, such as Ebola and Lassa fever, and why and how an African response may be a panacea to emerging infectious diseases in Africa. Section two addresses issues around the social determinants of health. It points to the varied social dimensions and cultural values that bear on the health of African populations, and largely determines the healthcare they get. The third section explores how approaches in global health affect healthcare in Africa and responses to African health issues. It focuses on issues around the politics, economics and strategic involvement of African governments in addressing local health problems. Section four considers the ethical and policy dimensions of healthcare. It points to the kind of ethic that should guide strategic healthcare approaches deployed on the continent, and determines ways in which ethics should guide African health policies. Finally, section five provides accounts of experiences emanating from the past Ebola outbreak in West Africa. It shows that African health and healthcare issues, beyond mere statistics, are everyday problems that affect human populations.

## References


Abdullah, I., & Rashid, I. (Eds.). (2017). *Understanding West Africa's Ebola epidemic: Towards a political economy*. London: Zed Books.

Bedford, J. (2018). *Socio-cultural considerations for vaccine introduction and community engagement*. Brief: Anthrologica.

Brouwer, S. B. (2011). *Revolutionary doctors: How Venezuela and Cuba are changing the world's conception of health care*. New York: NYU Press.

Carrión Martín, A. I., Derrough, T., Honomou, P., Kolie, N., Diallo, B., Koné, M., Rodier, G., Kpoghomou, C., & Jansà, J. M. (2016). Social and cultural factors behind community resistance during an Ebola outbreak in a village of the Guinean Forest Region, February 2015: A field experience. *International Health, 8*(3), 227–229. https://doi.org/10.1093/inthealth/ihw018.

Cha, J. (2017). Lives and livelihoods: The economic impact of Ebola in West Africa. *International Affairs Review*. http://www.iar-gwu.org/content/lives-and-livelihoods-economic-impact-ebola-west-africa

Daniels, N. (2000). Accountability for reasonableness: Establishing a fair process for priority setting is easier than agreeing on principles. *BMJ: British Medical Journal, 321*(7272), 1300.

Daniels, N. (2007). *Just health: Meeting health needs fairly*. New York: Cambridge University Press.

Elston, J. W. T., Cartwright, C., Ndumbi, P., & Wright, J. (2017). The health impact of the 2014–15 Ebola outbreak. *Public Health, 143*, 60–70.

Evans, N. G., Tara, C. S., & Maimuna, S. M. (2016). *Ebola's message: Public health and medicine in the twenty-first century*. Cambridge, MA: MIT Press.

Folayan, M. O., & Haire, B. (2016). History, culture and social norms: Implications for Ebola drug and vaccine clinical trials in affected region. In *Ebola's message: Public health and medicine in the 21st century*. Cambridge, MA: MIT Press.

Foster, G. M. (1987). Bureaucratic aspects of international health agencies. *Social Science & Medicine, 25*(9), 1039–1048.

Himelein, K., & Kastelic, J. G. (2015). *The socio-economic impacts of Ebola in Liberia* (World Bank Other Operational Studies 21893). The World Bank.

Himelein, K., Testaverde, M., Turay, A., & Turay, S. (2015). *The socio-economic impacts of Ebola in Sierra Leone* (Bank Other Operational Studies 22037), The World Bank.

Hofman, M., & Au, S. (2017). *The politics of fear: Médecins sans Frontières and the West African Ebola epidemic*. New York: Oxford University Press.

IHME, & The World Bank. (2013). *The global burden of disease: Generating evidence, guiding policy – Sub-Saharan Africa Regional Edition*. http://www.healthdata.org/policy-report/global-burden-disease-generating-evidence-guiding-policy-%E2%80%93-sub-saharan-africa-regional

Ikuomola, F. I. (2015). *The Ebola virus and West Africa: Medical and sociocultural aspects*. Bloomington: iUniverse.

Ippolito, G., Puro, V., & Piselli, P. (2015). Ebola in West Africa: Who pays for what in the outbreak. *The New Microbiologica, 38*(1), 1.

Kastelic, K. H., & Kastelic, J. G. (2015). *The socio-economic impacts of Ebola in Liberia: Results from a high frequency cell phone survey round five* (Working Paper Report No. 96196).

Katabarwa, N. M., Richards, F. O., Jr., & Ndyomugyenyi, R. (2000). In rural Ugandan communities the traditional Kinship/Clan system is vital to the success and sustainment of the African Programme for Onchocerciasis Control. *Annals of Tropical Medicine & Parasitology, 94*(5), 485–495.

Katabarwa, M. N., Habomugisha, P., Richards, F. O., & Hopkins, D. (2005). Community-directed interventions strategy enhances efficient and effective integration of health care delivery and development activities in rural disadvantaged communities of Uganda. *Tropical Medicine & International Health, 10*(4), 312–321.

Katabarwa, M. N., Habomugisha, P., Eyamba, A., Byamukama, E., Nwane, P., Arinaitwe, A., Musigire, J., Tushemereirwe, R., & AnnetKhainza. (2015). Community-directed interventions are practical and effective in low-resource communities: Experience of Ivermectin treatment for onchocerciasis control in Cameroon and Uganda, 2004–2010. *International Health, 8*(2), 116–123.

Ladu, I. M. (2012). Money spent on VIP treatment abroad can build 10 hospitals. *Daily Monitor*. http://www.monitor.co.ug/News/National/688334-1394344-9hmafbz/index.html

Liedong, T. A. (2017). African politicians seeking medical help abroad is shameful, and harms health care. The Conversation. http://theconversation.com/african-politicians-seeking-medical-help-abroad-is-shameful-and-harms-health-care 82771.

Logie, D. E., & Woodroffe, J. (1993). Structural adjustment: The wrong prescription for Africa? *BMJ: British Medical Journal, 307*(6895), 41.

Macklin, R. (2004). *Ethics and equity in access to HIV treatment: 3 by 5 initiative*. Geneva: World Health Organization.

Maconachie, R., & Hilson, G. (2015). Ebola and alluvial diamond mining in West Africa: Initial reflections and priority areas for research. *The Extractive Industries and Society, 2*(3), 397–400.

MSF. (2018). Democratic Republic of Congo: Ebola update June 2018. *MédecinsSansFrontières (MSF) International*. https://www.msf.org/democratic-republic-congo-ebola-update-june-2018

Musvanhiri, P. (2017). *World Health Organization blames Africa's health care inequality on lack of political will | DW | 30.08.2017*. DW.COM. 30 August 2017. http://www.dw.com/en/world-health-organization-blames-africas-health-care-inequality-on-lack-of-political-will/a-40283418

Nasir, J. (2017). Every year, Nigerians "spend $1bn" on medical treatment abroad. TheCable (blog). 14 April 2017. https://www.thecable.ng/every-year-nigerians-spend-1bn-medical-treatment-abroad.

Novelli, M., Burgess, L. G., Jones, A., & Ritchie, B. W. (2018). "No Ebola… Still Doomed" – The Ebola-induced tourism crisis. *Annals of Tourism Research, 70*, 76–87.

OPHI (Oxford Poverty & Human Development Initiative). (2018). *Global MPI 2017/2018*. https://ophi.org.uk/multidimensional-poverty-index/global-mpi-2016/

Ordaz-Németh, I., Arandjelovic, M., Boesch, L., Gatiso, T., Grimes, T., Kuehl, H. S., Lormie, M., Stephens, C., Tweh, C., & Junker, J. (2017). The socio-economic drivers of bushmeat consumption during the West African Ebola crisis. *PLoS Neglected Tropical Diseases, 11*(3), e0005450.

Pálsdóttir, B., Barry, J., Bruno, A., Barr, H., Clithero, A., Cobb, N., De Maeseneer, J., Kiguli-Malwadde, E., Neusy, A.-J., & Reeves, S. (2016). Training for impact: The socio-economic impact of a fit for purpose health workforce on communities. *Human Resources for Health, 14*(1), 49.

Parpia, A. S., Ndeffo-Mbah, M. L., Wenzel, N. S., & Galvani, A. P. (2016). Effects of response to 2014–2015 Ebola outbreak on deaths from Malaria, HIV/AIDS, and Tuberculosis, West Africa. *Emerging Infectious Diseases, 22*(3), 433.

Pellecchia, U., Crestani, R., Decroo, T., Van den Bergh, R., & Al-Kourdi, Y. (2015). Social consequences of Ebola containment measures in Liberia. *PLoS One, 10*(12), e0143036.

Ravi, S. J., & Gauldin, E. M. (2014). Sociocultural dimensions of the ebola virus disease outbreak in Liberia. *Biosecurity and Bioterrorism: Biodefense Strategy, Practice, and Science, 12*(6), 301–305.

Searcey, D., & Iyare, T. (2017). President Buhari Returns to Nigeria, Facing Serious Challenges. The New York Times, 22 December 2017, sec. World. https://www.nytimes.com/2017/08/21/world/africa/muhammadu-buhari-nigeria-boko-haram.html.

Steenhuysen, J. (2015). *Tuberculosis now rivals AIDS as leading cause of death: WHO | Reuters*. https://www.reuters.com/article/us-health-tuberculosis-global/tuberculosis-now-rivals-aids-as-leading-cause-of-death-who-idUSKCN0SM1Z520151028

Tangwa, G. B. (2017). Giving voice to African thought in medical research ethics. *Theoretical Medicine and Bioethics, 38*(2), 101–110.

The World Bank. (2016). *While poverty in Africa has declined, number of poor has increased*. Text/HTML. World Bank. http://www.worldbank.org/en/region/afr/publication/poverty-rising-africa-poverty-report

Ujewe, S. J. (2016). *Just health care in Nigeria – The Foundations for an African ethical framework*. Preston: University of Central Lancashire.

UNDG, United Nations Development Group. (2015). *Socio-economic impact of Ebola virus disease in West African countries: A call for national and regional containment, recovery and prevention*. Dakar: United Nations Development Group.

Whembolua, G. S., Kambamba, D., Conserve, D., & Tshiswaka, D. I. (2015). *Socio-cultural factors associated with epidemics: The case of 2014 Ebola outbreak* (MPRA Paper No. 83164).

WHO. (2017). *WHO | World malaria report 2017*. WHO. http://www.who.int/malaria/publications/world-malaria-report-2017/en/

WHO. (2018). *Ebola virus disease democratic Republic of Congo: External situation report 13*. 38. Geneva.

World Health Organisation. (2017). *World health statistics 2017: Monitoring health for the SDGs*. Geneva: World Health Organization.

World Health Organization. (2005). *The 3 by 5 initiative*. Geneva: WHO. Available from: http://www.who.int/3by5/en

World Health Organization. (2014a). *Noncommunicable diseases country profiles 2014*. Geneva: World Health Organization.

World Health Organization. (2014b). *WHO global health expenditure atlas: September 2014*. Geneva: World Health Organization.

Zane, D. (2017). Africa's "medical Tourist" Presidents. BBC News, 13 August 2017, sec. Africa. https://www.bbc.com/news/world-africa- 40685040.

# Part I
# Emerging Deadly Pathogens and Clinical Practice

# Chapter 2
# How and Why the Global Emerging Pathogens Treatment Consortium Was Created

**Akin Abayomi and Diran Makinde**

## 2.1 Introduction

Africa is making steady progress in the areas of food and nutrition security, health care delivery, energy, among others, resulting in positive impacts in the socio-economic development of its people. However, the challenges of increasing incidence of emerging and re-emerging infectious diseases (EIDs), the inadequate health care facilities and shortage of human capacity in medical and allied sciences and technologies, are perennial hurdles and constitute a biosecurity threat both locally and globally. The critically urgent need is that of harnessing and deploying science, technology and innovation to address some of these challenges. This need has been the subject of major policy and academic debates of late and Africa, like the rest of the world, has taken some steps towards realising this. Indeed, the critical importance of a nation's ability to create, acquire, accumulate, diffuse and utilize scientific and technological know-how is now widely acknowledged to be a major determinant of a nation's capacity for the industrial and socio-economic development needed to improve a people's quality of life (Mugwagwa et al. 2014).

On January 31st, 2017, African Heads of State and governments, as well as the leadership of the African Union Commission officially launched the Africa Centre

A. Abayomi (✉)
Global Emerging Pathogen Treatment Consortium (GET) Consortium, Lagos, Nigeria

Nigerian Medical Research Institute (NIMR), Lagos, Nigeria

Faculty of Medicine and Health Sciences, University of Stellenbosch, Stellenbosch, South Africa
e-mail: abayomi@sun.ac.za

D. Makinde
Global Emerging Pathogens Treatment Consortium, Lagos, Nigeria

New Partnership for Africa's Development Planning and Coordinating Agency, Midrand, South Africa



G. B. Tangwa et al. (eds.), *Socio-cultural Dimensions of Emerging Infectious Diseases in Africa*, https://doi.org/10.1007/978-3-030-17474-3_2

for Disease Control and Prevention (Africa CDC) in Addis Ababa, Ethiopia (Nkengasong et al. 2017). As detailed in the African Union's *Agenda 2063, a road map strategy for the development of the continent*, some of the concerns that justified the establishment and initiation of an Africa CDC include: a rapid population growth (estimated population 280 million in 1960 and 1.2 billion in 2016); increasing and intensive population movement across Africa, with increased potential for new or re-emerging pathogens to turn into pandemics; existing endemic and emerging infectious diseases, including antimicrobial resistance; threats posed by environmental toxins; among others (African Union 2015). In addition to these concerns, African countries are burdened with insufficient public health assets including inadequate surveillance, laboratory networks, competent workforce and research expertise, all of which hinder evidence-based decision-making. (Africa CDC: Enhancing Africa's Public Health Response through Innovation and Partnerships Concept Note, unpublished, 2017).

The challenges caused by emerging and re emergent infectious diseases have increasingly become exacerbated in their magnitude, in the way they spread and in the way they combine synergistically with other factors to present even bigger challenges (Abayomi 2013; Abayomi and Cowan 2014). Indeed, the health problems facing Africa are enormous and require massive investment and multi-sectorial, pragmatic approaches. Recent debates have focused on the need to build capacity in human capital, technology and infrastructure, to enable Africa make a significant contribution in finding lasting solutions for her own problems and limit overreliance on external donor funding and aid.

This chapter describes the process and outcome of the formation of an African-led initiative towards harnessing the science, technological advances and innovative ideas on the African continent in the quest towards increasing resilience and mitigating the impact of successive infectious disease outbreaks that are capable of causing public health emergencies in our communities.

In March 2014, the World Health Organization (WHO) and the Ministry of Health (MoH) of Guinea reported an outbreak of Ebola haemorrhagic fever in four south-eastern districts of Guinea Conakry (WHO 2015).What followed was an unprecedented loss and destruction of human life which brought into the fore the lack of ability and the inefficiency of African governments and health systems to handle such major health crises. Ebola Virus Disease (EVD) was identified in 1976 through two separate but almost simultaneous outbreaks in the Democratic Republic of Congo (DRC) and Sudan (WHO 2018). Subsequently EVD outbreaks have occurred in at least 12 African countries (Table 2.1), but mostly confined to Central Africa. The Ebola Virus Disease, while highly infectious, has generally been confined to small geographical communities with low total fatality numbers until the West African outbreak in 2014. Prior to that, the highest number of case fatalities was in 2000 when 425 people in Uganda were infected with a fatality rate of 53%. In the DRC, 264 people were infected with a fatality rate of 71% in 2007. EVD is mostly spread through direct contact with body fluids of symptomatic patients and can be stopped by an integrated approach including early diagnosis, contact tracing, patient isolation and care, infection control, and safe burial. Given that the number

**Table 2.1** Known cases and outbreaks of Ebola Hemorrhagic Fever in Africa, in chronological order

| Year | Country | Ebola subtype | Reported number of human cases | Reported number (%) of deaths among cases | Situation |
|---|---|---|---|---|---|
| 1976 | Zaire (Democratic Republic of the Congo – DRC) | Ebola virus | 318 | 280 (88%) | Occurred in Yambuku and surrounding area. Disease was spread by close personal contact and by use of contaminated needles and syringes in hospitals/clinics. This outbreak was the first recognition of the disease. |
| 1976 | Sudan (South Sudan) | Sudan virus | 284 | 151 (53%) | Occurred in Nzara, Maridi and the surrounding area. Disease was spread mainly through close personal contact within hospitals. Many medical care personnel were infected. |
| 1977 | Zaire | Ebola virus | 1 | 1 (100%) | Noted retrospectively in the village of Tandala. |
| 1979 | Sudan (South Sudan) | Sudan virus | 34 | 22 (65%) | Occured in Nzara, Maridi. Recurrent outbreak at the same site as the 1976 Sudan epidemic. |
| 1994 | Gabon | Ebola virus | 52 | 31 (60%) | Occured in Mékouka and other gold-mining camps deep in the rain forest. Initially thought to be yellow fever; identified as Ebola hemorrhagic fever in 1995. |
| 1994 | Ivory Coast | Taï Forest virus | 1 | 0 | Scientist became ill after conducting an autopsy on a wild chimpanzee in the Tai Forest. The patient was treated in Switzerland. |
| 1995 | Democratic Republic of the Congo (formerly Zaire) | Ebola virus | 315 | 250 (81%) | Occured in Kikwit and surrounding area. Traced to index case-patient who worked in forest adjoining the city. Epidemic spread through families and hospitals. |

(continued)

**Table 2.1** (continued)

| Year | Country | Ebola subtype | Reported number of human cases | Reported number (%) of deaths among cases | Situation |
|---|---|---|---|---|---|
| 1996 (January–April) | Gabon | Ebola virus | 37 | 21 (57%) | Occured in Mayibout area. A chimpanzee found dead in the forest was eaten by people hunting for food. Nineteen people who were involved in the butchery of the animal became ill; other cases occurred in family members. |
| 1996–1997 (July–January) | Gabon | Ebola virus | 60 | 45 (74%) | Occurred in Booué area with transport of patients to Libreville. Index case-patient was a hunter who lived in a forest camp. Disease was spread by close contact with infected persons. A dead chimpanzee found in the forest at the time was determined to be infected. |
| 1996 | South Africa | Ebola virus | 2 | 1 (50%) | A medical professional travelled from Gabon to Johannesburg, South Africa, after having treated Ebola virus-infected patients and thus having been exposed to the virus. He was hospitalized, and a nurse who took care of him became infected and died. |
| 2000–2001 | Uganda | Sudan virus | 425 | 224 (53%) | Occurred in Gulu, Masindi, and Mbarara districts of Uganda. The three most important risks associated with Ebola virus infection were attending funerals of Ebola haemorrhagic fever case-patients, having contact with case-patients in one's family, and providing medical care to Ebola case-patients without using adequate personal protective measures. |
| October 2001–March 2002 | Gabon | Ebola virus | 65 | 53 (82%) | Outbreak occurred over the border of Gabon and the Republic of the Congo. |

(continued)

**Table 2.1** (continued)

| Year | Country | Ebola subtype | Reported number of human cases | Reported number (%) of deaths among cases | Situation |
|---|---|---|---|---|---|
| October 2001–March 2002 | Republic of Congo | Ebola virus | 57 | 43 (75%) | Outbreak occurred over the border of Gabon and the Republic of the Congo. This was the first time that Ebola haemorrhagic fever was reported in the Republic of the Congo. |
| December 2002–April 2003 | Republic of Congo | Ebola virus | 143 | 128 (89%) | Outbreak occurred in the districts of Mbomo and Kéllé in Cuvette OuestDépartement. |
| November–December 2003 | Republic of Congo | Ebola virus | 35 | 29 (83%) | Outbreak occured in Mbomo and Mbandza villages located in Mbomodistric, Cuvette OuestDépartement. |
| 2004 | Sudan (South Sudan) | Sudan virus | 17 | 7 (41%) | Outbreak occurred in Yambio county of southern Sudan. This outbreak was concurrent with an outbreak of measles in the same area, and several suspected EHF cases were later reclassified as measles cases. |
| 2007 | Democratic Republic of Congo | Ebola virus | 264 | 187 (71%) | Outbreak occurred in Kasai Occidental Province. The outbreak was declared over November 20. Last confirmed case on October 4 and last death on October 10. |
| December 2007–January 2008 | Uganda | Bundibugyo virus | 149 | 37 (25%) | Outbreak occurred in Bundibugyo District in western Uganda. First reported occurrence of a new strain. |
| December 2008–February 2009 | Democratic Republic of the Congo | Ebola virus | 32 | 15 (47%) | Outbreak occurred in the Mweka and Luebo health zones of the Province of Kasai Occidental. |

(continued)

**Table 2.1** (continued)

| Year | Country | Ebola subtype | Reported number of human cases | Reported number (%) of deaths among cases | Situation |
|---|---|---|---|---|---|
| May 2011 | Uganda | Sudan virus | 1 | 1 (100%) | The Ugandan Ministry of Health informed the public that a patient with suspected Ebola Haemorrhagic fever died on May 6, 2011 in the Luwerodistrict, Uganda. The quick diagnosis was provided by the new CDC Viral Hemorrhagic Fever laboratory, Uganda Viral Research Institute (UVRI). |
| June–October 2012 | Uganda | Sudan virus | 11[a] | 4[a] (36.4%) | Outbreak occurred in the Kibaale District of Uganda. Laboratory tests of blood samples were conducted by the UVRI and the U.S. Centers for Disease Control and Prevention (CDC). |
| June–November 2012 | Democratic Republic of the Congo | Bundibugyo virus | 36[a] | 13[a] (36.1%) | Outbreak occurred in DRC's Province Orientale. Laboratory support was provided through CDC and the Public Health Agency of Canada (PHAC)'s field laboratory in Isiro, and through the CDC/UVRI lab in Uganda. The outbreak in DRC has no epidemiologic link to the near contemporaneous Ebola outbreak in the Kibaale district of Uganda. |
| November 2012–January 2013 | Uganda | Sudan virus | 6[a] | 3[a] (50%) | Outbreak occurred in the Luwero District. CDC assisted the Ministry of Health in the epidemiologic and diagnostic aspects of the outbreak. Testing of samples by CDC's Viral Special Pathogens Branch occurred at UVRI in Entebbe. |

(continued)

**Table 2.1** (continued)

| Year | Country | Ebola subtype | Reported number of human cases | Reported number (%) of deaths among cases | Situation |
|---|---|---|---|---|---|
| March 2014–Present | Guinea, Liberia, Sierra Leone, Nigeria, Senegal, Mali | Ebola virus | 1528[a] | 844 (55.2%)[a] | On-going outbreak across Guinea, northern Liberia, and now eastern Sierra Leone. Numbers of patients is constantly evolving due to the on-going investigation. |
| August 2014–Present | Democratic Republic of the Congo | Ebola virus | 70 | 42 | On August 26, 2014, the Democratic Republic of the Congo (DRC) Ministry of Health notified the World Health Organization of an outbreak of Ebola virus disease (EVD) in Equateur Province (in Lokolia, Boende, and Watshikengo). The index case was a pregnant woman from Ikanamongo Village who butchered a bush animal. She became ill with symptoms of EVD, reported to a private clinic in Isaka Village, and died on August 11, 2014. Local customs and rituals associated with death meant that several healthcare workers were exposed to Ebola virus. This outbreak is unrelated to the current outbreak of Ebola in West Africa. |

Source: NEPAD Agency (2015)
[a]Numbers reflect laboratory confirmed cases only

of cases involved in the past was low and isolated and that affected countries implemented safeguard measures based on their previous experiences of dealing with the epidemic, the EVD was controlled by rigorous interventions provided by national health systems which were effective in minimizing further transmissions.

Disease epidemics that spread regionally or globally and affect populations worldwide pose bio-security threats and are a cause for great concern among public health professionals and the general public alike. EVD outbreak in West Africa has demonstrated that events starting in one country can swiftly appear in another country. The threat of imported diseases has increased, owing to several factors, including increased opportunities for disease emergence due to the effects of globalization, international spread through human migration and international travel. The West African EVD outbreak caused significant loss of human lives way in excess of normal small outbreaks that we had been accustomed to. It became apparent that the first case was reported in Guinea in December 2013, but the outbreak was only confirmed by the WHO on March 23, 2014 (WHO 2014a). WHO declared the epidemic to be of "Public health emergency of international concern (PHEIC)" on August 6, 2014 (ibid). By September 14, 2014, there were a total of 4507 probable and confirmed cases of Ebola reported in Guinea, Liberia and Sierra Leone with 2296 deaths, the early wave of the outbreak being larger than the sum total of all the previous epidemics in terms of fatality (WHO Ebola Response Team 2014).EVD also spread to Senegal, Nigeria and Mali, where further infections were quickly halted by efficient public health interventions. It was estimated by the US Centres for Disease Control and Prevention (CDC) that, if not controlled, the cases of EVD could reach 1.4 million by late January 2015 (CDC 2016). Outside the continent, EVD was reported in Spain, Germany and USA that came about through international travels from infected areas (WHO 2014b; The Telegraph 2014). This resulted in further local infections limited to hospitals.

This initiative, the Global Emerging Pathogens Treatment Consortium (GET) was established with the aim of complementing existing and emerging efforts towards harnessing science, technology and innovation in the bio-security space on the African continent through creation and implementation of national, regional and cross-sectional policy dialogue, service and advice platforms. These platforms will endeavour to build on existing and new impetus towards integrated approaches at various levels, and to further build and/or strengthen synergies between key health and security sectors in which science, technology and innovation, in general, and bio-scientific research, in particular, have key roles to play in ensuring bio-threat management. It is our hope that this initiative will evolve into centres of excellence for real-time policy development, advice and oversight on matters of Bio-security in Africa. There are many individuals, institutions, sectors, nations, regions and international players in these efforts and their multiplicity and varying levels of involvement in the issue in space and time brings many dynamics to these efforts for developing countries.

## 2.2 Global Emerging Pathogens Treatment (GET) Consortium

The GET Consortium was established in the wake of the Ebola outbreak in 2014–2015 as an African-led multidisciplinary forum of experts with the ability to work together to build and strengthen Africa's preparedness and resilience in tackling public health crises caused by Emerging Infectious Diseases (EIDs). GET was formed in Lagos in 2014 by the Lagos State Commissioner of Health, Dr. Jide Idris, and Professor Akin Abayomi of Stellenbosch University, South Africa, who serves as the Principal Investigator for GET (Abayomi et al. 2016).The Consortium comprises experts from a wide spectrum of civil society, academia and the private sector. (Related reading: Peterson and Folayan 2017).

The Consortium, to this day, continues to partner with organizations globally to address some of the EIDs and public health and bio-security challenges faced on the Continent. Many partnerships have been formed between African intellectuals, African Governments, local non-governmental agencies and the International community. Our presence has been felt worldwide within a short time of existence; however, our work is mostly based in Africa where we focus on six key areas of the health system:

- New Emerging & Re-emerging Pathogens
- Research into areas that have been neglected or have potential threat of Infectious diseases
- Capacity development and appropriate technology
- Prevention and Education
- Bio-security and Bioethics
- Environmental integrity and surveillance.

As Africa has limited capacity to respond to public health crises, we feel that our focus should be on early warning and intelligence, policy and advocacy. Of paramount importance is public and community education and engagement. Currently we have offices in Accra, Ghana, Ibadan and Lagos, Nigeria, Freetown, Sierra Leone, and in Virginia, the United States of America. We work with more than 15 partners worldwide. The consortium also has a team of medical and project management experts from across. Our services are focused on indigenous human capital development, and where available, are tied to the national research agendas in the countries where the GET has a footprint. GET has partnered with a number of initiatives with the goal of providing high quality impact-focused results that would support African governments, health agencies and funders in the case of a public health emergency (https://www.getafrica.org/)

**The Objectives of GET Consortium Include the Following:**

- Anticipating in advance through surveillance and data gathering the possibility of the emergence of dangerous pathogens on the continent of Africa;
- Anticipating the entry of emerging pathogens into the continent and making appropriate recommendations to minimize risk;
- Identifying conditions that lead to the emergence of dangerous pathogens such as conflict and environmental perturbations and making necessary recommendations to mitigate such risk;
- Assessing the capacity, both in terms of infrastructure and human capital, that is necessary to respond with speed to early warning signs suggestive of the emergence of a dangerous pathogen outbreak;
- Conducting research into previous and current outbreaks in a harmonized fashion across the region;

- Developing a framework for ethical and community acceptable research and medical interventions cognizant of the culture and belief systems of the indigenous people of the continent, thereby engendering trust;
- Disseminating in a timely fashion, the findings of research;
- Acting as a conduit for access to expertise by international responders in scenarios where outbreaks create state of emergencies and facilitating collaborative relationships in a fashion that does not impose a threat to sovereignty and dignity of the continent;
- Promoting high level advocacy necessary for ensuring focused political will on appropriate spending on research and development necessary to fast-track all of the above;
- Ensuring capacity building for the effective development of bio-banking and biosecurity infrastructure.
- Developing the technology platforms for the monitoring and safety of patient data and bio-data.
- Facilitating global support for targeted vulnerable populations;
- Facilitating regulatory frameworks and guidelines for informing research into emerging pathogens on the continent. (see: https://www.getafrica.org/)

### *2.2.1 Governance of the GET Consortium*

Governance of the GET Consortium is designed to ensure that important decisions are identified optimally; that accountability exists to ensure important decisions are effectively implemented; and that problems can be quickly identified and escalated to the right parties for efficient and effective resolution. The Governance is multilayered and includes a core working group and several sub-working groups. These include:

**Plasmapheresis Working Group** This group is developing strategies to acquire convalescent apheresis plasma from survivors for treatment and/or prophylaxis of EIDs. The group will work out modalities of viral inactivation and fractionating appropriate for different technological environments in Africa. It will be involved in capacity building and training. Lyophilized plasma is also of interest.

**Bio-banking, Bio-containment and Bio-data Security** This group will define the consortium's approach to preserving samples safely from acutely ill patients and serial convalescent samples in all its research arms. Harmonizing SOPs and Laboratory Information Management Systems (LIMS) critical for good inventory accessioning and transportation as well Quality Assurance. All forms of data will require archiving and linking to samples in time and place in a bio-data repository. The working group will develop guidelines to engender trust in the science conducted by this consortium through providing levels of governance and minimizing risk to individuals, community and researchers.

**Communication, Public Relations and Sustainability Working Group** High level advocacy is critical to the long term success of this indigenous initiative to engender political will and also permit the right to ownership and risk mitigation and reduction. To do this the consortium needs to seek opportunities to present its objectives and mandate in all its ramifications to policy makers, strategic planners, senior academics and philanthropists in Africa and abroad. The image we portray as an indigenous-led organization with Africa's interests at the forefront of whatever happens on the continent during epidemic outbreaks and other such events is critical.

**Grant, Transcript and Publications Working Group** This working group will formulate a fair and equitable publication policy and guidelines for the Consortium inclusive of principles governing the collective intellectual Property Rights of data and information that resides within the Consortium. The working group will be responsible for identifying funding opportunities and bringing this to the attention of the Consortium and taking a lead in putting suitable members together to lead and generate a funding application. This working group can initiate manuscript ideas or review requests for manuscript generation from the body or within other working groups of the consortium and ensure that all Consortia output are in keeping with the agreed policy which should be in keeping with prevailing international publication guidelines and tailored to suit the African context.

**The Cultural, Anthropological, Social and Economic (CASE) Working Group** This working group focuses on African cultural practices and management of emerging infectious diseases (EIDs); community engagement and the fight against EIDs; determinants and impact of EIDs in Africa; ethics and the management of EIDs in Africa; contextualizing policy approaches and intervention strategies to fit local responses to EIDs and capacity building for public health emergencies in Africa. In short, the CASE WG is concerned with all that can be bracketed with what is commonly called ELSI (ethics, law and social issues) and strives to ensure that the GET consortium remains convincingly focused on Africa.

**Ethics, Community Engagement, Patient Advocacy and Support Working Group (ECEPAS)** This group is critical to the success of all the above sub working groups objectives. Thousands of persons have been infected and affected by EIDs and require an intense amount of psychosocial support and medical follow up to ascertain long term effects.

**Some of GET's On-Going Initiatives and Future Activities Include:**

- An indigenous Bio-data IT infrastructure and secured server;
- Scientific advisors for the collection of convalescent plasma from survivors in West Africa;
- Establishment of Community Advisory Boards for ethical research and medical interventions taking into consideration culture and belief systems;

- Promoting advocacy necessary for ensuring political will and creating a focus on research and development to fast track GET's objectives;
- Bio-banking and Bio-Security gap analysis projects in Freetown, Sierra Leone and Lagos, Nigeria;
- Memorandum of Understanding (MOU)signed with Lagos State Ministry of Health to support their Ebola Core research group and developing a CDC-like facility to serve the megacity of Lagos;
- MOU in development with Noguchi Memorial Medical Centre, Accra, Ghana;
- Facilitating development of policy guidance and frameworks for effective response to emerging pathogens in West Africa;
- MOU in development with the West African Task Force for research into emerging and re-emerging infections;
- Developing recommendations on the ethical conduct of research in emergency and epidemic situations and drawing up rules for the use of experimental drugs in clinical trials;
- Facilitating philanthropic support by Africans, thereby ensuring early and culturally acceptable indigenous responses to future humanitarian crises in African countries; (see: https://www.getafrica.org/) and
- Organizing an annual Conference on EIDs and Biosecurity in Africa. To date, the GET has organized three such conferences in Dakar, Senegal, (2015); Lagos, Nigeria, (2016); and Accra, Ghana, (2017). The next conference will be held in Freetown, Sierra Leone, in September 2018.
- GET Consortium Participation in the United Nations Security Council Resolution (UNSCR 1540) and the Biological Weapons Convention (BWC).

GET was invited as a resource organization meetings organized by the African Union for Member States in 2015, April 2016 and October 2017 in Addis Ababa to adopt legislation to prevent the proliferation of nuclear, chemical and biological weapons and to establish appropriate domestic controls to prevent any member state territories from being used as potential sources for non-State actors to acquire or transfer nuclear, chemical or biological weapons. AU Member States are committed to both the UNSCR 1540 and the BWC, but are hindered in their implementation and domestication by constraints such as lack of financial and human resources, limited infrastructure, limited technological capabilities and knowledge to harness the benefits of chemical, biological and nuclear sciences and technology in the areas of health, agriculture and energy. UNSCR 1540 and BWC establish obligations and provide assistance for all Member States to develop and enforce appropriate legal and regulatory measures in their respective countries. Open Consultation at the UN is calculated to provide participants with an opportunity to inform the 1540 Committee of their views on the implementation of Resolution 1540(2004) and to recommend practical ideas for the improvement of the implementation of the Resolution. GET Consortium was invited to the open consultation on UNSCR 1540 and made a statement at the UN Headquarters. GET organized a side event during this 1540 Comprehensive Review process which was held on the 22nd of June 2016 in New York. In the statement, GET expressed concerns on these among others: *A public health crises caused by a highly pathogenic emerging infectious disease outbreak is a source of biological material that can easily be diverted to non-peaceful uses, if appropriate measures are not in place to counter this opportunity; The West African region has thousands of Ebola samples located in facilities set up by international partners who are now withdrawing from the region, without a clearly defined plan for handover, safe keeping or destruction of these samples.*

Ebola Virus Disease has not been a top health priority because historically it has been sporadic in remote locations, permitting control measures mounted by national governments in collaboration with international partners alone to keep the fatalities low. Although the disease has been there for close to 40 years, it has not received much investment for research. Being a disease of the poor, as it were, it has not held the attention of the large drug manufacturers.

Our purpose at the GET is to define African strategies in a global context to curtail EID outbreaks by developing improved awareness, preparedness, preventive measures, capacity building and a deeper scientific understanding of the root-cause relationship between expanding human footprints and environmental integrity. GET is now working closely with the regional body, West African Health Organization, to assist in the development of a regional bio-banking network and bio-security framework. During the 47th Session of the Economic Community of West African States (ECOWAS), held in Accra on the 19th of May 2015, Heads of State agreed, given the inadequate diagnostic capacity for epidemic prone diseases, to establish the ECOWAS regional network for Regional Reference Laboratories and a Regional Bio-bank. This decision was triggered by the massive West African Ebola outbreak and the devastation it caused in its wake. Against this background, GET is providing significant support in the development of the first Multidisciplinary Technical Committee to define mechanisms for the operationalization of the regional Bio-bank in Abidjan and national mirror Bio-banks across the 15 States of West Africa. For more information please visit our website: https://www.getafrica.com

## 2.3 Conclusion

Given the high mortality and economic loss that the EVD outbreak in West Africa has brought about, it is important that African countries develop their own capacity and invest funding into research and innovation to address biosecurity and public health emergencies. Ebola is just a case in-point, but there are many other conditions that are prevalent on the African continent that are not priorities in "global health" and that do not attract attention and funding. These will have to be covered by each of the countries themselves, hence the need for each country to develop institutional and human capacity for conducting research on such tropical diseases which are currently receiving low global attention.

A search on Medical Publications (PubMed) database shows 1136 scientific research publications on Ebola Virus and its disease with more than 85 papers published as at 2014. EVD has been widely studied mainly by foreign scientists outside

Africa. Most of those Africans involved in Ebola research have studied the disease and its pathogen in overseas laboratories. It is however worthwhile to note that scientific research into the Ebola in Africa will require special facilities, up-to standard protective equipment, special protocols and special training of those involved. The GET consortium continues to grow and to impact the bio-security landscape in Africa and the diaspora, providing much needed expert support to governments to enhance resilience and to diminish vulnerability to EIDs and the risk of public health crises in general.

GET Consortium is there to complement existing and emerging efforts towards harnessing science, technology and innovation on the African continent through creation and implementation of national, regional and cross-sectional policy dialogue, service and advice platforms. These platforms will endeavour to build on existing and new impetus towards integrated approaches aimed at mitigating and adapting to the increasing incidence of emerging infectious diseases. The Consortium is committed to strengthening synergies between key sectors in which science, technology and innovation, in general, and bio-scientific research, in particular, have key roles to play. This initiative, we hope will evolve into centres of excellence for real-time policy development, advice and oversight that will be of immense benefit to African policy-makers in the health care delivery systems.

## References

Abayomi, E. A. (2013). HIV/AIDS disease burden complex in South Africa: Impact on health and environmental resources, and vulnerability to climate change. In *Climate vulnerability: Understanding and addressing threats to essential resources* (pp. 125–143). Amsterdam: Elsevier/Academic. ISBN:9780123847034.

Abayomi, A., & Cowan, M. N. (2014). The HIV/AIDS epidemic in South Africa: Convergence with tuberculosis, socioecological vulnerability, and climate change patterns. *South African Medical Journal/Suid-AfrikaanseTydskrifVirGeneeskunde, 104*(8), 583. https://doi.org/10.7196/samj.8645.

Abayomi, A., Gevao, S., Conton, B., Deblasio, P., & Katz, R. (2016). African civil society initiatives to drive a biobanking, biosecurity and infrastructure development agenda in the wake of the West African Ebola outbreak. *Pan African Medical Journal, 24*. https://doi.org/10.11604/pamj.2016.24.270.8429.

Africa CDC. (2017). *Enhancing Africa's public health response through innovation and partnerships concept note* (unpublished).

African Union. (2015). *Agenda 2063: The Africa we want*. Addis-Ababa: African Union Commission.

CDC. (2016). *Ebola: 2014–2016 Ebola outbreak in West Africa*. https://www.cdc.gov/vhf/ebola/history/2014-2016-outbreak/index.html. Accessed 11 Jan 2019.

Kamradt-Scott, A. (2016). WHO's to blame? The World Health Organization and the 2014 Ebola outbreak in West Africa. *Third World Quarterly, 37*(3), 401–418.

Mugwagwa, J. T., Kingiri, A., Muraguri, L., & Wamae, L. (2014). Understanding policy trajectories in Sub-Saharan Africa: The policy kinetics model. *International Journal of Technology Management and Sustainable Development, 13*(1), 37–52.

Nkengasong, J. N., Maiyegun, O., & Moeti, M. (2017). Establishing the Africa centres for disease control and prevention: Responding to Africa's health threats. *The Lancet Global Health, 5*(3), e246–e247.

Peterson, K., & Folayan, M. (2017). *How Nigeria defeated Ebola*. https://africasacountry.com/2017/12/how-nigeria-defeated-ebola/. Accessed 11 Jan 2019.

The Telegraph. (2014). *Ebola: Germany accepts infected patient for treatment*. https://www.telegraph.co.uk/news/worldnews/europe/germany/10998367/Ebola-Germany-accepts-infected-patient-for-treatment.html. Accessed 11 Jan 2019.

WHO. (2014a, August 8). *Statement on the 1st meeting of the IHR Emergency Committee on the 2014 Ebola outbreak in West Africa*.

WHO. (2014b). *Ebola virus disease – Spain*. https://www.who.int/csr/don/09-october-2014-ebola/en/. Accessed 11 Jan 2019.

WHO. (2015). *Emergency preparedness, response: Key events in the WHO response to the Ebola outbreak*. https://www.who.int/csr/disease/ebola/one-year-report/who-response/en/. Accessed 11 Jan 2019.

WHO. (2018). *Ebola virus disease: Key facts*. https://www.who.int/news-room/fact-sheets/detail/ebola-virus-disease. Accessed 11 Jan 2019.

WHO Ebola Response Team. (2014). Ebola virus disease in West Africa: The first 9 months of the epidemic and forward projections. *The New England Journal of Medicine, 371*, 1481–1495.

# Chapter 3
# Emerging Infectious Diseases: A Historical and Scientific Review

**Gibril Ndow, J. Radeino Ambe, and Oyewale Tomori**

## 3.1 Overview and History

Emerging Infectious Diseases (EIDs) are diseases caused by an infectious pathogen that has recently evolved and entered a given population for the first time; or a disease that had occurred before but whose incidence, impact and/or geographic range has increased or is expected to increase within a given time-frame (Jones 2008; CDC 1994; Morse and Schluederberg 1990). EIDs include novel infections in human, animal and plant populations.

Although the phrase "emerging diseases" has been used in scientific literature and publications since the early 1960s (Maurer 1962), it was not until after outbreaks of genital herpes and HIV/AIDS in the 1970s (Fleming et al. 1997) and early 1980s respectively that concern over EIDs and the use of the term became more widespread. Key landmark events and publications, notably the first conference on the prediction and prevention of EIDs jointly hosted by the Rockefeller University and National Institute for Health (NIH) in May 1989, and publication by the Institute of Medicine (IOM) in 1992 identifying the significance of EIDs and providing a

G. Ndow (✉)
Medical Research Council Unit The Gambia at London School of Hygiene & Tropical Medicine, Banjul, The Gambia

Institute of Global Health Innovation, Division of Integrative Systems Medicine & Digestive Diseases, Faculty of Medicine, Imperial College London, London, UK
e-mail: gndow@mrc.gm; g.ndow@imperial.ac.uk

J. R. Ambe
Department of Public Health, School of Nursing and Health Sciences, Capella University, Minneapolis, MN, USA

The Global Emerging Pathogens Treatment Initiative, Lagos, Nigeria

O. Tomori
Nigerian Academy of Science, University of Lagos, Lagos, Nigeria



G. B. Tangwa et al. (eds.), *Socio-cultural Dimensions of Emerging Infectious Diseases in Africa*, https://doi.org/10.1007/978-3-030-17474-3_3

guide for their recognition and prevention, stirred interest and attention towards EIDs and opened doors for more research, funding and publications (IOM 1992). The establishment of the Program for Monitoring Emerging Diseases (ProMED), devoted to rapidly disseminate information on infectious disease outbreaks and promote communication and collaboration amongst the international infectious diseases community during EID outbreaks, shortly followed this conference and publication. The Centres for Disease Control (CDC), in 1995, launched the Emerging Infectious Diseases journal, dedicated to rapidly disseminate reliable information on the emergence, prevention and elimination of EIDs.

Preceding these developments in EID dedicated programs and journals, research centres spread across the globe were developing vaccines and conducting trials to prevent various emerging infectious threats throughout history. The Institut Pasteur (IP), established in Paris in 1888, is one of the oldest of such centres for research on EIDs. The Institut, which conducts research at the frontline of EID outbreaks, aims to make discoveries to prevent, control, diagnose and treat EIDs. Soon after its creation, in 1896, Emile Marchoux established a microbiology laboratory in Saint-Louis, Senegal – the site where the first outbreak of yellow fever was reported in 1778 (Augustine 1909). This laboratory in Saint-Louis studied the epidemiology of malaria and sleeping sickness, and developed vaccines against smallpox, rabies and the plague. The laboratory was later transferred to Dakar in 1924 following an agreement with IP Paris, and was renamed the Institut Pasteur of Dakar. It is now a World Health Organisation (WHO) reference centre and a partner in the WHO Global Outbreak Alert and Response Network (GOARN). In addition to Senegal, Institut Pasteur is present in 9 other African countries: Guinea Conakry, Ivory Coast, Niger, Cameroon, Central African Republic, Madagascar, Morocco, Algeria and Tunisia; making the Institut Pasteur International Network a major player in almost every EID outbreak today.

In the 1920s, the West African Yellow Fever Commission was formed, run by a colonial research team from the Rockefeller Foundation. The Foundation build research centres and laboratories in Nigeria (Yaba, Lagos) and Ghana where significant studies and discoveries were made including the isolation of the yellow fever virus (Bigon 2014) and the eventual development of the yellow fever vaccine in 1937 by Max Theller (McNeill 2004). These centres would also pave the way for the establishment of the West African Council for Medical Research (WACMR) in 1954 by the British colonial government. Following independence in 1960, Nigeria took over the facilities of the WACMR and established the Medical Research Council (MRC). The facilites of this MRC were, in 1977, used by the Federal Military Government to establish the National Institute for Medical Research (NIMR) through the Research Institute Establishment Order 1977, pursuant to the National Science and Technology Development Agency Decree (No 5) of 1977.

The most developed of these early research establishments was perhaps the Medical Research Council (MRC) Unit in The Gambia. Established in 1947, it has since led infectious disease and public health research, making significant contributions in the prevention of endemic and emerging pathologies in the region including malaria, tuberculosis and *Haemophilus influenza*. It remains a beacon of excellence in bench, field and clinical research on infectious diseases, training and hosting some of Africa's leading scientists and producing a significant proportion of the region's research output. During the peak of the HIV epidemic in West Africa, the Unit supported the establishment of a field station in Caio, Guinea Bissau dedicated to the study and prevention of HIV infection. The MRC Unit in The Gambia is now incorporated within the London School of Hygiene & Tropical Medicine, and continues to forge partnerships with several other institutions in the West African region.

In the mid-1950s to 1970s, some African nations through national assembly acts, created what are perhaps the oldest indigenous government supported research centres in sub-Saharan Africa, tasked purposely to improve the health and quality of life of their respective populations. The National Research Centre (NRC) of Egypt, the South African Medical Research Centre (SAMRC), Kenya Medical Research Institute (KEMRI), the Medical Research Council of Zimbabwe (MRCZ), the National Institute for Medical Research (NIMR) in Tanzania and the Medical Research Council of Nigeria represent such indigenous centres created between 1956 and 1979. KEMRI, in 1989, went on to form a partnership with the Wellcome Trust and the University of Oxford to create the KEMRI-Wellcome Trust Research Programme. This world-renowned health research unit trains scientific leaders and champions innovative and novel ideas to improve healthcare in Africa. Its Genomics and Infectious Diseases platform studies the transmission of infectious diseases, including EIDs, in order to inform disease outbreak policies and understand the evolution of resistance.

Both the NIMR and the Noguchi Memorial Institute for Medical research, respectively the leading medical research institutes in Nigeria and Ghana, focus on preventing and controlling infectious diseases of the highest priority to their respective populations and the regions. Their research work includes studies to control and eradicate malaria, onchocerciasis, schistosomiasis, childhood diarrhoeal diseases, tuberculosis, HIV, leprosy, guinea worm, Ebola virus disease, yellow fever and Lassa fever.

In 1988, at the height of the HIV epidemic in sub-Saharan Africa, an agreement between the governments of Uganda and Britain led to the establishment of the MRC Unit in Uganda. This unit, hosted by the Uganda Virus Research Institute (UVRI), primarily conducts research to investigate the determinants of HIV and related infections, their subsequent disease progression, and evaluate new preventive strategies and interventions for their control in Africa. The UVRI also hosts a CDC supported laboratory for rapid diagnosis of haemorrhagic fever viruses. This diagnostic infrastructure, coupled with other public health measures, has helped in a more rapid detection and control of outbreaks in Uganda. Now a hotspot for Ebola experts, Uganda and its centres of excellence have assisted in controlling outbreaks within the region.

In 2004, the CDC in coordination with the WHO, established a Global Disease Detection (GDD) Regional Centre in Kenya, co-located with KEMRI. The GDD regional centre connects regions and countries throughout Africa, and assists in detecting and responding to disease outbreaks. A similar GDD regional centre was established in Thailand that year to address the complexity of EIDs in the Asia-Pacific region. Between 2005 and 2011, eight additional GDD centres were established in Bangladesh, Guatemala, Kazakhstan, China, Egypt, India, South Africa and Georgia, with all centres aiming to detect and stop disease outbreaks at their source thereby limiting spread and preventing epidemics. These centres, combined, have responded to hundreds of outbreaks; detected and identified scores of novel strains and pathogens; and improved regional capacity in personnel, diagnostics and surveillance.

In addition to the GDD program, the WHO created the Global Outbreak Alert and Response Network (GOARN) to facilitate harnessing of international resources at the request of WHO member states during outbreaks. This network augments country and regional responses to ongoing or potential public health emergencies. GOARN, in 2014, facilitated the deployment of nearly 900 experts to West Africa during the Ebola outbreak. The WHO and CDC publish recommendations to guide the coordination of national surveillance and response standards for EIDs and communicable diseases.

## 3.2 Stages in the Emergence of an Infectious Disease

An EID outbreak occurs in stages, the first of which is often the introduction of the new pathogen into the host population, or in the case of a previously existing pathogen, its establishment and dissemination within the new population and beyond. Whilst most of the EID outbreaks in recent history have resulted from zoonotic infections, only a few of the many zoonotic pathogens that periodically infect humans become adept at transmitting or propagating themselves. Human activity, however, is making this transition increasingly easy by creating efficient pathways for pathogen transmission around the globe.

Woolhouse and Gaunt (2007), following careful examination of dozens of newly identified human pathogens, noted four characteristics that they expect will describe most EIDs:

1. Caused by an RNA virus
2. Caused by pathogen with non-human (animal) reservoir
3. Caused by pathogen with a broad host range
4. Have potential for human-to-human transmission

In the presence of these four characteristics, changes in climate and human behaviour are key elements in the promotion of most EID outbreaks. With the on-going global ecological change, it is estimated that new pathogens and EIDs will continue to be introduced into the human population at or near the rate of three per year (Woolhouse and Gaunt 2007). Box 3.1 summarises the key factors that promote EIDs.

**Box 3.1: Factors That Drive EIDs**
1. PATHOGEN FACTORS
Adaptation to new host
Virulence
Short incubation period
Rate of mutation
Mode, speed and ease of transmission
Replication cycle
Mortality rate
2. HUMAN FACTORS
Demographics and behaviour
Susceptibility to new infection (lack of immunity)
International travel
Poverty
Dependence on livestock for food and labour
3. ENVIRONMENTAL FACTORS
Weather and climate change
Changing ecosystem
Drought
Famine
4. POLITICAL FACTORS
Lack of political will
Poor healthcare infrastructure
Lack of adequate public health measures
Economic development
Instability (war, civil unrest)
Social inequality
5. OTHER FACTORS
Bioterrorism
Technology

## 3.3 Reported EID Outbreaks

Despite the systems in place for preventing EIDs, the frequency of outbreaks have remained stable over the past decades. Between 1980 and 2017, more than two dozen EID outbreaks have been reports. Whilst some of these were re-emerging pathogens, there were more than ten newly emerging infectious diseases reported for the first time in humans during this time (Table 3.1). Unsurprisingly, most of these newly reported EIDs are new zoonotic viral infections or mutated forms of previously circulating viruses. Discussions of the epidemiology, the pathogen characteristics, and clinical features of these EIDs is beyond the scope of this chapter.

**Table 3.1** Emerging Infectious Diseases between 1980 and 2017

| Newly emerging | Re-emerging | Deliberately emerging |
|---|---|---|
| HIV | West Nile virus | Anthrax (bioterrorism) |
| Cryptosporidiosis | Methicillin-resistant *Staph aureus* | |
| Hepatitis C virus | Marburg hemorrhagic fever | |
| E coli O157:H7 | Human monkeypox | |
| E coli O104:H4 | Plague | |
| H1N1 influenza | Chikungunya fever | |
| H5N1 influenza | Cholera | |
| H7N9 influenza | Human African trypanosomiasis | |
| H3N2v influenza | Yellow fever | |
| SARS | Dengue | |
| MERS-CoV | Adenovirus | |
| SFTSV bunyavirus | Listeriosis | |
| Hantavirus pulmonary syndrome | Ebola hemorrhagic fever | |
| Zika virus | Drug resistant malaria | |
| Nipah virus | Diphtheria | |
| Hendra virus | Rift valley fever | |
| | Typhoid fever | |
| | Drug resistant tuberculosis | |

The increase in EID outbreaks in part reflects advances in medical and technological capabilities to detect and diagnose infections. However, increased globalisation, changes in global climate and human behaviour, natural and man-made disasters (poverty, war), weak healthcare systems, and lapses in public health measures all contribute to the increase in EIDs. The importance of these factors is borne in the fact that the majority of EIDs represent changes in the epidemiology, virulence or adaptation of previously known pathogens, with novel pathogens accounting for a minority of EID outbreaks.

## 3.4 Animal Diseases of Economic and/or Zoonotic Impact

Human activities, including war, poor health systems, international travel, increasing population, and dependence on livestock for food and labour, have promoted the emergence, expansion, and rapid spread of EIDs. With the majority of recent EID outbreaks caused by zoonotic viral infections, initiatives and response mechanisms have been established to curb, control and prevent the emergence and spread of animal and botanical EIDs that could have adverse impact on human lives and livelihood:

### 3.4.1 One Health Program, South Africa

As previously mentioned, the WHO had set up GDD Centers in Kenya and other African countries. There are 12 offices in all, one of which is in South Africa. The One Health Program was founded as a collaborative effort to bring the best possible conditions for health to people, animals and the environment. It pulls together professionals from international, national and local regions in agreement with the objectives of the WHO. The One Health Program focuses on public health and zoonotic diseases in an effort to curtail zoonotic outbreaks that affect morbidity and mortality of people and animals alike. The South Africa Regional Global Disease Detection Center (GDD) provides support for the training and human capital development to prepare health officials in the detection and response to zoonotic diseases according to the GHS initiatives. The strengthening of laboratory surveillance, research programs and an enhanced surveillance infrastructure are objectives of the GDD and One Health. Priority Zoonotic diseases are:

- Viral, endemic zoonotic diseases: Rabies, Ebola, Marburg
- Bacterial diseases: Anthrax, Brucellosis, Bovine Tuberculosis. Leptospirosis, Rickettsial diseases and food borne bacteria like Salmonella
- WHO neglected diseases: Toxoplasmosis, Cysticercosis, Cryptosporidium

### 3.4.2 Rinderpest

Rinderpest is German for "cattle plague". It is a highly infectious viral disease that can affect domesticated and wild, cloven-hoofed mammals. African cattle and buffalo are extremely susceptible to the disease while sheep and goats experience a mild form that is not as acute, resulting in lower fatalities. In susceptible animal, Rinderpest infection has a fatality rate greater than 90% and a mortality rate of 100%. In the 1890's, an outbreak of Rinderpest South of the River Zambezi killed about 5.2 million cattle, sheep, goats and oxen, and an unknown number of wild giraffe, buffalo and wildebeest. This Rinderpest epidemic, happening at a time of much historical tumult, was the most devastating epidemic to hit southern Africa in the late nineteenth century. There is no conclusive evidence on how Rinderpest was brought to Africa. It is thought to have been brought through Indian cattle by Italian colonial masters who introduced the cattle to the Horn of Africa. The disease is spread through ingested contaminated matter and/or through direct contact. Endemic areas have caused animals to develop immunity through exposure or vaccinations. In sub-Saharan Africa, Rinderpest outbreaks resulted in the death of 90% of domestic oxen. The resulting famine, both from loss of livestock and diminished agricultural produce, led to significant mortality among Ethiopian and Masai populations. European nations gradually eliminated Rinderpest in the early twentieth century through surveillance, early detection and culling of sick and exposed animals. It however continued to afflict developing African and Asian countries well into the second half of the twentieth century, re-emerging after several eradication campaigns were prematurely shut down due to mistaken belief that the virus had been eradicated. It was not until 2011 that Rinderpest was eradicated, marking one of the greatest veterinary achievements in recent history.

### *3.4.3 Rift Valley Fever*

Rift Valley Fever (RVF) is a virus from the Phlebovirus genus, first identified in the Rift Valley of Kenya in 1931. RVF primarily infects animals but has the ability to also affect humans. Since 1931, there have been repeated outbreaks in sub-Saharan Africa. Infected cattle along the River Nile and its irrigation system caused an outbreak of RVF in Egypt in 1977 that killed approximately 600 people. In 1987 there was an outbreak in West Africa that was connected with the Senegal River Project construction. In 1997–98, there was another outbreak due to El Nino in Tanzania, Kenya and Somalia amidst extensive flooding. Humans can get RVF through the bites of infected insects and contact with blood of infected animals.

### *3.4.4 Peste de Petits Ruminants (PPR)*

Also known as Ovine Rinderpest, PPR is a disease that affects smaller ruminants (primarily sheep and goats) in Central and Southern Africa, North Africa, the Middle East and the Indian subcontinent. It is a highly contagious and fatal disease, making its impact on livestock and human livelihood very important, and its global eradication an urgent need (Baron et al. 2011).

## 3.5 Control of EIDs and Deadly Outbreaks in Humans

Data and countermeasures to control and treat most EIDs are insufficient, often resulting in significant morbidity and mortality during outbreaks. This is especially problematic in resource-limited countries, where healthcare infrastructure for disease surveillance and rapid response to emerging outbreaks are weak. This urgent problem was brought to the forefront during the Ebola virus outbreak of 2014 in West Africa. As a result, the WHO has, since December 2015, maintained a list of EIDs that pose major public health threats and for which there are no effective countermeasures, and advocates the prioritization of these EIDs for research and vaccine/drug development.

An effective global prevention of EID outbreaks will require multidisciplinary collaboration and will include the following:

### 3.5.1 *Surveillance*

(a) Establishment and/or standardization of national disease surveillance systems
(b) Improvement of hospitals and laboratories to be able to identify, characterise and contain EIDs
(c) Establishment of strong EID databases and pathways to notify local and regional authorities of emerging or suspected EIDs
(d) Alignment of primary health care structures with surveillance systems
(e) Development of easy algorithms for detecting clusters of new or unusual diseases, especially in rural parts of low- and middle-income countries.

### 3.5.2 *Response Mechanism*

(a) Rapid, efficient response mechanisms to emerging outbreaks
(b) Well-funded emergency response systems able to mobilise investigative and control efforts of local agencies

### 3.5.3 *Research and Training*

(a) Develop national research agenda prioritizing EID research
(b) Dedicated EID research funding to drive and address local priorities
(c) Promote research on EID control measures, surveillance methods, and development of vaccines and drugs
(d) Train competent field epidemiologists, scientists, clinicians and other relevant personnel for EID surveillance and control.
(e) Create stockpiles of vaccines and drugs for known EIDs, ready for deployment in the event of an outbreak.

### 3.5.4 *Public Health Control Measures*

(a) Public health training to interrupt transmission of known pathogens, and reduce ongoing transmission during outbreaks
(b) Public engagement and collaboration during EID outbreaks
(c) Understanding cultural practices of relevance to EID outbreaks and disease transmission, and considering such practices when designing control and response mechanisms
(d) Good governance, policy and political will to prevent

## 3.6 Conclusion

It has been 50 years or more since many African countries became independent. During this period, Africa has experienced numerous disease outbreaks, many of which have become endemic and uncontrolled. It is sorrowful and painful to note that Africa remains the verdant pasture for EIDs despite global improvements in disease surveillance systems and better reliable laboratory diagnostic facilities. Behind Africa's failure to successfully control EID outbreaks is the pervasive state of poor governance in many African countries, with governments continuing to pay lip service to health issues including disease control, and African healthcare systems remaining weak despite repeated EID outbreaks. In the absence of good governance, priorities get misplaced and an atmosphere of poor planning and corruption is easily promoted resulting in poor allocation and mismanagement of funds for disease control and surveillance. It is essential for African governments to note that a healthy population is a sine qua non for orderly economic and social development, and that EID outbreaks negatively impact national economies and other development plans. It is only through good governance and political/economic stability that African countries can improve health security and prevent EIDs and preventable loss of life.

## References


Augustine, G. (1909). *History of yellow fever*. New Orleans: Searcy and Pfaff.

Baron, M. D., Parida, S., & Oura, C. A. (2011). Peste des petits ruminants: A suitable candidate for eradication? *The Veterinary Record, 169*(1), 16–21.

Bigon, L. (2014). Translational networks of administering disease and urban planning in West Africa: The inter-colonial conference on yellow fever, Dakar, 1928. *GeoJournal, 79*(1), 103–111.

Centers for Disease Control and Prevention; Atlanta. (1994). *Addressing emerging infectious diseases threats: A prevention strategy for the United States* (MMWR 43-RR-5).

Fleming, D. T., et al. (1997). Herpes simplex virus type 2 in the United States, 1976 to 1994. *The New England Journal of Medicine, 337*, 1105–1111. https://doi.org/10.1056/NEJM199710163371601.

IOM (Institute of Medicine). (1992). *Emerging infections: Microbial threats to health in the United States*. Washington, DC: National Academy Press.

Jones, K. E. (2008). Global trends in emerging infectious diseases. *Nature, 451*, 990–993.

Maurer, F. D. (1962). Equine piroplasmosis – Another emerging disease. *Journal of the American Veterinary Medical Association, 141*, 699–702.

McNeill, J. R. (2004). Yellow jack and geopolitics: Environment, epidemics, and the struggles for empire in the American tropics, 1650–1825. *OAH Magazine of History, 18*(3), 9–13.

Morse, S. S., & Schluederberg, A. (1990). Emerging viruses: The evolution of viruses and viral diseases. *The Journal of Infectious Diseases, 162*, 1–7.

Woolhouse, M., & Gaunt, E. (2007). Ecological origins of novel human pathogens. *Critical Reviews in Microbiology, 33*(4), 231–242.

# Chapter 4
# Epidemiology and Management of Lassa Fever in the West African Sub-Region: Overcoming the Socio-cultural Challenges

**Godsent Chichebem Isiguzo and Michael Onyebuchi Iroezindu**

## 4.1 Case Vignette

In August 2009, a 23-year-old lady on national service who recently returned from her place of primary assignment in north central Nigeria presented to the emergency room in a tertiary centre in Abakaliki, south-east Nigeria. She gave a 3-day history of malaise, headache, fever, diarrhoea, abdominal pain with swelling and one episode of hematemesis. Examination revealed a toxic-looking young lady, pale, febrile (axillary temperature 39.2 °C) with periorbital oedema and hepatomegaly. She had tachycardia with a pulse rate of 120 beats per minute; Blood pressure was 100/60 mmHg. A clinical diagnosis of acute abdomen was made most likely from typhoid perforation.

Emergency laparotomy was carried out, and intra-operatively, no bowel perforation was visualized. Rather there was evidence of gut oedema with purpuric lesions on the intestines and inflamed spleen. Delayed clotting was noticed, and the patient received two units of fresh whole blood during the operation. Unfortunately, 24 h after surgery the patient died, and relatives declined autopsy to ascertain the cause of death.

Four days later the surgical registrar who carried out the operation developed a high-grade fever with pharyngitis and dysphagia, this he blamed on exhaustion following a long weekend call and self-prescribed antimalarial drugs. The next day his condition worsened, and he was admitted to the hospital with features of hypovolemia

G. C. Isiguzo (✉)
Department of Medicine, Federal Teaching Hospital Abakaliki, Ebonyi State, Nigeria

Department of Medicine, Faculty of Health Sciences, University of Cape Town, Cape Town, South Africa

M. O. Iroezindu
College of Medicine, University of Nigeria, Enugu, Nigeria

Department of Internal Medicine, University of Nigeria Teaching Hospital, Enugu, Nigeria



G. B. Tangwa et al. (eds.), *Socio-cultural Dimensions of Emerging Infectious Diseases in Africa*, https://doi.org/10.1007/978-3-030-17474-3_4

and shortly became unconscious. Meanwhile, two other staff involved in the management of the index patient also reported fever and malaise. There was pandemonium in the hospital at what could be responsible for this and in the course of the confusion, the surgeon subsequently developed epitasis and 2 h later died. It was then obvious that the hospital may be dealing with a viral haemorrhagic fever. Blood samples collected from the surgeon and two sick healthcare workers (HCWs) were sent off to the National Lassa fever reference laboratory at Irrua, Edo State, and contact tracing commenced to identify all persons involved in the management of the index patient. The result of the blood samples collected from the Surgeon and one of the HCW returned positive for Lassa fever. The cloud of dismay that besieged the hospital in the aftermath of these events was unprecedented.

## 4.2 Introduction

Lassa fever is an acute zoonotic viral haemorrhagic fever caused by the Lassa virus which leads to significant morbidity and mortality in some cases. It is endemic in West Africa. The disease derives its name from Lassa town in Yerdseram river valley of northeast Nigeria where the virus was first isolated in 1969 following illness and death of two missionary nurses in Jos Nigeria (Frame et al. 1970). However, before this, there has been a report of the disease in Sierra Leone in the 1950s.

Following these initial reports, and characterization of the illness, (Buckley and Casals 1970) there have been outbreaks of Lassa fever with resultant mortality in several towns in Nigeria (Ogbu et al. 2007; Ajayi et al. 2013; Iroezindu et al. 2015) as well as epidemics in several West African countries like Liberia, Sierra Leone, Guinea, Mali and Senegal (Bausch et al. 2001). Serological evidence of the disease has also been reported in Ivory Coast, Togo and Ghana (Dzotsi et al. 2012; Sogoba et al. 2012) while importation to Europe and America is well recognized (Atkin et al. 2009; Günther et al. 2000).

## 4.3 Epidemiology

Lassa fever is caused by a single-stranded RNA virus belonging to the arenavirus family. The disease vector is the rodent *Mastomyces natalensis,* a ubiquitous rat seen commonly in rural communities in West, Central and East Africa (Wulff et al. 1977; Salazar-Bravo et al. 2002). The Lassa virus (LASV) is shed in the rat's faeces, urine, respiratory secretions and found also in the blood. Human infections occur through direct contact with the rat's excretions, or inhalation of contaminated dust, and eating of the rat as seen in some of the communities in West Africa. Infection can also occur from person to person through handling of secretions. The virus can be shed in the urine for 3–6 weeks, and in semen for 3 months, so sexual transmission is a possibility.

The incubation period of 3–21 days which favours importation of Lassa fever outside the endemic regions as has occurred in USA, South Africa, Germany, United Kingdom and the Netherlands (Holmes et al. 1990; Günther et al. 2000; Atkin et al. 2009; Macher and Wolfe 2006). This potential for importation makes LASV a candidate for bioterrorism, and it is arguably the most common biosafety Level (BSL) four agent and a prominent threat to human health worldwide (Sogoba et al. 2012).

Lassa fever is endemic in most countries in West Africa, Benin (first diagnosed in November 2014), Ghana (first diagnosed in October 2011), Guinea, Liberia, Mali (first diagnosed in February 2009), Sierra Leone, and Nigeria. But probably the disease also exists in other West African countries with varying degrees of seropositivity. There have also been reports of seropositivity in the Central African Republic and the Democratic Republic of Congo (Organization 2017; Ogbu et al. 2007; Childs et al. 2007; Safronetz et al. 2010).

It has been shown that the degree of seroprevalence of LASV specific antibodies is higher among populations in rural areas. However, this is highly variable depending on the geographical location, ranging from 1.8% to 55% (Lukashevich et al. 1993; McCormick et al. 1987b; Tomori et al. 1988; Keenlyside et al. 1983). This finding supports the assumption that up to 80% infections are mild or possibly asymptomatic and not resulting in hospitalization. The assertion underpins the conclusion that 5–20% of the nonimmune population per year have a high incidence of LASV-specific seroconversion (McCormick et al. 1987b). The prevalence of LASV antibodies in the general population is 8–52% in Sierra Leone, (Frame et al. 1984) 4–55% in Guinea, (Frame et al. 1984) and 21% in Nigeria (Ogbu et al. 2007).

Estimated annual incidence is 100,000–300,000 cases with up to 5000 fatalities (Grove et al. 2011; Shaffer et al. 2014). The overall case-fatality rate is 1% (Organization 2017). However, the observed case fatality rate for hospitalized patients ranges from 15% to 20%, further increasing to 50% during epidemics (Branco et al. 2011b) and up to 90% in third-trimester pregnancies for both the expectant mother and the foetus (Branco et al. 2011a; Shaffer et al. 2014). In Nigeria, there have been several epidemics almost on a yearly basis, (Fisher-Hoch et al. 1995) and in August 2017 the Federal Ministry of Health reported that for the year 2017, a total of 718 cases were recorded including 217 confirmed cases and 68 deaths (Ojosipe 2017).

### *4.3.1 Factors That Promote the Epidemics*

In most West African communities, cereals and grains form the staple source of carbohydrate. These are usually dried in the open spaces either for preservation or as part of processing during the dry season of December to March. These open spaces are accessible to the rodents which in the process of helping themselves to these exposed grains contaminate same with their excreta (Monath et al. 1974; McCormick 1987). The practice of drying of food which as stated above occurs in the hot, dry season of December to March coincides with harvest time and had been shown to be the period with the highest presentations in most cases seen in West Africa compared to the wet season of April to November (Wilson 1995). However, some reports from Kenema in Sierra Leone showed that transmission was highest during the period of change from dry to the wet season (Richmond and Baglole 2003; Wilson 1995). This phenomenon is related to the civil war in Sierra Leone and the migration of people in search of food with congestion and unhealthy living conditions (McCormick and Fisher-Hoch 2002).

Some other communities use the rats as a source of meat and so are exposed to the body fluid (Ter Meulen et al. 1996). Also, practices such as bush burning, either done as part of farming or to aid catching of the rats for meat, destroy their natural habitat and force them to seek shelter within the households, hence at proximity with humans and heightened risk of infection.

The clinical presentation of Lassa fever is non-specific, like other common illnesses such as malaria and typhoid fever, so the unsuspecting healthcare workers (HCWs) are usually at grave risk. This situation is further promoted by the lack of requisite diagnostic and management infrastructure, with ill-equipped laboratories and poorly motivated/trained staff. There is also a lack of an organized and structured system for disease notification, contact tracing and surveillance. These factors work together unfortunately in most endemic areas to drive the Lassa fever infection and outbreaks (Fig. 4.1).

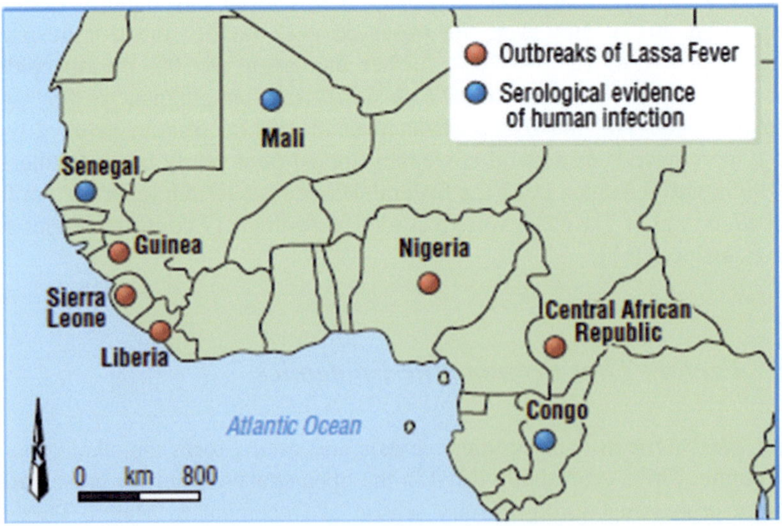


**Fig. 4.1** Distribution of Lassa fever in West Africa. Outbreaks have occurred in the Central African Republic, Guinea, Liberia, Nigeria, and SierraLeone; serological evidence of human infection has been found in the Democratic Republic of the Congo, Mali, and Senegal. (Picture was taken with permission from Richmond and Baglole 2003)

## 4.4 Virology

Lassa virus (LASV) is an enveloped single-stranded bi-segmented RNA virus of the Arenaviridae family. Phylogenetically, the virus has a close relation to other segmented nsRNA viruses belonging to *Bunyaviridae* and *Orthomyxoviridae*. The three virus families share the primary feature of the intracellular replication cycle. All arenaviruses based on serological cross-reactivity, (Wulff et al. 1978) phylogenetic relations (Bowen et al. 1997) and geographical distribution are further subdivided into the New World and the Old World virus complexes (Yun and Walker 2012). Arenavirus seen in South America (i.e., Tacaribe (TACV), Junin (JUNV), Machupo (MACV), Guanarito (GTOV), Sabia (SABV) viruses) and North America (i.e., Bear Canyon (BCNV) viruses), Whitewater Arroyo (WWAV), Tamiami (TAMV), make up the New World arenavirus complex. The Old-World complex includes arenaviruses that circulate in Africa, Europe, and Asia (i.e., lymphocytic choreomeningitis (LCMV) and Lassa (LASV) viruses).

The LASV lacks the conventional negative strand coding arrangement, and there is a difference in genetic serological and pathological characteristics of isolates of the virus (Jahrling et al. 1985). The envelope of the virus is smooth with T-shaped spikes of between 7 and 10 nm in length made of the glycoprotein (Ruo et al. 1991). This envelope encloses the genome which has helical and nucleocapsid measuring between 400 and 1300 nm in length (Yun and Walker 2012). The name ‘arena’ meaning sandy is derived from its appearance as granules in the centre of the host cell ribosome when viewed by electron microscopy (McCormink et al. 1986). The virus can be inactivated by ultraviolet radiation or heating from 50 to 100 °C. Also, chemical agents like 0.5% sodium hypochlorite, 0.5% phenol and 10% formalin can be used to inactivate LASV (McCormick 1987).

## 4.5 Pathogenesis

Following infection, LASV proliferates mainly in macrophages, dendritic and endothelial cells, leading to uninhibited viral proliferation and host immune suppression. The inhibition of the host immune response occurs in two ways. The usual rate of endothelial trafficking crucial for innate immunity recognition is bypassed (Brosh-Nissimov 2016). Interferon production is directly suppressed by LASV, and the infected immune cells are unable to secrete other proliferating cytokines such as TNFα, IL-6, and IL-1β. So unlike other viral haemorrhagic fevers, LASV does not manifest with cytokine storm (McLay et al. 2014; Brosh-Nissimov 2016).

There is increased capillary permeability leading to oedema and hypovolemic shock; peripheral vasoconstriction follows with disseminated intravascular coagulation leading to the hemorrhagic syndrome (Ogbu et al. 2007; Frame et al. 1970). Bleeding may involve the intestine, liver, myocardium, lungs, and brain. Other changes include hepatitis, hepatic necrosis, splenic and adrenal necrosis (McLay et al. 2014; Ogbu et al. 2007). There may also be thrombocytopenia, hematemesis, and watery diarrhoea which further contributes to hypotension (Fisher-Hoch et al. 1988).

Survivors show high cellular immunity with strong T cell response with antibody response less important despite the production of specific antibodies seen in the disease. (Yun and Walker 2012) Neutralizing antibodies appear only after weeks with low titre and avidity (Bennett et al. 2014).

## 4.6 Clinical Presentation

Lassa virus infection causes symptomatic disease in only about 20% of cases with the remaining 80% demonstrating serological evidence of infection without symptoms. Diagnosis of Lassa fever based on clinical features alone could be quite challenging especially among relatively inexperienced and unsuspecting clinicians. This is because Lassa fever presents with symptoms and signs indistinguishable from those of several other febrile illnesses in the tropics such as malaria, typhoid fever, influenza and sepsis especially in the early phase of the disease. It is also difficult to convincingly differentiate Lassa fever from other African haemorrhagic fevers such as Ebola virus disease and Dengue in the absence of strong epidemiological evidence.

Lassa fever often manifests gradually, following an incubation period of 3–21 days (average 10 days), as an acute illness of one to 4 weeks duration. The classical progression of the disease when uninterrupted by treatment are summarised in Table 4.1. Survivors show improvement within 8–10 days, while fatal cases progress to shock, coma, and death during the third week.

Some of the clinical features of Lassa fever deserve further description. Fever is almost always present occurring in 90–100% of cases; with peaks of 39–41 °C (McCormick et al. 1987a; Ehichioya et al. 2012; Ajayi et al. 2013). However, body temperature within or even below the normal range has been observed in some patients (Asogun et al. 2012). A sore throat may occur with or without pharyngitis.

**Table 4.1** Clinical stages of Lassa fever

| Stage | Symptoms |
|---|---|
| 1 (Days 1–3) | General weakness and malaise. High fever >39 °C, constant with peaks of 40–41 °C |
| 2 (Days 4–7) | A sore throat (with white exudative patches); a headache; back, chest, side, or abdominal pain; conjunctivitis; nausea and vomiting; diarrhoea; a productive cough; proteinuria; low blood pressure (systolic <100 mm Hg); anaemia |
| 3 (After 7 days) | Facial oedema; convulsions; mucosal bleeding (mouth, nose, eyes, e.t.c); internal bleeding; confusion or disorientation |
| 4 (After 14 days) | Coma and death |

Adapted from McCarthy (2002)

If present, pharyngitis is frequently exudative. Conjunctival injection is usually devoid of itching and discharge and subconjunctival haemorrhages may be present. Maculopapular or petechial rash which tends to appear over the thorax, face and arms is difficult to decipher in black Africans. Overdependence on bleeding from body orifices for diagnosis may be misleading as it occurs in less than 20% of hospitalised cases and it may not be externally visible (Ajayi et al. 2013; McCormick et al. 1987a; Ehichioya et al. 2012). In women, bleeding may be responsible for prolonged menstruation or postpartum haemorrhage (Ajayi et al. 2013; Dahmane et al. 2014). Nervous system symptoms including confusion, seizures, meningism and coma occur late and could easily be misdiagnosed as bacterial meningitis. In a prospective case-control study of 441 hospitalised Lassa fever patients in Sierra Leone, the combination of features that were found to be most predictive of Lassa fever was fever, pharyngitis, retrosternal pain and proteinuria with a positive predictive value of 81% (McCormick et al. 1987a).

Clinical complications of Lassa fever include: deafness, spontaneous abortion, transient hair loss, pericarditis/pericardial effusion especially in males, arrhythmia, pancytopenia, renal failure, cerebellar ataxia and depression (McCormick et al. 1987a; Ogbu et al. 2007). Majority of these sequelae could occur even during convalescence and may be immune-mediated. Deafness is sensorineural, could be unilateral or bilateral and affects about 30% of cases. It is irreversible in two-thirds of cases and not related to the severity of the illness or the level of viremia (Cummins et al. 1990).

### 4.6.1 The Case Definition for Suspected Lassa Fever

The use of case definition for Lassa fever enhances epidemiological surveillance and increases the index of clinical diagnosis among healthcare workers. The adapted WHO case definition for suspected Lassa fever summarized in Table 4.2 is widely used in several settings in West Africa.

### 4.6.2 Socio-cultural Challenges in Clinical Diagnosis and Management of Lassa Fever

There are many socio-cultural challenges that need to be surmounted in order to achieve early diagnosis of Lassa fever and possibly more favourable outcomes. A study in Sierra Leone identified the following key socio-cultural issues that impact on the clinical diagnosis of Lassa fever:(Richmond and Baglole 2003)

- Stigmatization: people understand that Lassa fever can be contracted through contact with an affected person which leads to patients and their families being stigmatised.

**Table 4.2** Adapted WHO Case definition for suspected Lassa fever

| |
|---|
| Fever >38 °C for less than 3 weeks ***and***<br>The absence of signs of local inflammation (i.e. the illness is systemic) ***and***<br>The absence of a clinical response after 48 h of anti-malaria treatment and/or a broad-spectrum antibiotic ***and***<br>Two major signs ***or*** one major sign and two minor signs described below: |
| **Major signs**<br>Bleeding (including from the mouth, nose, rectum, or vagina)<br>Swollen neck or face<br>Conjunctivitis or subconjunctival haemorrhage<br>Spontaneous abortion<br>Petechial or hemorrhagic rash<br>New onset of tinnitus or altered hearing<br>Persistent hypotension<br>Elevated liver transaminases, especially aspartate aminotransferase (AST) > alanine aminotransferase (ALT)<br>Known exposure to a person suspected to have Lassa fever |
| **Minor signs**<br>A headache<br>A sore throat<br>Vomiting<br>Diffuse abdominal pain/tenderness<br>Chest/retrosternal pain<br>A cough<br>Diarrhoea<br>Generalized myalgia or arthralgia<br>Profuse weakness<br>Proteinuria<br>Leucopenia<4000/L |

Dahmane et al. (2014)

- Early clinical diagnosis is impeded by difficulties reaching health facilities.
- Many people are unlikely to seek medical care if they suspect they have Lassa fever as they consider the treatment expensive and could only be afforded by sacrificing necessities such as food and school fees.
- Belief in traditional (herbal) remedies for acute febrile illness.
- Mistrust of treatment offered at the hospital: some people do not go to medical facilities because of the unfounded belief that injections administered at the hospital could kill them.
- Spontaneous abortion (miscarriage) is blamed on the woman; it is often attributed to witchcraft and may lead to divorce.
- Deafness has been described as a social embarrassment and as having a catastrophic effect on family relationships.

These cultural practices are not peculiar to Sierra Leone but are similar in most endemic countries and communities in Africa. In Nigeria, most farming communities dry their food substances such as maize, cassava flour and beans either on abandoned roads or on concrete surfaces in the open exposed to rodents and the element. Also, in most markets, traders leave their food commodities exposed overnight with minimal covering. Eating of rats is still a local practice in some communities, in such instances bush burning to capture these rodents is employed. This not only exposes humans to the blood and fluids from the dead rats but also the process of pursuing the rodents from their natural habitat in the bushes usually translocate them to living homes, thereby increasing the exposure and contact with humans and perpetuating the cycle of epidemics.

A visit to hospitals and health centres in most rural communities in West Africa reveal that pre-colonial health infrastructures are still in use with little or no upgrading. There are either no electricity or where such exist are epileptic, so laboratory facilities are at most rudimentary. These hospitals lack even the most basic facilities for treatment of common disease, and the poorly trained health facilities are disillusioned and unmotivated. The sad situation is aptly captured by a recent pronouncement of a Health Minister of one of the countries in West Africa who while answering questions concerning facilities for specialization of health workers from reporters in 2018 was proud to advise that some doctors consider farming and politics as alternative professions rather than continue with the Medical practice. In situations such as this, the sad outcome of cases as shown in our case vignette becomes the norm.

Another socioeconomic factor that could be driving the epidemics of Lassa fever and other hemorrhagic endemic diseases is the urbanization of the rural communities in sub-Saharan Africa. This has led to two things; extreme spatial and technological connectivity of the population and enlarging urbanization that overwhelm the health infrastructure of the resource-poor countries (Dudas et al. 2017). Other important factors identified as drivers of the geographical spread of emerging infectious disease such as Lassa and Ebola are road construction for mining, logging and hydroelectric activities (Potapov et al. 2017). These open hitherto inaccessible and remote locations leading to human movement between previously isolated communities. So, road construction and other anthropogenic disturbance directly alter the ecosystem in which pathogens reside (Allen et al. 2017).

These activities in themselves are for the general good of the communities and could be rightly so if the economic gains are used to strengthen public health preparedness for emerging diseases (Munster et al. 2018). One way this could be achieved could include training and education of health care workers, especially in the rural areas. This training could focus on identification, reporting and proper handling of cases of emerging diseases, diagnostic capacity and access to healthcare (Munster et al. 2018). There is also a need to invest in research empowerment through training of research scientist to strengthen clinical research infrastructure for vaccine development and therapeutics.

To confront the challenge of Lassa fever and other endemic diseases, responsible government and local communities must brace up to the challenges of development. There is a need for education and enlightenment of the populace on abandoning of inimical practices such as bush burning, provision of modern food processing and preservation methods. In addition to efforts at improving the road network and provision of sustainable sources of power, there should be upgrading of available health facilities and provision of incentives to the health workers to enable them to consider rural practice. Development must go beyond urban centres and spread urbanization to rural communities. Politicians such as the honourable Minister who advised health workers to take up farming should in addition to the well-intended counsel, seek ways to harness the abundant human resources in the continent to make our communities better and comparable to those countries where they and their families go to seek healthcare. One such way could be by investing in health research and manpower development into endemic diseases. That way the teeming young health workers instead of queuing for non-existent specialization training can pick up careers in health-related research that will ultimately improve the well-being of the population and improvement in our practice.

## 4.7 Laboratory Diagnosis

Laboratory diagnosis of Lassa fever can be made based on any of the following:

- Positive IgM serology or seroconversion (IgG antibody) in paired serum specimens or
- Demonstration of Lassa virus antigen in serum by ELISA or in autopsy tissues by immunohistochemistry
- Positive Reverse Transcriptase Polymerase Chain Reaction (RT-PCR) from serum or autopsy tissues
- Isolation of virus (only in the laboratory of biosafety level 4) from blood, urine or throat washings.

Laboratory diagnosis of Lassa fever has traditionally been by the indirect fluorescent-antibody (IFA) test. Recently, more sensitive enzyme-linked immunosorbent assays (ELISAs) for Lassa virus antigen and immunoglobulin M (IgM) and G (IgG) antibodies were developed and are now preferred for serological diagnosis. However, the specificity (77%) and sensitivity (57%) of the IgM serological assay as a screening tool for early detection of Lassa fever appear weak while the negative and positive predictive values were 63% and 72% respectively according to findings in a large referral centre in Nigeria (Ibekwe et al. 2012). Taken together, Lassa virus antigen and IgM ELISAs have been reported to be 88% sensitive and 90% specific for acute infection (Bausch et al. 2000). The RT-PCR test on viral antigen isolate by immunofluorescence has proven a reliable diagnostic tool with specificity and sensitivity of near 100% by the third day of illness. It is considered the gold standard for laboratory diagnosis of Lassa fever (Bausch et al. 2000; Ogbu et al. 2007).

In West Africa, confirmatory diagnosis of Lassa fever is usually made at reference laboratories which are few in most countries and far away from most communities and health facilities where individuals suspected to have Lassa fever are cared for. Before the confirmatory laboratory result becomes available, experienced clinicians have found findings of some of the routine laboratory investigations useful in strengthening the resolve to commence empirical ribavirin therapy. Although not peculiar to Lassa fever, these laboratory abnormalities are sometimes referred to as "surrogate markers" and they include presence of anaemia, leucopenia (leucocytosis may also occur) thrombocytopenia, coagulopathy such as prolonged international normalized ratio (INR), proteinuria, haematuria, elevated transaminases (AST greater than ALT), hyperbilirubinemia and azotemia (Ajayi et al. 2013; Richmond and Baglole 2003; McCormink et al. 1986).

### *4.7.1 Logistic Challenges in Laboratory Diagnosis of Lassa Virus Infection*

Laboratory diagnosis of Lassa fever in West Africa suffers a lot of setbacks due to logistic and socio-economic challenges. Several leading teaching hospitals in countries affected by Lassa fever do not have the diagnostic capacity to confirm Lassa virus infection due to various reasons including lack of biosafety level 3 or 4 system, lack of PCR machines and/or other equipment, lack of trained laboratory personnel or consumables. In most countries, indigenous government commitment/funding of Lassa fever reference laboratories is sub-optimal leading to overdependence on international donor agencies and research collaborators. In regions where reference laboratories exist, most of the primary, secondary and sometimes tertiary health facilities in endemic communities still have difficulties getting samples across to the reference laboratories. Coordination of sample collection from Lassa fever suspects, subsequent storage and dispatch between health facilities and government public health departments have frequently been inefficient. In the absence of appropriate personal protective equipment, laboratory workers are wary of collecting or processing blood samples of patients with suspected Lassa fever. On occasions, patient relatives have resorted to travelling long distances to the reference laboratories with Lassa fever suspects or their blood samples in public vehicles which constitutes a big public health risk. Sometimes, samples dispatched to reference laboratories are poorly preserved or mishandled in transit and get rejected on arrival. There are also difficulties with repeat sample collection/dispatch for an RT-PCR assay for Lassa fever suspects with initial negative RT-PCR results following sample analysis too early during the illness unless the patients were admitted at the reference centre.

## 4.8 Treatment

Individuals diagnosed to have Lassa fever should be managed in isolation facilities, away from general wards under the care of health personnel who are provided with appropriate personal protective equipment (PPE) and other basic requirements. The mainstay of treatment is supportive care and ribavirin therapy.

The major goal of supportive care is fluid and electrolyte replacement. More often than not, intravenous fluid replacement is preferred especially in patients with excessive fluid loss or haemodynamic instability. Transfusion of blood and/or blood products is beneficial; more so if there is bleeding. Other supportive treatments include respiratory support, broad-spectrum antibiotic therapy, antipyretics and nutritional support. Patients with Lassa fever usually have transient immunosuppression which increases their risk of nosocomial bacterial infections hence the need for broad-spectrum antibiotics. Paracetamol is the preferred antipyretic. The use of aspirin and non-steroidal anti-inflammatory drugs (NSAIDS) is discouraged due to their antiplatelet effects. Antimalarial therapy can also be administered especially if there is laboratory evidence of parasitaemia.

Ribavirin, a guanosine analogue antiviral drug, is effective in the treatment of Lassa fever especially if administered early in the course of the illness. Although intravenous ribavirin in standard doses has a much higher bioavailability than the oral form, both preparations have been observed to be beneficial in Lassa fever treatment, with the former showing a stronger effect in higher risk cases (McCormink et al. 1986). It is usually administered slowly in an infusion. In the landmark study in Sierra Leone, it was observed that patients with a high risk of death who were treated for 10 days with ribavirin, begun within the first 6 days after the onset of fever were significantly more likely to survive; with a case-fatality rate of 5% compared to case fatality rate of 26% in those whose treatment began seven or more days after the onset of fever (McCormink et al. 1986). The study confirmed the efficacy of ribavirin in the treatment of Lassa fever and recommended that it should be used at any point in the illness, as well as for post-exposure prophylaxis. The commonly recommended regimen is a loading dose of 33 mg/Kg body weight (up to maximum dose of 2.4 g stat) followed by 16 mg/kg (up to 1 g) 6 hourly for 4 days, then 8 mg/kg (up to 500 mg) 8 hourly for 6 days (McCormink et al. 1986). Although empiric therapy with ribavirin is said to be undesirable due to its expense, need for intravenous administration, potential toxicity and teratogenicity, (McCormink et al. 1986; Fisher-Hoch et al. 1992; Kochhar 1990) withholding ribavirin in the management of Lassa fever suspects with strongly suggestive clinical features is often impractical in the absence of readily available Lassa virus diagnostic laboratory capacity. Similarly, it is difficult to discontinue ribavirin therapy in such patients if clinical improvement is observed during treatment but Lassa virus RT-PCR and/or serology eventually turn out negative.

Management of some complications of Lassa fever such as acute kidney injury (AKI) is key to favourable outcomes. Prompt institution of haemodialysis for patients with AKI non-responsive to conservative management could be life-saving. This is a big challenge in treatment centres where there is no dedicated haemodialysis machine bearing in mind that most health facilities in resource-limited settings may not be sufficiently equipped to dedicate a haemodialysis machine for Lassa fever patients with renal failure. In addition, sub-optimal infection control mechanisms make it difficult to use haemodialysis machines that serve general renal patients for Lassa fever cases with renal failure in order to limit the risk of secondary transmission.

Treatment of Lassa fever outside designated reference/treatment centres in West Africa is challenging but inevitable considering the logistic demands and enormous out-of-pocket expenditures encountered in accessing reference centres. Despite the periodic outbreaks of Lassa fever in West Africa, the majority of hospitals in the region do not have purpose-built isolation facilities or hardly have a regular supply of essential consumables required for the proper running of make-shift isolation facilities. Regular use of appropriate PPE is unattainable due to limited supplies. Stock out of government or donor supplied ribavirin coupled with the heavy financial burden of procuring the drug out-of-pocket continues to be a problem in several settings. Probably worrisome is the occasional apathy among healthcare workers for management of suspected viral haemorrhagic fever due to fear of nosocomial transmission.

In a survey of 146 medical officers in South East Nigeria, the factors that were perceived to constitute challenges to Lassa fever management were low index of suspicion among health-care workers, lack of diagnostic facilities, lack of PPE, poor awareness of Lassa fever in communities, late presentation, lack of isolation facilities, low government commitment and lack of ribavirin (Unigwe et al. 2016).

## 4.9 Prognosis

The overall case-fatality rate of Lassa fever is 1%. However, the observed case-fatality rate among patients hospitalized with severe cases of Lassa fever is 15%. Death rates are particularly high for women in the third trimester of pregnancy, and for fetuses, about 95% of which die in the uterus of infected pregnant mothers. Other poor prognostic factors include high viral load, serum AST level greater than 150 IU/L, the presence of bleeding and encephalitis.

## 4.10 Prevention and Control

Prevention of primary transmission of Lassa fever depends on control of *Mastomys* rodents, especially in endemic communities. This can be effectively achieved by storing grain and other foodstuffs in rodent-proof containers, refuse disposal far from homes, regular cleaning of households and keeping cats. Prolonged drying of grains on exposed surfaces should be discouraged especially in communities with heavy rodent population. Additional efforts should be made to keep homes free of rats during farming seasons when rodents are displaced from the bushes following bush burning. Use of rodents as meat should be highly discouraged. Trapping in and around homes can help reduce rodent populations. However, due to the wide distribution of *Mastomys* in Africa, complete elimination of rodent reservoir from the environment is impractical (Ogbu et al. 2007; Keenlyside et al. 1983). Health education and community sensitization to prevent transmission in endemic areas is beneficial and should focus on rodent control, minimising contact with rodent excreta, early presentation to health facilities and safe burial practices.

Prevention of secondary transmission of Lassa fever in communities and health facilities is very important. Caring for sick persons at home should be discouraged and family members should always avoid contact with blood and body fluids while caring for sick persons. Optimal management of patients with Lassa fever can only be guaranteed in isolation facilities. Health-care workers should always observe standard infection prevention and control precautions when caring for patients, irrespective of the presumed diagnosis. Air-borne transmission of Lassa fever is not proven. Guidelines from the WHO focus on contact and droplet-based precautions. These include basic hand hygiene, respiratory hygiene, use of PPE (to block splashes or other contacts with infected materials), safe injection practices and safe handling of corpses (WHO 2017). Health-care workers caring for patients with suspected or confirmed Lassa fever should apply extra infection control measures to prevent contact with the patient's blood and body fluids and contaminated surfaces or materials such as clothing and bedding. When in close contact (within 1 m) of patients with Lassa fever, health-care workers should wear face protection (a face shield or a medical mask and goggles), a clean, non-sterile long-sleeved gown, and gloves (sterile gloves for some procedures) (WHO 2017).

Laboratory workers are also at risk. Inexperienced personnel should not be asked to obtain blood samples. The correct procedure for transporting materials suspected to contain a highly virulent virus or micro-organisms must be observed (McCormick 1987). In addition, samples taken for diagnosis of Lassa virus infection or ancillary investigations should only be handled by trained staff and processed in suitably equipped laboratories under maximum biological containment conditions (WHO 2017).

Contact tracing, risk categorization and monitoring should be instituted following an outbreak or nosocomial spread. Beyond observation for compatible clinical features, blood samples of contacts may need to be sent for diagnosis of Lassa virus infection, and/or surrogate markers where possible. High-risk contacts should receive ribavirin post-exposure prophylaxis.

Cremation is about the safest way to dispose of the remains of viral haemorrhagic fever cases. In Africa, this is generally difficult to implement due to cultural reasons. Nevertheless, direct contact with dead bodies of individuals suspected or confirmed to have Lassa fever should be avoided.

To avoid export of Lassa fever from West Africa to non-endemic regions including Europe and the Americas, diagnosis of Lassa fever should be entertained in febrile patients returning from areas of recent outbreaks or individuals with a history of contact with anyone whose illness is suggestive of viral haemorrhagic fever.

Indigenous government commitment in the West African region is important for effective prevention/control and overall management of Lassa fever. Key government roles include health education, regular supply of PPE, ribavirin; as well as the establishment of purpose-built isolation/treatment centres and laboratory diagnostic support. Funding for research that is aimed at improving Lassa fever prevention and management should be encouraged.

Despite some research work for vaccine candidates, (Ölschläger and Flatz 2013) no effective vaccine for Lassa virus is currently available.

**Dedication** This chapter is dedicated to the memory of Dr. Udenna Ama (1970–2009) and all health care workers in Africa who have lost their lives treating patients with Lassa fever.

## References


Ajayi, N. A., Nwigwe, C. G., Azuogu, B. N., Onyire, B. N., Nwonwu, E. U., Ogbonnaya, L. U., Onwe, F. I., Ekaete, T., Günther, S., & Ukwaja, K. N. (2013). Containing a Lassa fever epidemic in a resource-limited setting: Outbreak description and lessons learned from Abakaliki, Nigeria (January–March 2012). *International Journal of Infectious Diseases, 17*(11), e1011–e1016.

Allen, T., Murray, K. A., Zambrana-Torrelio, C., Morse, S. S., Rondinini, C., Di Marco, M., Breit, N., Olival, K. J., & Daszak, P. (2017). Global hotspots and correlates of emerging zoonotic diseases. *Nature Communications, 8*(1), 1124.

Asogun, D. A., Adomeh, D. I., Ehimuan, J., Odia, I., Hass, M., Gabriel, M., Ölschläger, S., Becker-Ziaja, B., Folarin, O., & Phelan, E. (2012). Molecular diagnostics for Lassa fever at Irrua specialist teaching hospital, Nigeria: Lessons learnt from two years of laboratory operation. *PLoS Neglected Tropical Diseases, 6*(9), e1839.

Atkin, S., Anaraki, S., Gothard, P., Walsh, A., Brown, D., Gopal, R., Hand, J., & Morgan, D. (2009). The first case of Lassa fever imported from Mali to the United Kingdom, February 2009. *Euro Surveillance: Bulletin European sur les maladies transmissibles= European Communicable Disease Bulletin, 14*(10), 19145.

Bausch, D. G., Rollin, P. E., Demby, A. H., Coulibaly, M., Kanu, J., Conteh, A. S., Wagoner, K. D., McMullan, L. K., Bowen, M. D., & Peters, C. J. (2000). Diagnosis and clinical virology of Lassa fever as evaluated by enzyme-linked immunosorbent assay, indirect fluorescent-antibody test, and virus isolation. *Journal of Clinical Microbiology, 38*(7), 2670–2677.

Bausch, D. G., Demby, A. H., Coulibaly, M., Kanu, J., Goba, A., Bah, A., Condé, N., Wurtzel, H. L., Cavallaro, K. F., & Lloyd, E. (2001). Lassa fever in Guinea: I. Epidemiology of human disease and clinical observations. *Vector Borne and Zoonotic Diseases, 1*(4), 269–281.

Bennett, J. E., Dolin, R., & Blaser, M. J. (2014). *Principles and practice of infectious diseases*. London: Churchill Livingstone.

Bowen, M. D., Peters, C. J., & Nichol, S. T. (1997). Phylogenetic analysis of the Arenaviridae: Patterns of virus evolution and evidence for cospeciation between arenaviruses and their rodent hosts. *Molecular Phylogenetics and Evolution, 8*(3), 301–316.

Branco, L. M., Boisen, M. L., Andersen, K. G., Grove, J. N., Moses, L. M., Muncy, I. J., Henderson, L. A., Schieffellin, J. S., Robinson, J. E., & Bangura, J. J. (2011a). Lassa hemorrhagic fever in a late term pregnancy from northern Sierra Leone with a positive maternal outcome: Case report. *Virology Journal, 8*(1), 404.

Branco, L. M., Grove, J. N., Boisen, M. L., Shaffer, J. G., Goba, A., Fullah, M., Momoh, M., Grant, D. S., & Garry, R. F. (2011b). Emerging trends in Lassa fever: Redefining the role of immunoglobulin M and inflammation in diagnosing acute infection. *Virology Journal, 8*(1), 478.

Brosh-Nissimov, T. (2016). Lassa fever: Another threat from West Africa. *Disaster and Military Medicine, 2*(1), 8.

Buckley, S. M., & Casals, J. (1970). Lassa fever, a new virus disease of man from West Africa. *The American Journal of Tropical Medicine and Hygiene, 19*(4), 680–691.

Childs, J. E., Mackenzie, J. S., & Richt, J. A. (2007). *Wildlife and emerging zoonotic diseases: The biology, circumstances and consequences of cross-species transmission* (Vol. 315). Berlin: Springer.

Cummins, D., McCormick, J. B., Bennett, D., Samba, J. A., Farrar, B., Machin, S. J., & Fisher-Hoch, S. P. (1990). Acute sensorineural deafness in Lassa fever. *JAMA, 264*(16), 2093–2096.

Dahmane, A., van Griensven, J., Van Herp, M., Van den Bergh, R., Nzomukunda, Y., Prior, J., Alders, P., Jambai, A., & Zachariah, R. (2014). Constraints in the diagnosis and treatment of

Lassa fever and the effect on mortality in hospitalized children and women with obstetric conditions in a rural district hospital in Sierra Leone. *Transactions of the Royal Society of Tropical Medicine and Hygiene, 108*(3), 126–132.

Dudas, G., Carvalho, L. M., Bedford, T., Tatem, A. J., Baele, G., Faria, N. R., Park, D. J., Ladner, J. T., Arias, A., & Asogun, D. (2017). Virus genomes reveal factors that spread and sustained the Ebola epidemic. *Nature, 544*(7650), 309.

Dzotsi, E. K., SA Ohene, F., Asiedu-Bekoe, J., Amankwa, B., Sarkodie, M. A., Thouphique, A. M., Ofei, A., Oduro, J., & Atitogo, D. (2012). The first cases of Lassa fever in Ghana. *Ghana Medical Journal, 46*(3), 166–170.

Ehichioya, D. U., Asogun, D. A., Ehimuan, J., Okokhere, P. O., Pahlmann, M., Ölschläger, S., Becker-Ziaja, B., Günther, S., & Omilabu, S. A. (2012). Hospital-based surveillance for Lassa fever in Edo state, Nigeria, 2005–2008. *Tropical Medicine & International Health, 17*(8), 1001–1004.

Fisher-Hoch, S. P., McCormick, J. B., Sasso, D., & Craven, R. B. (1988). Hematologic dysfunction in Lassa fever. *Journal of Medical Virology, 26*(2), 127–135.

Fisher-Hoch, S. P., Gborie, S., Parker, L., & Huggins, J. (1992). Unexpected adverse reactions during a clinical trial in rural West Africa. *Antiviral Research, 19*(2), 139–147.

Fisher-Hoch, S. P., Tomori, O., Nasidi, A., Perez-Oronoz, G. I., Fakile, Y., Hutwagner, L., & McCormick, J. B. (1995). Review of cases of nosocomial Lassa fever in Nigeria: The high price of poor medical practice. *BMJ: British Medical Journal, 311*(7009), 857–859.

Frame, J. D., Jr, J. M. B., Gocke, D. J., & Troup, J. M. (1970). Lassa fever, a new virus disease of man from West Africa. *The American Journal of Tropical Medicine and Hygiene, 19*(4), 670–676.

Frame, J. D., Yalley-Ogunro, J. E., & Hanson, A. P. (1984). Endemic Lassa fever in Liberia. V. Distribution of Lassa virus activity in Liberia: Hospital staff surveys. *Transactions of the Royal Society of Tropical Medicine and Hygiene, 78*(6), 761–763.

Grove, J. N., Branco, L. M., Boisen, M. L., Muncy, I. J., Henderson, L. A., Schieffellin, J. S., Robinson, J. E., Bangura, J. J., Fonnie, M., & Schoepp, R. J. (2011). Capacity building permitting comprehensive monitoring of a severe case of Lassa hemorrhagic fever in Sierra Leone with a positive outcome: Case report. *Virology Journal, 8*(1), 314.

Günther, S., Emmerich, P., Laue, T., Kühle, O., Asper, M., Jung, A., Grewing, T., ter Meulen, J., & Schmitz, H. (2000). Imported Lassa fever in Germany: Molecular characterization of a new Lassa virus strain. *Emerging Infectious Diseases, 6*(5), 466–476.

Holmes, G. P., McCormick, J. B., Trock, S. C., Chase, R. A., Lewis, S. M., Mason, C. A., Hall, P. A., Brammer, L. S., Perez-Oronoz, G. I., & McDonnell, M. K. (1990). Lassa fever in the United States. *New England Journal of Medicine, 323*(16), 1120–1123.

Ibekwe, T. S., Nwegbu, M. M., Asogun, D., Adomeh, D. I., & Okokhere, P. O. (2012). The sensitivity and specificity of Lassa virus IgM by ELISA as a screening tool at the early phase of Lassa fever infection. *Nigerian Medical Journal: Journal of the Nigeria Medical Association, 53*(4), 196–199.

Iroezindu, M. O., Unigwe, U. S., Okwara, C. C., Ozoh, G. A., Ndu, A. C., Ohanu, M. E., Nwoko, U. O., Okoroafor, U. W., Ejimudo, E., & Tobin, E. A. (2015). Lessons learnt from the management of a case of Lassa fever and follow-up of nosocomial primary contacts in Nigeria during Ebola virus disease outbreak in West Africa. *Tropical Medicine & International Health, 20*(11), 1424–1430.

Jahrling, P. B., Frame, J. D., Smith, S. B., & Monson, M. H. (1985). Endemic Lassa fever in Liberia. III. Characterization of Lassa virus isolates. *Transactions of the Royal Society of Tropical Medicine and Hygiene, 79*(3), 374–379.

Keenlyside, R. A., McCormick, J. B., Webb, P. A., Smith, E., Elliott, L., & Johnson, K. M. (1983). Case-control study of Mastomys natalensis and humans in Lassa virus-infected households in Sierra Leone. *The American Journal of Tropical Medicine and Hygiene, 32*(4), 829–837.

Kochhar, D. M. (1990). Effects of exposure to high concentrations of ribavirin in developing embryos. *The Pediatric Infectious Disease Journal, 9*(9), S88–S90.

Lukashevich, I. S., Clegg, J. C. S., & Sidibe, K. (1993). Lassa virus activity in Guinea: Distribution of human antiviral antibody defined using enzyme-linked immunosorbent assay with recombinant antigen. *Journal of Medical Virology, 40*(3), 210–217.

Macher, A. M., & Wolfe, M. S. (2006). Historical Lassa fever reports and 30-year clinical update. *Emerging Infectious Diseases, 12*(5), 835–837.

McCarthy, M. (2002). USA moves quickly to push biodefence research. *The Lancet, 360*(9335), 732.

McCormick, J. B. (1987). Epidemiology and control of Lassa fever. *Arenaviruses: Biology and Immunotherapy, 134*, 69–78.

McCormick, J. B., & Fisher-Hoch, S. P. (2002). Lassa fever. In *Arenaviruses I* (pp. 75–109). Berlin: Springer-Verlag.

McCormick, J. B., King, I. J., Webb, P. A., Johnson, K. M., O'Sullivan, R., Smith, E. S., Trippel, S., & Tong, T. C. (1987a). A case-control study of the clinical diagnosis and course of Lassa fever. *Journal of Infectious Diseases, 155*(3), 445–455.

McCormick, J. B., Webb, P. A., Krebs, J. W., Johnson, K. M., & Smith, E. S. (1987b). A prospective study of the epidemiology and ecology of Lassa fever. *Journal of Infectious Diseases, 155*(3), 437–444.

McCormink, J. B., King, Y. L., & Webb, P. A. (1986). Lassa fever: Effective therapy with ribavirin. *The New England Journal of Medicine, 314*, 2–26.

McLay, L., Liang, Y., & Ly, H. (2014). Comparative analysis of disease pathogenesis and molecular mechanisms of New World and Old World arenavirus infections. *Journal of General Virology, 95*, 1):1–1)15.

Monath, T. P., Newhouse, V. F., Kemp, G. E., Setzer, H. W., & Cacciapuoti, A. (1974). Lassa virus isolation from Mastomys natalensis rodents during an epidemic in Sierra Leone. *Science, 185*(4147), 263–265.

Munster, V. J., Bausch, D. G., de Wit, E., Fischer, R., Kobinger, G., Muñoz-Fontela, C., Olson, S. H., Seifert, S. N., Sprecher, A., & Ntoumi, F. (2018). Outbreaks in a rapidly changing Central Africa – Lessons from Ebola. *New England Journal of Medicine, 379*, 1198–1201.

Ogbu, O., Ajuluchukwu, E., & Uneke, C. J. (2007). Lassa fever in west African sub-region: An overview. *Journal of Vector-Borne Diseases, 44*(1), 1–11.

Ojosipe, D. (2017, August 27). Nigeria: Lassa fever kills 68, 718 cases recorded. *Leadership*. Accessed 28 Aug 2017. http://leadership.ng/2017/08/22/lassa-fever-kills-68-718-cases-recorded/

Ölschläger, S., & Flatz, L. (2013). Vaccination strategies against highly pathogenic arenaviruses: The next steps toward clinical trials. *PLoS Pathogens, 9*(4), e1003212.

Potapov, P., Hansen, M. C., Laestadius, L., Turubanova, S., Yaroshenko, A., Thies, C., Smith, W., Zhuravleva, I., Komarova, A., & Minnemeyer, S. (2017). The last frontiers of wilderness: Tracking loss of intact forest landscapes from 2000 to 2013. *Science Advances, 3*(1), e1600821.

Richmond, J. K., & Baglole, D. J. (2003). Lassa fever: Epidemiology, clinical features, and social consequences. *BMJ: British Medical Journal, 327*(7426), 1271.

Ruo, S. L., Mitchell, S. W., Kiley, M. P., Roumillat, L. F., Fisher-Hoch, S. P., & McCormick, J. B. (1991). Antigenic relatedness between arenaviruses defined at the epitope level by monoclonal antibodies. *Journal of General Virology, 72*(3), 549–555.

Safronetz, D., Lopez, J. E., Sogoba, N., Traore, S. F., Raffel, S. J., Fischer, E. R., Ebihara, H., Branco, L., Garry, R. F., & Schwan, T. G. (2010). Detection of Lassa virus, Mali. *Emerging Infectious Diseases, 16*(7), 1123.

Salazar-Bravo, J., Ruedas, L. A., & Yates, T. L. (2002). Mammalian reservoirs of arenaviruses. In *Arenaviruses I* (pp. 25–63). Berlin: Springer.

Shaffer, J. G., Grant, D. S., Schieffelin, J. S., Boisen, M. L., Goba, A., Hartnett, J. N., Levy, D. C., Yenni, R. E., Moses, L. M., & Fullah, M. (2014). Lassa fever in post-conflict Sierra Leone. *PLoS Neglected Tropical Diseases, 8*(3), e2748.

Sogoba, N., Feldmann, H., & Safronetz, D. (2012). Lassa fever in West Africa: Evidence for an expanded region of endemicity. *Zoonoses and Public Health, 59*(s2), 43–47.

Ter Meulen, J., Lukashevich, I., Sidibe, K., Inapogui, A., Marx, M., Dorlemann, A., Yansane, M. L., Koulemou, K., Chang-Claude, J., & Schmitz, H. (1996). Hunting of peridomestic rodents and consumption of their meat as possible risk factors for rodent-to-human transmission of Lassa virus in the Republic of Guinea. *The American Journal of Tropical Medicine and Hygiene, 55*(6), 661–666.

The organization, World Health. (2017). Lassa fever-Nigeria. In *Factsheet*. Geneva: World Health Organization (WHO).

Tomori, O., Fabiyi, A., Sorungbe, A., Smith, A., & McCormick, J. B. (1988). Viral hemorrhagic fever antibodies in Nigerian populations. *The American Journal of Tropical Medicine and Hygiene, 38*(2), 407–410.

Unigwe, U. S., Iroezindu, M. O., Umenzekwe, C. C., Chima, E. I., & Isiguzo, G. C., (2016, November 25–27). Knowledge, attitude and practices of medical officers in south-east Nigeria regarding Lassa fever management. In *Annual general scientific conference of the Nigerian infectious diseases society*. Abuja Nigeria.

WHO. (2017). *Lassa fever factsheet*. Geneva: World Health Organization.

Wilson, M. E. (1995). Infectious diseases: An ecological perspective. *BMJ: British Medical Journal, 311*(7021), 1681.

Wulff, H., Bruce M, M. I., Hamner, D. B., & Johnson, K. M. (1977). Isolation of an arenavirus closely related to Lassa virus from Mastomys natalensis in South-east Africa. *Bulletin of the World Health Organization, 55*(4), 441.

Wulff, H., Lange, J. V., & Webb, P. A. (1978). Interrelationships among arenaviruses measured by indirect immunofluorescence. *Intervirology, 9*(6), 344–350.

Yun, N. E., & Walker, D. H. (2012). Pathogenesis of Lassa fever. *Viruses, 4*(10), 2031–2048.

# Part II
# Social Determinants of EID

# Chapter 5
# Socio-cultural and Economic Concerns on Use of Convalescent Blood or Plasma for the Management of Ebola Virus Disease in Africa

**Nchangwi Syntia Munung, Godfrey B. Tangwa, David Houeto, Awa Keita, J. Radeino Ambe, and Akin Abayomi**

## 5.1 Introduction

Africa continues to be the unenviable epicenter of most epidemics in human history. Some of the unforgettable epidemics that have ravaged the continent in recent times include: Small pox, meningitis, tuberculosis, HIV/AIDS and Ebola Virus Disease (EVD) (Kebede et al. 2010; Shears 2000). Africa, on the other hand, is endowed

N. S. Munung (✉)
Department of Medicine, University of Cape Town, Cape Town, South Africa

Global Emerging Pathogen Treatment Consortium (GET) Consortium, Lagos, Nigeria

G. B. Tangwa
Department of Philosophy, University of Yaounde 1, Yaounde, Cameroon

Cameroon Bioethics Initiative (CAMBIN), Yaounde, Cameroon

Global Emerging Pathogen Treatment Consortium (GET) Consortium, Lagos, Nigeria

D. Houeto
School of Public Health, University of Parakou, Parakou, Republic of Benin

A. Keita
Centre for Research on SCD, Bamako, Mali

J. R. Ambe
Department of Public Health, School of Nursing and Health Sciences, Capella University, Minneapolis, MN, USA

The Global Emerging Pathogens Treatment Initiative, Lagos, Nigeria

A. Abayomi
Global Emerging Pathogen Treatment Consortium (GET) Consortium, Lagos, Nigeria

Nigerian Medical Research Institute (NIMR), Lagos, Nigeria

Faculty of Medicine and Health Sciences, University of Stellenbosch, Stellenbosch, South Africa
e-mail: abayomi@sun.ac.za



G. B. Tangwa et al. (eds.), *Socio-cultural Dimensions of Emerging Infectious Diseases in Africa*, https://doi.org/10.1007/978-3-030-17474-3_5

with enormous natural resources and a recognized, sophisticated level of social development, characterized as "Ubuntu"-a cohesive "WE" philosophy (Tutu 1999), yet the continent, paradoxically, remains the least technologically developed; and most exploited continent in the world. This situation has had devastating effects in Africa especially on health and human life. The EVD outbreak has been endemic in Central Africa since 1976 and attained epidemic proportions in some West African countries in 2014 (WHO 2015c). The 2014 Ebola epidemic in West Africa was eventually brought under control in 2015 with the declaration of Liberia being "Ebola free", first on May 9th 2015 (WHO 2015a), and for a second time on September 3, 2015 (WHO 2015b). By the end of September 2015, the figures had dropped to four new cases in Guinea and no new recoded case in Liberia or Sierra Leone.

Following the devastating effects of the EVD outbreak in West Africa, some African scientists and allied health experts, in the typical African philosophy of Ubuntu, decided not to continue standing by, hands akimbo, while the rest of the world, through altruism philanthropy or for other motives, responded to an African situation. They decided to form the "GET" (Global Emerging-Pathogens Treatment) consortium to provide an indigenous response to the 2014 epidemic and as a platform that African experts could use to play their requisite role in responding, in a timely manner, to health emergencies in Africa. In a bid to find a lasting solution to the Ebola crisis in West Africa, the consortium supported the use of convalescent plasma as a means of managing EVD in the absence of a proven prophylactic. To this effect, clinical trials on the efficacy of convalescent plasma were kick started in Liberia and Sierra Leone.

## 5.2 Discussion

From a scientific point of view, understanding the cause of a disease or epidemic would ideally be a first step in its control and elimination. The second, arguably, would be to find an antidote. This has, to a large extent, been the case with EVD with a number of clinical trials for potential drugs/therapy options currently on the rail. However, irrespective of the actual or perceived cause(s) of a disease or infection, treatment would have to be culture-congruent for it to be effective and satisfactory. A population's perception of the disease and its possible remedies is deeply anchored in its culture, social organization and practices. This is because culture, basically, is the way of life of a group of people and it is underpinned by adaptation to a particular environment, worldview, similar ways of thinking and acting and doing, similar attitudes, expectations and practices (Tangwa 2010). Also, different socio-cultural contexts offer opportunities for discovering and appreciating different perspectives, paradigms and frameworks (Tangwa 2004) especially as pertains to healthcare. Therefore, addressing cultural issues linked to the control of the disease would be crucial in the fight against EVD. For example, manipulating human biological samples from Ebola infected persons requires strict isolation facilities and level 4 bio-containment laboratories (of which there are currently two in Africa). Care for patients requires strict isolation from the healthy through the use of containment facilities. Burial of those who die from EVD is performed in isolation and by persons wearing personal protective equipment (suits, boots, face masks, gloves and goggles). Based on this approach of managing EVD, it is understandable why the EVD outbreak in some West African countries caused a lot of panic, given cultural life-styles, beliefs regarding disease and care for the sick, cultural practices on the handling of corpses and burial ceremonies.

### 5.2.1 Use (Standard or Experimental) of Blood as a Form of Therapy in Africa

The use of blood, blood components and convalescent plasma for therapy is not new. As far back as the 1920s, studies had documented the use of convalescent plasma as a means of achieving passive immunization in epidemic situations and for the treatment of typhoid, measles and poliomyelitis (Jensen 1935; Zingher 1924; Dewar 1946). More recently, the effectiveness of convalescent plasma for the treatment of severe acute respiratory syndrome was reported in a systematic review (Mair-Jenkins et al. 2015) with the recommendation that a well-designed trial is required. In Africa, the use of blood or its components for therapy has been documented, mostly in the form of small scale research. An example is a Cameroon-based study on the use of blood components for the treatment of HIV/AIDS patients (Ngu and Ambe 2001; Ngu et al. 2002, 2007). In the 2014 EVD outbreak, the use of convalescent blood/plasma therapy also made headlines as a possible method of therapy especially as there was no proven therapy or vaccine at the time.

### 5.2.2 Feasibility of Using Plasma Component Therapy in Africa

Convalescent blood therapy and convalescent plasma (CP) is particularly attractive as a modality of intervention when there are risks of epidemics caused by emerging pathogens for which there is little known therapy or any vaccine (Lachmann 2012). It allows the health care system to combine treatment and vaccine modalities, thereby theoretically preventing the transition from epidemic to pandemic. The scientific principles underlying the use of convalescent blood therapy are based on the harvesting of components, known as antibodies. Antibodies reside in the blood and are generated by the convalescent patient, who has recovered from a particular infective episode. Blood or its components are harvested from a convalescent patient and transferred, by a parenteral route to another individual either to protect them from infection or, if already exposed to the pathogen, to ameliorate the natural infective process that would ensue. The cellular components of blood are red blood cells, white blood cells and platelets. These components circulate in a medium of clear fluid called plasma. Plasma is rich in proteins and chemical metabolites. Antibodies are a collection of proteins derived from white blood cells, which through a miracle of human physiology, recognize any known pathogen. It is these antibodies in plasma that constitute the main interest of harvesting convalescent blood for therapy.

Convalescent plasma therapy will therefore require antibodies to be obtained from a convalescing patient. There are three procedures involved in this form of therapy. The simplest and cheapest is to harvest whole blood as is normally done for a blood transfusion and use the whole blood as an infusion to an infected patient. Alternatively, the convalescing patient can be placed on an Apheresis machine which has the capacity to separate the clear plasma from the red and white cells and return the cellular compartment back to the patient while harvesting just plasma which is rich in the antibodies. CP can be given to a patient with the same infection that the convalescent survivor recovered from. A step further would be to process the plasma into different components such as: antibodies (immuno globulin) or in the case of EVD, Hyper Immune Ebola Globulin (HIEG); proteins like albumen; and blood clotting factors. This is called plasma fractionation and requires meticulous attention to blood transfusion principles, especially in view of the fact that large numbers of plasma volumes derived from multiple donors are pooled and processed in large biotechnology infrastructures that cost a lot of money to develop and maintain (Burnouf and Seghatchian 2014).

While whole blood is viable for a few weeks when stored in a fridge, CP can be stored at minus 30 degrees for approximately 3 years without losing potency. Fractionated hyperimmune globulin, on the other hand, can be stored at room temperature or in a fridge in small volumes for years and does not need cross matching to administer. It may be given by intramuscular or intravenous routes and used either prophylactically or therapeutically. In the case of EVD, there is an interest in using both whole blood and CP for treatment; the argument being that these modalities are quite feasible in an epidemic situation in Africa and could permit rapid stocks of donation within a relatively short period.

The use of either whole blood or CP therapy would therefore require efficient and well coordinated transfusion services. However, blood transfusion services in sub-Saharan Africa tend to be too decentralized, making it difficult to form a coordinated activity of best practices, while taking into consideration the socio-cultural factors relating to blood and blood transfusion (Ala et al. 2012). Although it is thought that in the time of an epidemic, convalescent plasma is preferable (Butler 2014) economic factors come into play as the equipment needed to enable the donation of plasma is not the same as with whole blood donation where blood flows into a plastic bag and when the bag is full, the needle is removed and the tubing clamped off, while the capacity to obtain CP requires a fairly sophisticated piece of equipment and expertise that is not readily available on the continent.

### 5.2.3 Historical Cases of Use of Plasma in Ebola or Other Viral Hemorrhagic Fever Outbreaks in Africa

Despite the above mentioned challenges, human CP has been widely used for post-exposure prophylaxis or treatment of some types of viral hemorrhagic fevers (VHF). As early as 1984, a study in Jos, Nigeria (Frame et al. 1984), used CP for the treatment of Lassa fever (a close relative of EVD). In the context of EVD, convalescent therapy was first documented in Zaire, in 1976, where a patient, who later died, was transfused with plasma from a survivor of the Ebola-related Marburg Virus. Close to 20 years after, eight EVD patients in the DRC were treated with whole blood collected from recovered patients (Mupapa et al. 1999). While seven out of the eight patients recovered, a firm conclusion could not be reached as to whether their recovery was based on the use of convalescent blood. In the 2014 EVD outbreak, a few patients were managed using convalescent blood or CP therapy, though mainly as an experimental form of treatment, in combination with an experimental drug and supportive care (Pollack 2014). Additionally, there is fairly convincing evidence from nonhuman primate (NHP) studies conducted at the United States Army Reference Institute for Infectious Diseases, where CP from NHP that had recovered from EVD was used to provide 100% protection to a set of unexposed NHP that were challenged with infective doses of EVD (Dye et al. 2012).

It was partly on the strength of the above evidence that GET proposed blood based therapy for EVD as a plausible solution to the EVD outbreak in West Africa, particularly as there was no other proven intervention. In December 2014, it was reported that the first ever clinical trial on the use of convalescent plasma (CP) in Africa would kick off in Liberia (Butler 2014). This was made possible by a collaboration between GET and a Clinical Research Organization, with funding from a number US and European donor agencies. The concept for the use of CP was first evidenced by GET in Lagos during the arrival of the first Ebola index case into the 23 million dense population of Lagos. At the time, it appeared that, in the absence of any known treatment, CP was probably the only hope Lagos had of preventing a major catastrophic epidemic in the overcrowded metropolis. Simultaneously, investigators in Freetown, Sierra Leone, had started using convalescent whole blood as a treatment modality, as well as subjecting this to a home grown clinical trial which arguably, would be the first comprehensive trial in Africa (Personal Communication with Prof Gevao). The use of CP therapy in Africa is therefore not new but would require subjection to robust clinical trial modalities while paying attention to socio-cultural and economic factors on the use of blood (and/or its components) as a form of therapy.

### 5.2.4 Socio-Cultural, Determinants of EVD and Implications for Behavior and Disease Control in Epidemic Situations

The concept of socio-cultural determinants to health emerged in the 1990s and are so strong that neither policy makers nor health systems planners can ignore them. They are important in planning infectious disease control therefore should be taken into consideration when designing interventions (research or health care) aimed at fighting EVD and other similar diseases. For example, in some communities in Mali, there is a belief that washing hands with soap could bring poverty. Therefore, it was not easy to sensitize the population on the importance of basic rules of hygiene like regularly washing hands with soap, as a means of avoiding EVD, without first tackling such belief. It is therefore not surprising that during the epidemic there was a preference for hand sanitizers in such communities and those who could afford it, paid for anti-bacterial formulations. The prices of these products instantly increased and unsurprisingly so especially as people thought this was more effective than washing hands, let alone washing hands with soap and risking poverty.

The conditions in which people are born, grow, live, work, and age, as wel as the systems put in place to deal with illness (Marmot et al. 2008) constitute their 'social determinants of health' (SDH). These SDH are the major part of the general determinants of health which are factors or characteristics that bring about a change in health' either for better or for worse (Reidpath 2004). Some of the determinants are of a socio-ecological, environmental, cultural, or biological-genetic nature, but they are all interrelated. That interrelatedness is concerned with questions such as 'how social forces act on individuals to affect their biological processes and change disease risk' (Marmot 2000) or how behavior affects both social processes and disease risk; and how social, political and economic structural conditions could enhance or diminish opportunities for populations to be healthy.

A focus on these health determinants would help improve understanding on individual and population health issues, especially as they pertain to the EVD. This is based on a notion of health that recognizes the range of social, economic, and environmental factors that contribute to health and that understands health in terms of people's capacity to have access to the resources that they need in order to be healthy, to adapt, respond to, or control the challenges and changes in the environments that surround them. In epidemic situations like EVD, this approach enables us to shift our focus from making the state of health itself our object of interest or measurement, to making the determinants our object of analysis and the basis of our interventions and responses to it, in order to control it in a sustainable way (Reidpath 2004). For instance, the geography, socio-cultural patterns and political situations of the countries most affected by the recent EVD outbreak must have had a great influence in the spread and management of the disease. Some of these factors include the sexual patterns and activities of the population, food (especially bush meat) consumption, migration for social reasons (to visit friends, relatives and attend ceremonies like funerals, weddings and naming ceremonies or for business purposes) and the role of caregivers, especially women, in society.

Political factors like poor health systems, limited educational support and state of preparedness cannot be overlooked. For example, at the peak of the outbreak, when a number of aid agencies and organizations were in Liberia and Sierra Leone to help fight the disease, a lot of rumors widely spread about the disease having been introduced into Liberia by the USA for the purpose of biological weapon experimentation. This was also the case in Mali, where people believed more in the conspiracy theory that EVD is a weapon used by the western world against Africans to make them abandon certain cultural practices, like shaking hands, embracing loved ones, and their manner of caring for the sick or burying the dead etc. These rumors and conspiracy theories are neither easily provable nor disprovable and therefore constitute a dangerous distraction in the face of a deadly epidemic. They ought firmly but provisionally to be set aside until the epidemic is convincingly completely over.

In Nigeria, false information spread on social media platforms that EVD could be prevented by bathing with, and drinking a salt and water mixture. Such misinformation, spread beyond the affected countries and could have prevented the formulation of policies and strategies necessary for curbing the spread of the disease. In Mali, the lack of adequate and coordinated public health messages on EVD resulted in a scandal involving one of the country's most respected health institutions. The clinic had hospitalized a patient from Guinea, who later died of EVD. It is reported that the clinic never publicly reported the death of the patient until one of their staff allegedly died of Ebola (Souké 2014). The intention behind the clinic's decision not to report the death of the patient is unclear might have been to avoid causing panic in a population that was already scared of what was happening to their neighbours. Perhaps it was also to cover up some negligence, which they could no longer do, when their own staff died. It took two deaths and rumors in the community for the hospital authorities to make a statement and when they eventually did, it was said that the staff who is reported to have died was a student on internship and had presented with symptoms of pneumonia and not Ebola (Souké 2014). The above scenarios demonstrate the impact rumours and false information can have in an outbreak situation. The recommendation for health authorities to always have a coordinated public health messaging strategy (Ravi and Gauldin 2014) can therefore not be overlooked. As Ravi and Gauldin (2014) would argue, a coordinated public health response would ensure that policymakers, the public and health care workers have access to timely, accurate, and reliable information about EVD. This will be also be an advantage to research and clinical trials for potential therapies and vaccines against EVD.

The 2014 EVD epidemic also had a huge socio-economic impact on entire communities and, in some cases, the national economy. Governments in the countries most hit by Ebola are yet to recover, financially and politically, from the investments they made in the fight against the disease. Introducing a relatively new technology, first in the form of clinical trials may meet an ill prepared social, political and economic set-up in the affected countries. Of course, there are clear advantages if these clinical trials take place in the affected areas; however, it would require some background work both at the social, political and economic levels, to ensure that the goodwill of all stakeholders is not mistaken;

and that the vulnerability of the people and communities of the affected countries is not exploited. An instructive example of such a scenario is Pfizer's 1996 trial of a meningitis vaccine in Kano state, Nigeria, (http://www.pfizer.com/files/news/trovan_statement_defense_summary.pdf). Leaving aside issues connected with informed consent, this trial took place in an epidemic situation. Affected communities were still struggling to come to terms with a strange disease that was ravaging their community, threatening lives and causing deaths. There were no existing policies or regulations in place and the political system, at the time, was more concerned about bringing the situation under control. Most did not realize that Pfizer was conducting a clinical trial. Pfizer faced a number of court cases because of the trials. Today, the Muslim leaders in the north of Nigeria have welcomed the court actions against Pfizer, saying it confirmed their views that those (of the western world) who pretended that they wanted to help were actually killing them and that they were happy the Nigerian government had finally seen this (http://www.irinnews.org/report/72601/nigeria-government-blames-polio-vaccine-boycott-on-pfizer-trials). This highlights the lack of trust and suspicion that could develop if a proper, well intentioned trial does not allow communities to buy into and fully support the trial. Setting up a trial for the use of convalescent therapy for EVD would undoubtedly need to consider all these socio-cultural and economic factors. There would be an undeniable need to actively engage the community (Folayan et al. 2015) and this would require lots of public-private partnerships and a strong commitment from community leaders, African governments and international aid or humanitarian agencies.

### 5.2.5 Socio-Cultural Challenges in Managing Outbreaks of Emerging Infectious Disease in African Countries

There are a number of socio-cultural practices in certain african countries that may present as challenges in the management of outbreaks of EIDs. Generally, different communities tend to have different perceptions and representations about disease and ill-health, some of which are shaped by the existential conditions in which the majority of the African populations live including: illiteracy, ignorance, ill-health and chronic poverty. Also, during disease outbreaks (e.g. cholera, meningitis, Ebola), some communities tend to first seek care from traditional healers. This can compromise public health strategies because in such cases, the communal by beliefs on the causality and by extension, the management of the disease, goes beyond what modern medicine cannot address such as, witchcraft, breaking a taboo or pleasing angry ancestors or the gods of the land (Houéto and Deccache 2007).

Low health literacy levels in many African communities also present as a challenge in the management of outbreaks of emerging infectious diseases. This is because, whilst providing print information on the outbreak and public health measures may be a quicker approach to sensitising the population, there is a likelyhood that some communities may not read or easily comprehend information provided in print. An extra effort would have to put in designing posters with appropriate and contextually suitable images so that people with low literacy levels may easily understand. Television and radio messages may be more appropriate, yet public health programs must ascertain that populations, especially in rural areas have access to radio and television services they aim to use to improve public health literacy on the disease. Surely, during a disease outbreak, social media, radio and posters on bill boards can serve as effective mechanisms for conveying public health messages that could help curb the spread of the disease; however, close collaboration with communities through a genuine community engagement approach should not be overlooked. This is because people can easily understand a disease outbreak and the public health measures when time is taken to orally explain things clearly. People who have witnessed cases of Ebola deaths, for instance, get really scared and are more suitably disposed to do what is necessary to avoid infection and to shake-off log held prejudices on the disease, especially after watching a relation or neighbour die and they could offer little or no help.

### *5.2.6 Cultural Concepts and Perceptions of Blood and Blood Donation in Africa: Implications for Blood-Based Therapy in Epidemic Situations*

Biologically, the use of convalescent blood for the treatment of EVD is possible, pending conclusive scientific evidence. However, a potential challenge, besides infrastructure, for the use of convalescent blood for therapy or treatment of EVD in Africa, would be the willingness of EVD survivors to donate blood and for potential beneficiaries to accept the donated blood. This could be due to a number of reasons related to cultural perceptions and beliefs about blood. Although clinically, there is acceptance of blood transfusion by patients in need, little is known if convalescent blood would be easily accepted by patients in need of treatment. The good news is that, although the practice of blood donation in Africa is low (Tapko et al. 2007), it has also been documented that a major motivating factor for blood donors is the desire to is to save the life of a friend or a relative (Olaiya et al. 2004; Nebie et al. 2007; Osaro and Charles 2011), otherwise, blood donation is often associated with a strong feeling of mistrust and discrimination (Agasa and Likwela 2014; Jacobs and Berege 1995; Umeora et al. 2005).

In most African communities, blood is considered mystical and sacred. Therefore, any attempt to use blood or its components for therapy would therefore have to be accompanied by community engagement activities with the aim of building trust between healthcare workers, researchers and communities. This would ensure that the altruistic donation of blood is matched by a feeling of strong ownership and commitment to help patients. Moreover, in the case of Ebola, survivors are sometimes viewed as having special supernatural powers and in some instances have been accused of being witches or a wizards (Kinsman 2012). This has lead to some survivors concealing their identity for fear of being treated like a "plague". For example, an Ebola survivor in Guinea said: "Revealing my identity is to run a big risk, especially of rejection by the population, we are ghosts" (http://www.africaguinee.com/articles/2014/08/10/en-guinee-les-survivants-d-ebola-ont-la-joie-discrete accessed 12 August 2015). In such a situation it may be culturally problematic to propose that blood from a witch, a ghost or a wizard be given to other members of the community, even if it is for the treatment of a deadly condition. But the fear of witches and wizards is not the same as the fear of becoming a witch or wizard. Therefore, the realization or belief that a blood transfusion might give a person supernatural powers (and immunity against Ebola infection might be viewed as one such power) might lead people not only to accept but to seek this particular type of power. For example, a study in south-Eastern Nigeria showed socio-cultural barriers (not feeling well, loss of libido, exposure of blood to witchcraft,) to voluntary blood donation were associated with misconception, misinformation and ignorance about blood donation (Umeora et al. 2005). Similar perceptions have also been recorded in the Democratic Republic of Congo, including that freely donated blood could be sold by the hospitals storing the blood (Agasa and Likwela 2014). These different perceptions of blood donation and acceptance of blood from persons with "supernatural" powers would have to be taken into consideration when designing programs (research or healthcare) on treatment based on convalescent blood.

Considering the examples provided above, a western-styled model of blood donation drives will certainly not be appropriate for use in plasma therapy in Africa. For instance, whilst financial remuneration for blood donors may tend to be unduly inducive particularly in epidemic situations, some form of compensation would be necessary to achieve a successful blood donation drive. It should be noted that whilst blood donors usually consider blood donation as voluntary, studies in different African countries have shown that blood donors usually expect some form of compensation (Koster and Hassall 2011; Nebie et al. 2007; Umeora et al. 2005; Jacobs and Berege 1995). Celebrating the gift of blood donation, the provision of cash and non-cash incentives and the recognition of voluntary blood donors has been listed as one of the ways of motivating blood donation in Africa (Osaro and Charles 2011; Olaiya et al. 2004). Equally, in an outbreak, some form of recognition, for example giving certificates to blood or plasma donors, may be exciting as this could highlight their roles as heroes in the fight against Ebola.

The success of using convalescent plasma for post exposure treatment of EVD or for clinical trials would largely depend on the ability to recruit and retain voluntary EVD survivors, despite the prevailing stigma associated with having been an EVD patient. Stigma is one issue that needs to be seriously addressed. The needs of treatment and clinical trials would definitely require repeat blood donors. The altruism of these donors would have to be matched by active community engagement and establishing a feeling that they are doing something worthy, that is, saving lives in an epidemic situation. A lot of work would have to be done to ensure successful use of convalescent plasma in epidemic situations in Africa. This would require active community engagement and public education. It would require the appropriate use of media (radio, TV, newspapers) to convey messages on blood/plasma donation for use in therapy, in ways that are culturally acceptable. It would also benefit from the effective use of mobile phone services (e.g. ring tones and broadcast messages) and effective social media communication with the aim of actively engaging the community on the benefits of blood donation.

The use of socially adapted methods and mass media for blood donation campaigns has been effective in Ghana for increasing blood donation at a little extra cost (Allain et al. 2008; Owusu-Ofori et al. 2010). While this scenario may be different from an epidemic situation, a lot could be learned from the Ghanaian experience. Of course, this implies that while we learn from experiences in other African countries, we also take into consideration the values, beliefs, customs, communication styles, behaviors, practices, of the different communities as well as show respect for local institutions and community leaders.

### *5.2.7 Socio-Cultural Issues in CP Trials for EVD*

With regards to clinical trials for convalescent therapy for EVD, many social and ethical issues have been considered (Kombe et al. 2016). This includes the ethical appropriateness of procedural options, proper constitution of data and safety monitoring board and extensive community engagement aimed at addressing stigma and to aid the process of healing. A number of workshops, in Freetown and Monrovia have educated survivors on the use of CP, the promise it has for containing EVD and the possible adverse effects. Cultural issues were also addressed and community leaders were challenged to help reverse stigmatization while embracing survivors as champions of the community. The spiritual connotation of life in blood was entertained for discussion and understanding (GET Manuscript in development) and emphasis was laid on the fact that GET and the national ethics authorities would safeguard the interests of the people and ensure that Africans would not be exploited or used as guinea pigs by any commercial or external entity without a clear understanding and ownership of the research and data by Africans. While this promise maybe difficult to ascertain till the end of the trials, all stakeholders would have a key role and responsibility to ensure that is upheld and that the communities do not end up feeling that an unfortunate epidemic situation was used as a means of exploitation by those in the research industry as, this would not augur well for biomedical research in Africa.

## 5.3 Conclusion

Africa's generosity for social development mostly manifested through collective welfare for the community, synergistically and symbiotically aligned to the environment, could arguably have made Africa vulnerable to exploitation and extractive abuse. This is evident in the management of epidemic situations in Africa. The recent EVD outbreak in West Africa has roused the conscience of African scientists and intellectuals from lethargic slumber in the face of health catastrophes on the continent. In the 2014 epidemic, the African-led GET Consortium sought to find a permanent solution to the epidemic and explored studying the feasibility of using convalescent blood and products as therapy for EVD and similar diseases. This was done mostly with funding from partners in high income countries. While the use of convalescent plasma has firm basis in scientific history and has promising prospects as therapy for EVD and similar emerging infectious diseases, clinical tests to confirm this method of treatment are however up against a number of socio-cultural and economic concerns and challenges, some of which are peculiar to the African context. The good news is that these are addressable and most of them have been more or less satisfactorily addressed by the GET consortium. However, unexpected challenges, reminiscent of north-south dichotomy and inequity may emerge in the conduct of these clinical trials and would have to be addressed satisfactorily in a spirit of fairness and altruistic concern for future victims of EVD and other lurking future epidemics in Africa.

**Acknowledgement** We thank Alice Mungwa for inputs in the initial draft of the manuscript.

## References

Agasa, S. B., & Likwela, J. L. (2014). Barriers to voluntary blood donation in the population of Kisangani in the Democratic Republic of Congo. *The Pan African Medical Journal, 17*, 306. https://doi.org/10.11604/pamj.2014.17.306.2663.

Ala, F., Allain, J. P., Bates, I., Boukef, K., Boulton, F., Brandful, J., Dax, E. M., El Ekiaby, M., Farrugia, A., Gorlin, J., Hassall, O., Lee, H., Loua, A., Maitland, K., Mbanya, D., Mukhtar, Z., Murphy, W., Opare-Sem, O., Owusu-Ofori, S., Reesink, H., Roberts, D., Torres, O., Totoe, G., Ullum, H., & Wendel, S. (2012). External financial aid to blood transfusion services in sub-Saharan Africa: A need for reflection. *PLoS Medicine, 9*(9), e1001309. https://doi.org/10.1371/journal.pmed.1001309.

Allain, J. P., Sarkodie, F., Boateng, P., Asenso, K., Kyeremateng, E., & Owusu-Ofori, S. (2008). A pool of repeat blood donors can be generated with little expense to the blood center in sub-Saharan Africa. *Transfusion, 48*(4), 735–741. https://doi.org/10.1111/j.1537-2995.2007.01599.x.

Burnouf, T., & Seghatchian, J. (2014). "Go no go" in plasma fractionation in the world's emerging economies: Still a question asked 70 years after the COHN process was developed! *Transfusion and Apheresis Science, 51*(2), 113–119. https://doi.org/10.1016/j.transci.2014.10.002.

Butler, D. (2014). First trials of blood-based Ebola therapy kick off. *Nature News*. Accessed 18 May 2015. http://www.nature.com/news/first-trials-of-blood-based-ebola-therapy-kick-off-1.16564

Dewar, H. A. (1946). Treatment of typhoid fever with convalescent whole blood. *Journal of the Royal Army Medical Corps, 86*, 249–253.

Dye, J. M., Herbert, A. S., Kuehne, A. I., Barth, J. F., Muhammad, M. A., Zak, S. E., Ortiz, R. A., Prugar, L. I., & Pratt, W. D. (2012). Postexposure antibody prophylaxis protects nonhuman primates from filovirus disease. *Proceedings of the National Academy of Sciences of the United States of America, 109*(13), 5034–5039. https://doi.org/10.1073/pnas.1200409109.

Folayan, M. O., Brown, B., Haire, B., Yakubu, A., Peterson, K., & Tegli, J. (2015). Stakeholders' engagement with Ebola therapy research in resource limited settings. *BMC Infectious Diseases, 15*(1), 242. https://doi.org/10.1186/s12879-015-0950-8.

Frame, J. D., Verbrugge, G. P., Gill, R. G., & Pinneo, L. (1984). The use of Lassa fever convalescent plasma in Nigeria. *Transactions of the Royal Society of Tropical Medicine and Hygiene, 78*(3), 319–324.

Houéto, D., & Deccache, A. (2007). Child malaria in sub-saharan Africa: Effective control and prevention require a health promotion approach. *International Quarterly of Community Health Education, 28*(1), 51–62. https://doi.org/10.2190/IQ.28.1.e.

Jacobs, B., & Berege, Z. A. (1995). Attitudes and beliefs about blood donation among adults in Mwanza region, Tanzania. *East African Medical Journal, 72*(6), 345–348.

Jensen, C. (1935). The 1934 epidemic of poliomyelitis in Denmark. Preliminary report on the epidemiology, clinical features and convalescent serum therapy: (Section of pathology). *Proceedings of the Royal Society of Medicine, 28*(8), 1007–1026.

Kebede, S., Duales, S., Yokouide, A., & Alemu, W. (2010). Trends of major disease outbreaks in the African region, 2003–2007. *East African Journal of Public Health, 7*(1), 20–29.

Kinsman, J. (2012). "A time of fear": Local, national, and international responses to a large Ebola outbreak in Uganda. *Globalization and Health, 8*, 15. https://doi.org/10.1186/1744-8603-8-15.

Kombe, F., Folayan, M. O., Ambe, J., Igonoh, A., & Abayomi, A. (2016). Taking the bull by the horns: Ethical considerations in the design and implementation of an Ebola virus therapy trial. *Social Science & Medicine, 148*, 163–170.

Koster, J., & Hassall, O. W. (2011). Attitudes towards blood donation and transfusion in Bamenda, Republic of Cameroon. *Transfusion Medicine, 21*(5), 301–307. https://doi.org/10.1111/j.1365-3148.2011.01079.x.

Lachmann, P. J. (2012). The use of antibodies in the prophylaxis and treatment of infections. *Emerging Microbes & Infections, 1*, e11.

Mair-Jenkins, J., Saavedra-Campos, M., Baillie, J. K., Cleary, P., Khaw, F. M., Lim, W. S., Makki, S., Rooney, K. D., & Beck, C. R. (2015). The effectiveness of convalescent plasma and hyperimmune immunoglobulin for the treatment of severe acute respiratory infections of viral etiology: A systematic review and exploratory meta-analysis. *The Journal of Infectious Diseases, 211*(1), 80–90. https://doi.org/10.1093/infdis/jiu396.

Marmot, M. (2000). Multilevel approaches to understanding social determinants. In L. F. K. Berkman (Ed.), *Social epidemiology* (pp. 349–367). New York: Oxford University Press.

Marmot, M., Friel, S., Bell, R., Houweling, T. A. J., Taylor, S., & on behalf of the Commission on Social Determinants of Health. (2008). Closing the gap in a generation: Health equity through action on the social determinants of health. *The Lancet, 372*(9650), 1661–1669. https://doi.org/10.1016/S0140-6736(08)61690-6.

Mupapa, K., Massamba, M., Kibadi, K., Kuvula, K., Bwaka, A., Kipasa, M., Colebunders, R., & Muyembe-Tamfum, J. J. (1999). Treatment of Ebola hemorrhagic fever with blood transfusions from convalescent patients. *Journal of Infectious Diseases, 179*(Suppl 1), S18–S23. https://doi.org/10.1086/514298.

Nebie, K. Y., Olinger, C. M., Kafando, E., Dahourou, H., Diallo, S., Kientega, Y., Domo, Y., Kienou, K., Ouattara, S., Sawadogo, I., Ky, L., & Muller, C. P. (2007). Lack of knowledge among blood donors in Burkina Faso (West Africa); potential obstacle to transfusion security. *Transfusion Clinique et Biologique, 14*(5), 446–452. https://doi.org/10.1016/j.tracli.2007.12.005.

Ngu, V. A., & Ambe, F. A. (2001). Effective vaccines against and immunotherapy of the HIV: A preliminary report. *Journal of the Cameroon Academy of Science, 1*(1), 2–8.

Ngu, V. A., Ambe, F. A., & Boma, G. A. (2002). Significant reduction of HIV loads in the sera of patients treated with VANHIVAX. *Journal of the Cameroon Academy of Science, 2*(1), 7–12.

Ngu, V. A., Besong-Egbe, B. H., Ambe, F. A., Ngu, J. A., & Caspa, C. G. (2007). The conversion of HIV sero-positive to sero-negative following VANHIVAX. *Journal of the Cameroon Academy of Science, 7*(1), 17–20.

Olaiya, M. A., Alakija, W., Ajala, A., & Olatunji, R. O. (2004). Knowledge, attitudes, beliefs and motivations towards blood donations among blood donors in Lagos, Nigeria. *Transfusion Medicine, 14*(1), 13–17. https://doi.org/10.1111/j.0958-7578.2004.00474.x.

Osaro, E., & Charles, A. T. (2011). The challenges of meeting the blood transfusion requirements in sub-Saharan Africa: The need for the development of alternatives to allogenic blood. *Journal of Blood Medicine, 2*, 7–21. https://doi.org/10.2147/JBM.S17194.

Owusu-Ofori, S., Asenso-Mensah, K., Boateng, P., Sarkodie, F., & Allain, J. P. (2010). Fostering repeat donations in Ghana. *Biologicals, 38*(1), 47–52. https://doi.org/10.1016/j.biologicals.2009.10.021.

Pollack, A. (2014, October 3). A plan to use survivors' Blood for Ebola treatment in Africa. *The New York Times*. Accessed 19 May 2015. http://www.nytimes.com/2014/10/04/health/use-of-ebola-survivors-blood-as-possible-treatment-gains-support.html.

Ravi, S. J., & Gauldin, E. M. (2014). Sociocultural dimensions of the Ebola virus disease outbreak in Liberia. *Biosecurity and Bioterrorism: Biodefense Strategy, Practice, and Science, 12*(6), 301–305. https://doi.org/10.1089/bsp.2014.1002.

Reidpath, D. D. (2004). Social determinants of health. In H. Keleher & B. Murphy (Eds.), *Understanding health: A determinants approach* (pp. 9–22). Oxford: Oxford University Press.

Shears, P. (2000). Emerging and reemerging infections in africa: The need for improved laboratory services and disease surveillance. *Microbes and Infection, 2*(5), 489–495.

Souké, G. (2014). Propagation du virus Ebola au Mali: l'irresponsabilité de la Clinique Pasteur. *Mali24*, Last Modified 13 November 2014, Accessed 11 June. http://www.mali24.info/dossier/sante/831-propagation-du-virus-ebola-au-mali-l-irresponsabilite-de-la-clinique-pasteur.

Tangwa, G. B. (2004). Bioethics, biotechnology and culture: A voice from the margins. *Developing World Bioethics, 4*(2), 125–138. https://doi.org/10.1111/j.1471-8731.2004.00088.x.

Tangwa, G. B. (2010). *Elements of African bioethics in a Western Frame*. Mankon/Bamenda: Langaa Research & Publishing CIG.

Tapko, J., Mainuka, P., & Diarra-Nama, A. J. (2007). Status of blood safety in the WHO African region: Report of the 2006 survey. Accessed 12 May 2015. http://www.afro.who.int/en/divisions-a-programmes/dsd/health-technologies-a-laboratories.html.

Tapko, J. B., Toure, B., & Sambo, L. G. (2014). *Status of blood safety in the WHO African region: Report of the 2010 survey*. Brazzaville/Republic of Congo: WHO Regional Office for Africa.

Tutu, D. (1999). *No future without forgiveness*. New York: Doubleday.

Umeora, O. U., Onuh, S. O., & Umeora, M. C. (2005). Socio-cultural barriers to voluntary blood donation for obstetric use in a rural Nigerian village. *African Journal of Reproductive Health, 9*(3), 72–76.

WHO. (2015a). *The Ebola outbreak in Liberia is over*.

WHO. (2015b). *Ebola transmission in Liberia over*. Nation enters 90-day intensive surveillance period.

WHO. (2015c). *Ebola virus disease*. Fact sheet N°103.

Zingher, A. (1924). Convalescent whole blood, plasma and serum in prophylaxis of measles. *Journal of the American Medical Association, 82*(15), 1180–1187. https://doi.org/10.1001/jama.1924.02650410022011.

# Chapter 6
# The Impact of Ebola Virus Disease on Government Expenditure in Sierra Leone

**Fuein Vera Kum, Saheed Olayiwola, and Njong Mom Aloysius**

## 6.1 Introduction

Emerging infectious disease like EVD adversely affects government tax and expenditures in many affected African countries. This has the potential to indirectly threaten the lives and livelihoods of more than 22 million people in Ebola-affected areas (ACAPS 2014). The epidemic may also have a long-term socio-economic and political implications on the affected country's development trajectory (Piot 2014). The first episode of the disease was first recorded in the Democratic Republic of Congo in 1976. The most recent outbreak occurred in Sierra Leone, Liberia, and Guinea. The origin of EVD (the primary infectious event) is yet to be known in spite of various studies that have been carried out on the epidemic. According to Nadia, (2015) an index case was identified four times and hypothesized in two other instances among the twenty-one documented outbreaks of EVD in Africa. For instance, as at 2016, there were estimated 28,639 suspected, likely, and established cases of EVD and a projected 11,316 deaths from the 2014 epidemic of EVD in West Africa (CDC 2016). More so, there were 2427 reported cases and 1597 deaths in all other outbreaks of Ebola (CDC 2016). The Ebola outbreak began slowly in Sierra Leone and quickly degenerated to an epidemic between May and June, 2014. An ex-post examination indicated that the first case recorded in Sierra Leone was a woman who was a guest at the home of the index case in Meliandou, Guinea (WHO 2015).

F. V. Kum (✉)
Faculty of Economics and Management, University of Bamenda, Bamenda, Cameroon

Denis and Lenora Foretia Foundation, Yaounde, Cameroon

S. Olayiwola
Department of Economics, Federal University of Technology, Akure, Nigeria

N. M. Aloysius
Faculty of Economics and Management, University of Bamenda, Bamenda, Cameroon



G. B. Tangwa et al. (eds.), *Socio-cultural Dimensions of Emerging Infectious Diseases in Africa*, https://doi.org/10.1007/978-3-030-17474-3_6

The Ebola epidemic had a pronounced socio-economic impact in Guinea, Liberia, and Sierra Leone aside the devastating health effects (CDC 2016). According to a World Bank 2014 projection, *"an estimated $2.2 billion was lost in 2015 in the gross domestic product (GDP) of the three countries. The disease also resulted in lower investment and a substantial loss in private sector growth, declining agricultural production that led to concerns about food security, and a decrease in cross-border trade as restrictions on movement of goods and services increased"* (CDC 2016). Sierra Leone recorded the highest number of cases with 14,124 suspected and confirmed cases and a total of 3956 confirmed deaths among all the three most affected West African countries, (CDC 2016). It equally recorded a total government budget (deficit of about 3.10% of the country's Gross Domestic Product GDP) in 2015. Government budget in Sierra Leone averaged −4.46% of GDP from 1999 until 2015, reaching an all-time height of −0.98% of GDP in 2007 and a record low of about −9.47% of GDP in 1999 (World Bank 2016).

Available literature has enumerated different views of looking into the issue of Ebola and its impact on the country's growth and individual's welfare. For example, Hakon et al. (2014) *"noted that Ebola has strong and devastating effects on the health of the population and submitted that in addition to the direct health effects of the viral disease, the indirect effects on health service may lead to increased morbidity and mortality"*. More so, factors such as patient's fear of Ebola and death of health care staff has reportedly affected health-seeking behaviour and reduced the function of health service. Despite many studies on the Ebola-welfare transmission mechanism, decreasing government revenue resulting from the closure of most mining and food companies of the affected countries, makes investigation of the impact of the Ebola disease on the government expenditures of the affected country vital. This is because decreasing government revenue may impact negatively on the growth of the economy. This study therefore investigates the effect of Ebola outbreak on government capital expenditure of the Sierra Leonean government. The rest of this chapter is organized as follows: Sect. 6.2 reviews empirical literature on the effects of disease outbreak on government expenditures, Sect. 6.3 presents stylized facts on the effects of Ebola crisis on the Sierra Leone economy; Sect. 6.4 described the theory and method of analysis Sect. 6.5 while Sect. 6.6 presents the empirical results and discussion of results.

## 6.2 Conceptual Linkage Between Epidemic Diseases and Economic Growth

The manner of allocation of public expenditure has important impact on the development process of any nation. For example, budgetary allocations to key sectors such as health and education through its positive effects can enhance equity and reduce poverty (Gupta et al. 2001). Budgetary allocations to public sectors are classified into capital expenditure and recurrent expenditure. Capital expenditure can be classified as a payment for non-financial assets used in the production process while recurrent expenditure is payment for non-repayable transactions within one year. Gupta et al. (1998) suggested that public spending on health and education through its positive effects on the formation of human capital can boost economic development and reduce poverty. This is achieved through reduction and eradication of diseases and improvement in the health of the populace.

The need for an instant and substantial intervention from the government given any disease outbreak especially communicable disease is likely to divert public spending from investment in development projects to health and other social spending. Foreign and domestic private investments may also decline without government support to the investors (ECA 2014a, b, c, d). For example, the 2014 Economic Commission for Africa (ECA) report on Ebola crisis in Africa showed that EVD decreased public revenue and increased expenditure in health. This creates pressure on the fiscal stability and weakened state's capacity to manage the disease or protect the economy against spill over effects of the outbreak. Fiscal imbalance due to the outbreak may also force the country to depend on external support. ECA (2014a, b, c, d) argued that health crisis due to the epidemic may lead to a large health spending to manage the disease and provide social protection as a result of the number of deaths, increase in the number of orphans and number of poor. These unfavourable changes in revenue and expenditures of government may force a reallocation of resources in favour of the new needs against productive public investment.

Economic growth is strongly connected to the increase in living standard which inevitably leads to higher economic standard. But health appears to be a decisive factor for economic growth and the increasing overall health level in the population has a strong positive effect on economic growth (Birchenall 2007). A reasonable conclusion therefore is that epidemic diseases will hinder economic growth which may further negatively affect government revenue and spending. Despite many studies on the Ebola-welfare transmission mechanism, the dwindling government revenue of the affected countries due to the outbreak of Ebola disease makes investigation of the impact of the Ebola disease on the government expenditures of the affected country vital. Studies have attempted to study the cost of the EVD on the health sector and health workers of the countries affected, as well as on individuals and households of these countries but very little or nothing has been done on the impact of the disease on government expenditure of these countries especially on the Sierra Leonean economy. This study therefore, delves into this by looking at the resulting effect from such a scenario.

### 6.2.1 Empirical Review

There is little disagreement that the spread of EVD was aggravated by the poor health infrastructure in Sierra Leone. There are many problems facing the health sector in Sierra Leone before the outbreak of Ebola. According to "The Agenda for Prosperity' Sierra Leone health sector suffers from inadequate health infrastructure, shortage of skilled personnel, insufficient prevalence of trained doctors and nurses and weak supervision in the health system and high burden of disease. According to WHO (2010), Sierra Leone had only 132 community health workers as at 2010 and there are more Sierra Leonean doctors working in OECD countries. Which makes Sierra Leone be one of the African countries bedevilled with brain drain in the health sector. Curtis, (2015) observed that the challenges in the Sierra Leonean health sector, as outlined in the Agenda for Prosperity, include: poor health infrastructure, inadequate health care financing resulting in catastrophic health spending. Also included in this Agenda is low coverage in the provision of water and sanitation, high burden of communicable diseases and increasing non-communicable diseases, shortage of healthcare workers and weak human resource as well as poor health sector management.

Beside studies linking epidemic diseases and economic performance, other stream of literature have investigated the impact of public spending on the prevalence of diseases. Filmer and Pretchett (1999), for example, submitted that public spending on health is not significantly related to the overall health of the population and that factors such as income inequality, history of civil conflict, (female) education, ethnic and religious fragmentation and trade integration tend to be more appropriate explanation for cross-country variance in health levels than public spending on health (e.g. Castro-Leal et al. 2000; Evans et al. 2001; Ghobarah et al. 2004; Bor 2007). It was further pointed out that the effectiveness of health measures does not only rely on financial resources (i.e. public and private spending) but also on the political support or goals of the government (Cassels 1995; Hsiao and Heller 2007) and the efficient use of existing resources (institutional quality & good governance) (Walt and Gilson 1994; Evans et al. 2001; Ghobarah et al. 2004; Gauri and Lieberman 2006; McGuire 2006; Gilson and Raphaely 2008).

Thus, political and institutional features seem to play a crucial role in explaining the spread of epidemic diseases in terms of allocating funds effectively on combating infectious diseases. Also, differences in public spending patterns which can be observed between low- middle- and high-income countries may be related more to dissimilarities in health challenges as well as institutional designs of the health sector (Gerdtham et al. 1992). One major distinction between low-and high-income countries regarding health challenges, is that, while individuals in high-income countries suffer mostly from non-communicable diseases (e.g. stroke, cancer, heart attack), health systems in developing countries are used to finance the burden of communicable and infectious diseases such as Ebola and tuberculosis (Hsiao and Heller 2007).

In a study on the impact of epidemic outbreak on consumer expenditures for Middle East respiratory syndrome coronavirus (MERS) in South Korea, Hojin et al. (2016) found that the South Korean government was forced to cut the country's economic growth forecast for 2015 to 3.1%, a drop from the projected 3.8% in 2014. This was due to the government's inability to effectively control MERS. Consequently, and compared to the previous year, retail shops in South Korea faced a 3.4% decrease in sales, and department stores also experienced a 16.5% decrease in sales. The authors further asserted that the outbreak led to over 100,000 cancelled tourist visits to South Korea. As a result, a stimulus package of over $13.5 billion and a 0.25-percentage-point cut in interest rates was offered by the government to reduce the adverse economic effects of the outbreak. This stimulus package was a re-direction of government spending from productive sector to reduce the effects of the epidemic.

Thompson et al. (2003) on the economic costs of the foot and mouth disease (FMD) outbreak in the United Kingdom in 2001 shows that the losses to agriculture and the food chainamount to about £3.1 billion. Government incurred the majority of these costs through compensation for slaughter and disposal and clean-up costs which adversely affects government spending on productive investment. The surveys of tourism shows that tourist-related businesses lost about £2.7–3.2 billion due to reduced number of tourists. However, the overall costs to the UK economy are substantially less than the sum of these components. Much of what was gotten from tourists expenditure was moved to other sectors of the economy. According to the Thompson et al. (2003) the overall net effect of FMD was estimated to have reduced the gross domestic product in the UK by about 0.2% in 2001.

Therefore, literature, in general revealed that the overall effects of outbreak of disease such as Ebola, FMD etc. can have a depressing effect on economic growth and government expenditures and re-directs government spending away from productive sector to curtailing and eradicating disease outbreak.

## 6.3 Ebola Crisis and the Sierra Leone Economy

The 2014–2015 (EVD) outbreak in West Africa was the largest and most widespread in history. The pressures of the epidemic collapsed an already weak health system. Health workers were among the high risk group because, they were exposed to risk during routine patient care and community exposures. Piot, (2014) observed that healthcare workers were principally vulnerable to contracting the disease. This led to an increase in non-Ebola related mortality (ACAPS 2014; Piot 2014). Also, about 80% HIV/AIDS positive individuals living in the three most affected countries were unable to access treatment and pregnantwomen stopped giving birth in health facilities (ACAPS 2014; Glassman and Raghavan 2014). Muiderman, (2014) affirmed that the Ebola crisis had a significant negative impact on the economies of the countries it has affected and its impact can be felt in different sectors. This include loss of gross domestic output, threat to food security, and a fall in employment and decline in foreign investment (UNDP 2014).

The direct effects of EVD in Sierra Leone include over 8000 infected and 1820 deaths which include 106 health care workers. Ten out of the 124 medical doctors in the country died due to Ebola, equivalent to a risk ratio of 280 compared to the general population (Hakon et al. 2014). Many health centres and hospitals in the country were closed down due to the death or desertion of member of staff (Welthungerhilfe 2014; Glassman and Raghavan 2014). Health and burial workers also went on strike over hazard payment and in some cases no payment (ACAPS 2014). Thus, there was a general reversal of the gains made in the health sector in relation to child mortality, maternal mortality, HIV/AIDS, malaria, and other diseases as a result of the closure of health services and the diversion of resources to combatting Ebola (Glassman and Raghavan 2014). The EVD epidemic also had a devastating socio-economic impact in Guinea, Liberia, and Sierra Leone beside the adverse health effects. The disease resulted in low investment and a large loss in private sector growth and declining agricultural production, and a decrease in cross-border trade due to increased restrictions on movement of goods and services. The school children lost a total of 39 productive week in Sierra Leone and children experienced a gap in vaccination schedules due to a decrease in routine immunizations by 30% (CDC 2016).

Due to disruptions in most activities such as agriculture, mining, construction, manufacturing, trade, tourism and transport in Sierra Leone as a result of the Ebola outbreak, there was a slower economic growth in the preceding years (Glassman and Raghavan 2014; UNDP 2014). There were worrying signs for future growth from the drop-in sales in the manufacturing and construction sectors (Welthungerhilfe 2014; Glassman and Raghavan 2014). In December 2014, there was a drop of −2.0% in Sierra Leone economic growth compared to a pre-Ebola 8.9% estimated growth (World Bank 2015). The crisis culminated in increasing unemployment among the youth (GoSL et al. 2014). The government and donors agencies also diverted fund for different sectors to combat Ebola. This created a funding gap for non-Ebola related government services (Brigitte 2014). The emphasis on health versus social spending varies among the three countries. In Sierra Leone, EVD-related spending for 2014 and 2015 were about $36 million and $40.9 million respectively (IMF 2014a). In Liberia the authorities estimated direct EVD spending at $79.7 million, besides $20 million in cash transfers and $30 million in agricultural stimulus (Government of Liberia 2014). Therefore, EVD increase fiscal deficit. The fiscal deficit in Sierra Leone was forecast to widen by 1.5% and 1.7% points in 2014 and 2015 (IMF 2014a, b).

Containing EVD led to rises in government spending and reallocation of spending earmarked for long-term growth. The balance of payments suffered because of increased food and health-related imports (Government of Sierra Leone 2014). The IMF (2014a) estimated the balance of payments shifting from a programmed surplus of $38 million before the crisis to a deficit of $72.4 million in 2014. The currency depreciated relative to international currencies. Other studies indicated the revenue implications of EVD on Sierra Leone and have identified transmission channels. The preliminary country estimates shows that due to the EVD, the country experienced a 14.9% decline in revenue by the end of 2014 (National Revenue Authority of Sierra Leone 2014). The EVD-related revenue loss was around $45.7 million in 2014 and $91.3 million in 2015, or 1% and 1.6% of non-iron GDP In monetary terms (IMF 2014a). The negative effects of EVD in Sierra Leone include mortality of key health personnel, stretched health infrastructure and reversal of health gains as non-EVD health delivery was compromised. The education sector suffered due to school closures. Many students were forced to study via online platforms or through radio programs. Hence, EVD is a threat to social structure among vulnerable groups such as women and children. About 51% of women and 49% of men were infected including more women in agriculture and trade than men (Government of Sierra Leone 2014).

## 6.4 Theoretical Framework and Methodology

EVD like any outbreak of communicable disease puts budget under pressure due to its adverse effects on public revenue and spending thereby widening the fiscal deficit. There have been several criteria used in classifying public expenditure (Akpan 2005). Economists assumed that there should not be an absolute classification, but rather, a classification that is relative to the purpose which it intends to serve (Akpan 2005). However, the best classification of public expenditure is the economic categorization as shown below (Fig. 6.1).

Most studies carried out on the economic effects of diseases, have laid emphasis on forgone income as well as direct medical costs incurred by the population. This then results in greater morbidity and mortality of the ailment. Such costs borne by the burden of disease includes: both private and public expenditures incurred in managing the disease. All these costs are incurred or increased by the pressing need to sustain a free environment, implement better preventive measures and carry out research that can help curb the disease. (Commission on Macroeconomics and Health 2002). The immediate effect of epidemics is a negative shock on the popula-

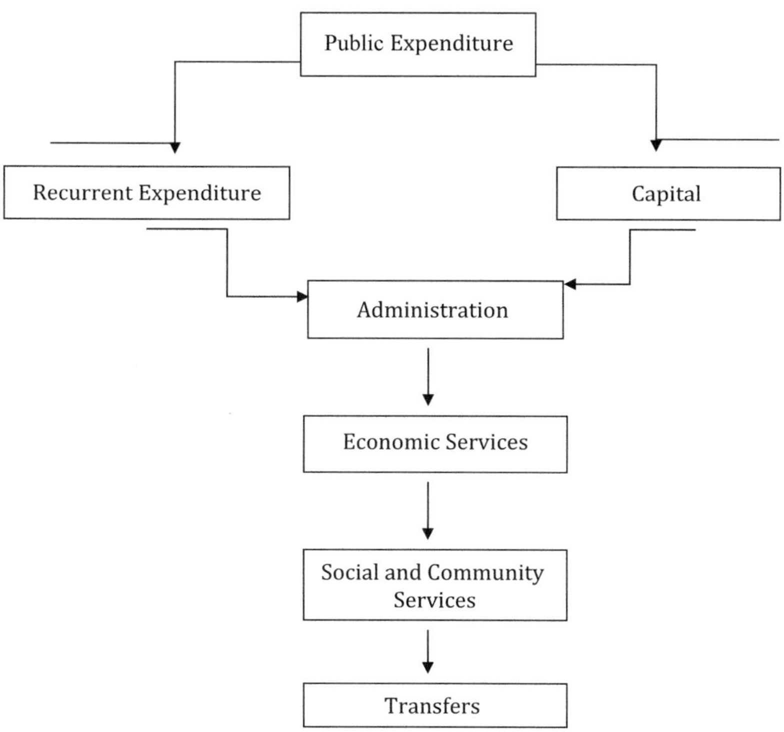


**Fig. 6.1** Classification of public expenditure. (Source: Aregbeyen 2006, p 12)

tion and labour force. Lee and McKibbin, (2004) argued the destruction of human capital is another transmission mechanism through which disease outbreak adversely affects the economy's long-term growth. However, in term of private costs and public spending, the direct consequences of the Ebola epidemic are high and have detrimental effects on productive sectors. Ebola influences the Sierra Leone economy in major three ways. First, fear of Ebola leads to a considerable decline in consumer demand, especially for travel since the fast rate of contagion makes people avoid social interactions. The decrease in consumption has a more detrimental effect on regions with more service industries and higher population densities and this negatively affects not only the revenue generation capacity of the government but also compel an inevitable diversion of public expenditure from productive industry and human capital development to Ebola epidemic. Second, uncertainty concerning any future epidemics reduces confidence in the future and this effect is very important for a developing country like Sierra Leone which required foreign investment for growth and development. Third, Ebola unquestionably increases the cost of disease prevention, especially in the most affected industries, such as travel, retail and the service industries.

The Government of Sierra Leone introduced the declaration of a State of Emergency and special security powers to separate the affected areas, place restrictions on internal movement, close markets and schools and reduce public gatherings among others as measures to control the epidemic. These measures had profound effects on people. The quarantine and other restrictions of movement had a noticeable effect on economic activity, including foregone output, higher fiscal deficits, rising consumer prices, depreciation of the national currency, loss of employment and increased levels of poverty. The agricultural sector also suffered significant declines in production and disruptions in the planting cycle with far reaching effect on household food security which may take several years to recover. Other impacts include distraction of efforts aimed at improving water and sanitation and reduced social cohesion that harms vulnerable groups.

The Endogenous Growth of Public Expenditure usually provides the theoretical framework for analyzing persistent Gross National Income (GNI) growth which is determined by forces governing the production process rather than by forces outside it. The theory assumes the existence of a single sector of production or all sectors are symmetrical, existence of increasing returns to capital and that, public and private investment in human and physical capital creates economies and productivity improvements and hence impacts positively on the growth of government expenditure which subsequently sustain long–term growth. Mathematically, endogenous growth theories can be expressed as:

$$Y = AK \tag{6.1}$$

where: Y represents gross national income or output

A represents any factor that affects technology while K represents both physical and human capital

The theory assumed that for income to grow, there must be continuous accumulation of factor of production. The implication is that government can influence long-run economics growth through its investment expenditure, education (human capital) and research and development (R&D) expenditure. But given an outbreak of a deadly communicable disease, all these expenditures may be absent. The exposition of work on endogenous growth has generated a number of models linking public spending with economic growth. A particular simple version is Barro's (1990), which takes government expenditure to be complementary with production. This framework assumes that all components of public expenditure are productive. This study considers a modification of simple model of endogenous growth assuming that the government imposes a proportional income tax rate and instead of using the public budget to furnish both households with public consumption and firms with productive investments, uses public budget to contain disease outbreak.

## 6.5 Methodology

Given the modification of the endogenous growth model, the functional form of the model for this study is expressed as follows:

$$GCE = f(EVD) \tag{6.2}$$

Equation (6.2) states that government capital expenditure is a function of Ebola disease outbreak. This means that EVD influences government capital expenditure. If EVD positively affects government capital expenditure, it implies the growth of government capital expenditure during the outbreak and hence, the growth of the economy. On the other hand, if EVD negatively impacts government capital expenditure, it indicates a dampening effect on the growth of the economy during the crises. Other variables that can impact positively on government capital expenditure include the quality of human capital measure by population growth, life expectancy, net migration, health expenditure per capita and GDP growth. Causes of death by communicable diseases were employed as a measure of EVD. Therefore, Eq. (6.2) can be modified as

$$\text{GCE} = f\ (\text{EVD,PG,LE,NM,HEP,GDP}) \tag{6.3}$$

Where: GCE represents Government Capital Expenditure,
EVD represents Ebola Virus Disease,
PG represents Population Growth,
LE represents Life Expectancy,
NM represents Net Migration,
HEP represents Health Expenditure Per capita and
GDP represents Gross Domestic Product

Equation (6.3) can be stated in explicit form as:

$$GCE_t = \beta_0 + \beta_1 EVD + \beta_2 PG + \beta_3 LE + \beta_4 NM + \beta_5 HEP + \beta_6 GDP + \mu_t \quad (6.4)$$

Equation (6.4) measures the impact of EVD and other variables as defined above on government capital expenditure in Sierra Leone. The apriori expectations in the above equation are: $B_1 < 0$; $\beta_2 > 0$; $\beta_3 > 0$; $\beta_4 > 0$; $\beta_5 > 0$ and $\beta_6 > 0$. That is an outbreak of disease such as EVD will reduce government capital expenditure and hence growth. An increase in life expectancy, population growth, net migration, health expenditure per capita, growth rate of GDP will increase government capital expenditure and thereby increase economic growth and a decrease in all these variables will have a dampening effect on the economy.

### 6.5.1 *Data and Estimation Technique*

The relevant data for the study covered the period 2006–2014. The data employed were obtained from the World Bank Data repository (World Bank 2017). The causes of death by communicable disease was from World Bank data bank including other variables like population growth, life expectancy, net migration, health expenditure per capita and GDP growth (World Bank 2017). Unit root test (Brown et al. 1975) was employed to test for the stationarity of the variables and also the use of the co-integration and error correction model (ECM) to test for both short-run and long-run effect of EVD on government capital expenditure.

## 6.6 Presentation and Discussion of Results

The Augmented Dickey Fuller test (ADF) was employed to test for the stationarity of the variables used in the analysis. In this analysis, three models were considered and they are with constant, linear trend and none (with no constant and trend). The null hypothesis in both the ADF is that there is the presence of unit root. Table 6.1 below reports the ADF results.

**Table 6.1** Augmented dickey fuller tests

| Variables | Levels | | | First difference | | |
|---|---|---|---|---|---|---|
| | Model 1 (constant) | Model 2 (linear trend) | Model 3 (no constant and trend) | Model 1(constant) | Model 2 (linear trend) | Model 3(no constant and trend) |
| GCE | −2.627490*** | −2.582746 | −1.48377*** | −4.746538* | −4.635601* | −4.853823* |
| EVD | −3.979727* | 4.455449* | −0.151322 | −5.935387* | −5.935387* | −6.030935* |

Lag length on ADF chosen by Akaike Criterion; *, ** and *** significant at 1%, 5% and 10%.
Source: Authors Computation

The results of the ADF tests reported in Table 6.1 show the behaviour of the variables in their levels and first difference form respectively. Model 1 includes a constant; model 2 includes a constant and a linear trend while model 3 includes none in the test regression as exogenous. The lags were selected based on the Schwartz Information Criterion for all the variables to ensure that the residual was white noise (i.e. it has zero mean and a constant variance). The result shows that GCE was stationary at levels for model 1 and model 3 and non-stationary at model 2 while it was stationary at the first difference in the three models. Also, EVD was stationary at levels for both models 1 and models 2 and also at first difference for the three models. Therefore, we can say that GCE and EVD are both integrated of order 0 and order 1 at different models. These results indicate that the series are I (0) variables. Hence, we can conduct co-integration tests on the variables. Tables 6.2 and 6.3 show the estimated results of the Engle-Granger co-integration test and the results of the residual-based test. It is clear from the results that we cannot reject co-integration (i.e. long-run relationship) between GCE and EVD.

Unit root test performed on the residuals in Table 6.3 shows the test statistic (−3.649) is less than the critical ($r$ tau) value (−3.082) at 5% significance level. Therefore, the null hypothesis of no co-integration was rejected in favour of the alternative. This indicates evidence of long-term relationship between GCE and EVD in Sierra Leone. However, the speed of this pre-shock adjustment depends on ECM result.

Table 6.4 shows the ECM estimates for the short-run and long-run movements and the speed of adjustment. From the table, EVD has negative effect on GCE in the short-run and this is statistically significant at 5% level. This suggests that EVD negatively affects GCE in the short-term in Sierra Leone. Table 6.4 further shows the long-run relationship between GCE and EVD. The equilibrium adjustment coefficient (−0.8044) shows the correct sign (negative). This suggests that GCE and EVD converge to long-run equilibrium and deviations from this equilibrium relationship as a result of shocks will be corrected over time. It can also be observed that $\alpha_2$ tends to one, indicating that the speed of adjustment to equilibrium is fast. It follows that about 80% of the deviation from equilibrium path is corrected

**Table 6.2** Estimation of the long run relationship ($GCE = \alpha_0 + \alpha_1 EVD + \mu_1$)

| Variables | Co-efficient | Std error | Significance | D.W Stat |
|---|---|---|---|---|
| Constant | 0.8106 | 0.573 | 0.051 | 1.956 |
| EVD | −0.7665 | 0.487 | 0.097 | |

Source: (Author's Computation)

**Table 6.3** Residual based unit root test ($\Delta \mu t = \alpha \mu_{t-1} + \epsilon_t$)

| Variables | Critical value 10% | Critical value 5% | Critical value 1% | Test statistic |
|---|---|---|---|---|
| Residuals ($\mu_t$) | −2.68288 | −3.08179 | −3.963 | −3.649** |

Lag length on ADF chosen by Akaike Criterion. Source: (Author's Computation)
*, **, *** indicates significance at 1%, 5% and 10% significance level

**Table 6.4** Error correction mechanism ($\Delta GCE = \alpha_1 + \alpha_2 \Delta EVD + \epsilon_{t-1}$)

| Variable | Co-efficient | Std error | t-Stat | Significance level |
|---|---|---|---|---|
| $\alpha$ | −0.175728 | 0.26558 | 0.66168 | 0.5217 |
| $\alpha_1$ | −0.043532 | 0.495276 | 0.8789 | 0.03** |
| $\alpha_2$ | −0.8044 | 0.3440 | −3.5885 | 0.01* |
| $R^2 = 0.54192$ | | | | |
| Adjusted $R^2 = 0.45865$ | | | | |
| DW = 1.975 | | | | |

Lag length on ADF chosen by Akaike Criterion. *, **, *** indicates significance at 1%, 5% and 10% significance level. Source: (Author's Computation)

**Table 6.5** The regression result of the impact of Ebola on government capital expenditure

| Government capital expenditure | Coeff[a] | SE[b] |
|---|---|---|
| EVD (Ebola Virus Disease) | −0.87*** | 0.49 |
| PG (Population Growth) | 4.36* | 1.20 |
| LE (Life Expectancy) | 4.25* | 1.15 |
| NM (Net Migration) | 2.47 | 5.53 |
| HEP (Health Expenditure Per capita) | 0.89 | 0.69 |
| GDP (Gross Domestic Product) | 0.12 | 0.45 |
| Constant | 0.43*** | 0.23 |
| $R^2 = 0.991702$; | | |
| Durbin Watson (DW) = 1.550248; | | |
| F-statistics = 866.4929; P-value = 0.0000 | | |

[a]Estimated Parameters *, **, ***, Significant at 1%, 5% and 10%, [b] Robust Standard Errors

per annum. The ECM results therefore show a long-run relationship between GCE and EVD.

The result of the Ordinary Least Square result is presented in Table 6.5 further shows that the coefficient of EVD conforms to our apriori expectation. It shows that EVD impacted negatively on government capital expenditure and hence on growth. The transmission mechanism involves the redirection of government capital expenditures which are supposed to be spent on investment and infrastructural facilities to containing the spread of the disease and treating the infected individuals. More so, much of the foreign assistance to the country will also be targeted at attacking the epidemic rather than economic growth and development. These will conspicuously have a dampening effect on growth in Sierra Leone. Therefore, EVD or outbreak of any communicable disease will affect government capital expenditure negatively and by implication dampen the economic growth of any affected country. Also, population growth and life expectancy are directly related to government capital expenditure. This also implies that both can aid growth of the economy with an increase in capital expenditure. Both results are also significant at 1% level. Net migration, health expenditure per capita and GDP are also positively related to government capital expenditure but not significant. The non-significance of net migration, health expenditure per capita and GDP may be as a result of the outbreak of the disease during this period.

The F-statistic result shows that Ebola disease (EVD), population growth (PG), life expectancy (LE), net migration (NM), health expenditure per capita (HEP), and GDP are jointly statistically related to government capital expenditure and the Durbin-Watson statistics shows absence of autocorrelation. The result of the $R^2$ implies that about 99% of the variation in the government capital expenditure in Sierra Leone can be explained by EVD and other covariates.

## 6.7 Conclusion

The occurrence of the Ebola Virus Disease between 2013 and 2015 has so far had far reaching and devastating socio- economic and political effects on the general population of Sierra Leone. As highlighted earlier, the disease did not only infected and killed people in this country, but had the greater impact of affecting the economic situation of the country leading to a deficit in government budget of about 3.1%. This study examined the impact of EVD on government capital expenditure in Sierra Leone. This is important for the implication of disease outbreak on economic growth. The study shows that EVD impacted negatively on government capital expenditure, hence economic growth. EVD impacted negatively on growth due to diversion of government spending on curtailing the spread of the disease, treating the affected individuals and caring for the orphans and widows who lost their parents and husbands due to the outbreak of the disease. Equally, the restriction of movement of people to and from affected zones also led to many more people not being able to work and thus leading to a decline in productivity and growth. Minimizing the impact of communicable diseases vs reducing their occurrence is to prioritize investment in human capital development through e.g. education for all, water and sanitation for all, settings approaches (healthy cities, Health promoting schools, health promoting hospitals, health promoting working places and markets), etc. Emergency funds also needs to be created to spend on possible future occurrence of this nature, so as to prevent spending funds meant for growth on containing outbreak of diseases. Finally, since economic growth and development are the main objectives of public expenditure, issues of growth policy should emphasize quality and adequate levels of investment in social and economic infrastructure.

## References

ACAPS. (2014). *Ebola outbreak in West Africa: Update (Briefing note – 26 November 2014)*. ACAPS Retrieved http://www.acaps.org/img/documents/bacaps_briefing_note_ebola_west_africa_update_26 nov_2014.pdf

Akpan, N. I. (2005). Government expenditure and economic growth in Nigeria: A disaggregated approach. *CBN Economic and Financial Review, 43*(1), 51–69.

Aregbeyen, O. (2006). Public expenditure and economic growth in Africa. *Nigerian Journal of Economic and Social Studies, 68*(160).
Barro, R. (1990). Government spending in a simple model of endogenous growth. *Journal of Political Economy, 98*(5), 103–125.
Birchenall, J. A. (2007). Escaping high mortality. *Journal of Economic Growth, 12*, 351–387.
Bor, J. (2007). The political economy of AIDS leadership in developing countries: An exploratory analysis. *Social Science & Medicine, 64*, 1585–1599.
Brown, R. L., Durbin, J., & Evans, J. M. (1975). Techniques for testing the constancy of 442 regression relations over time. *Journal of the Royal Statistical Society, 37*, 149–192.
Cassels, A. (1995). Health sector reform: Key issues in less developed countries. *Journal of International Development, 7*(3), 329–347.
Castro-Leal, F., Dayton, J., Demery, L., & Mehra, K. (2000). Public spending on health care in Africa: Do the poor benefit? *Bulletin of the World Health Organization, 78*(1), 66–74.
CDC. (2016, January 20). 2014. *Ebola outbreak in West Africa – case counts*. https://www.cdc.gov/vhf/ebola/outbreaks/2014-west-africa/case-counts.html
Commission on Macroeconomics and Health. (2002). *Macroeconomics and health: Investing in health for economic development*. Geneva: Report of the Commission on Macroeconomics and Health to the World Health Organization.
Curtis, M. (2015). *Three lessons from the Ebola crisis for Sierra Leone's government and investors*. Policy Brief for the Budget Advocacy Network.
ECA. (2014a, November 12–18). *Rapport de mission de l'Équipe de la CEA en Guinée*. Addis Ababa.
ECA. (2014b, October 6–15). *Report of the ECA team mission to Liberia*. Addis Ababa.
ECA. (2014c, October 6–15). *Report of the ECA team mission to Sierra Leone*. Addis Ababa.
ECA. (2014d, October). *Report of the executive secretary on the joint AUC/AfDB/ECA visit to West Africa* (Guinea, Liberia, Sierra Leone). Addis Ababa.
Evans, D. B., Tandon, A., Murray, C. J. L., & Lauer, J. A. (2001). Comparative efficiency of national health systems: Cross national econometric analysis. *British Medical Journal, 323*(7308), 307–310.
Filmer, D., & Pritchett, L. (1999). The impact of public spending on health: Does money matter? *Social Science & Medicine, 49*, 1309–1323.
Gauri, V., & Lieberman, E. S. (2006). Boundary institutions and HIV/AIDS policy in Brazil and South Africa. *Studies in Comparative International Development, 41*(3), 47–73.
Gerdtham, U., Sogaard, J., Andersson, F., & Jönsson, B. (1992). An econometric analysis of health care expenditure: A cross-section study of the OECD countries. *Journal of Health Economics, 11*, 63–84.
Ghobarah, H. A., Huth, P., & Russett, B. (2004). Comparative public health: The political economy of human misery and well-being. *International Studies Quarterly, 48*, 73–94.
Gilson, L., & Raphaely, N. (2008). The terrain of health policy analysis in low and middle income countries: A review of published literature 1994–2007. *Health Policy and Planning, 23*, 294–307.
Glassman, A., & Raghavan, S. (2014). *How much is actually being spent on Ebola?* Washington, DC: Center For Global Development. http://www.cgdev.org/blog/how-much-actually-being- spentebola
Government of Liberia. (2014). *Potential impacts of the Ebola crisis on the Liberian economy (draft)*. Monrovia.
Government of Sierra Leone. (2014, October). *The economic and social impact of Ebola virus disease in Sierra Leone, A preliminary assessment*. Freetown/undp_sle_The%20Agenda%20for%20Prosperity%20.pdf
Government of Sierra Leone (GoSL), United Nations Development Programme, International Monetary Fund, the World Bank, & African Development Bank. (2014). *The economic and social impact of Ebola virus disease in Sierra Leone: Joint preliminary assessment report*. Retrieved from http://reliefweb.int/sites/reliefweb.int/files/resources/Joint%20preliminary%20assessment%20socioeconomic%20impact%20of%20EVD%20in%20Sierra%20Leone.pdf

Gupta, et al. (1998, September). Public spending on human development. *Finance & Development, 35*(3).

Gupta, S. B., Clement, B., Guen-siu, M. T., & Leruth, L. (2001). Debt relief and health. *Spending in Heavily Indebted Poor Countries: IMF Finance and Development, 38*(3), 10–13.

Hakon, A. B., Donald, A. B., Mohammed, S., Martin, G., & Johan, S. (2014). *Ebola and indirect effects on health service function in Sierra Leone*. Freetown.

Hojin, J., Minjae, P., Kihoon, H., & Eunjung, H. (2016). The impact of an epidemic outbreak on consumer expenditures: An empirical assessment for MERS Korea. *Sustainability, 8*(5):454.

Hsiao, W. C., & Heller, P. S. (2007). *What macroeconomists should know about health care policy*. Washington, DC: IMF.

International Monetary Fund (IMF). (2014a). *Adhoc review under the extended credit facility arrangement and request for augmentation of access, modification of performance criteria and financing assurances review – staff report; Press release; and statement by the Executive Director for Sierra Leone. no. 14/300*. Washington, DC. http://www.imf.org/external/pubs/ft/scr/2014/cr14300.pdf

International Monetary Fund (IMF). (2014b). *Adhoc review under the extended credit facility and request for augmentation of access and modification of performance criteria – staff report; press release; and statement by the Executive Director for Liberia. no. 14/199*. Washington, DC. http://www.imf.org/external/pubs/ft/scr/2014/cr14299.pdf

Lee, J.-W., & Mckibbin, W. (2004). Globalization and disease: The case of SARS. *Asian Economic Papers, 3*, 113–131.

McGuire, J. (2006). Basic health care provision and under-5 mortality: A Cross-National study of developing countries. *World Development, 34*(3), 405–425.

Muiderman, K. (2014). Ebola's international impact: Analysis of the dynamics of a region in crisis. *The Broker*. Retrieved from: http://www.thebrokeronline.eu/content/view/pdf/15084

Nadia, W. (2015). *Understanding the emergence of Ebola virus disease in Sierra Leone: Stalking the virus in the threatening wake of emergence*.

National Revenue Authority of Sierra Leone. (2014). *The current Ebola outbreak in Sierra Leone and its potential revenue implication*. Freetown

Piot, P. (2014). *The West African Ebola crisis: Beyond short-term consequences and responses (Africa Programme Transcript)*. Chatham House. Retrieved from: http://www.chathamhouse.org/sites/files/chathamhouse/field/field_document/20141126EbolaConsequences Responses Update.pdf

Thompson, D. K., Muriel, P., Russell, D., Osborne, P., Bromley, A., Rowland, M., Creigh- Tyte, S., & Brown, C. (2003). Economic costs of the foot and mouth disease outbreak in the United Kingdom in 2001. *Revue scientifique et technique (International Office of Epizootics)., 21*, 675–687. https://doi.org/10.20506/rst.21.3.1353

UNDP. (2014). *Socioeconomic impact of the Ebola virus disease in Guinea, Liberia and Sierra Leone* (Policy notes volume 1, Numbers 1–5). Retrieved from: http://www.africa.undp.org/content/dam/rba/docs/Reports/UNDP%20Policy%20note%20EN_web.pdf

Walt, G., & Gilson, L. (1994). Reforming the health sector in developing countries: The central role of policy analysis. *Health Policy and Planning, 9*(4), 353–370.

Welthungerhilfe. (2014). *The non-medical impacts of the Ebola crisis in Sierra Leone*. Bonn: Deutsche Welthungerhilfe. Retrieved from: http://www.welthungerhilfe.de/fileadmin/user_upload/Mediathek/Mediathek_int/Fachpapiere/Sierr a-Leone-Ebola-Study-Non-Medical-Impacts-Welthungerhilfe-October2014.pdf

WHO. (2010). *Increasing access to health workers in remote and rural areas, through improved retention*. Geneva: WHO.

WHO. (2015). *How is the end of an Ebola outbreak decided and declared?*. http://www.who.int/csr/disease/ebola/declaration-ebola-end/en

World Bank. (2014). *Update on the economic impact of the 2014 Ebola epidemic on Liberia, Sierra Leone, and Guinea*. World Bank Group. Retrieved from: http://www.worldbank.org/content/dam/Worldbank/document/Economic%20Impact%20Ebola%20 Update%202%20Dec%202014.pdf

World Bank. (2015). *Summary on the Ebola recovery plan: Sierra Leone*. http://www.worldbank.org/en/topic/ebola/brief/summary-on-the-ebola-recovery-plan-sierra-leone
World Bank. (2016). *World Bank Group Ebola response fact sheet*. From http://www.worldbank.org/en/topic/health/brief/world-bank-group-ebola-fact-sheet
World Bank. (2017). *World development indicators, 2017*.

# Chapter 7
# Public Health Emergencies: The Role of Science Education and Communication in Africa

**Elizabeth Rasekoala and African Gong**

## 7.1 Introduction

'What we've got here is…failure to communicate'

This legendary line from the Classic Film -'***Cool Hand Luke***'- with which the Prison Captain repeatedly taunts a recalcitrant prisoner – played by Actor Paul Newman…is an appropriate charge to put to Africa's scientists, academics and researchers, in the face of the repeated outbreaks of health pandemics, longstanding 'knowledge gaps' and developmental challenges on the continent. The film plot poignantly illustrates how this 'failure of communication' in no small measure, ultimately leads to the unfortunate death of the prisoner. In a similar vein, the failure of Africa's scientists and researchers, to communicate, disseminate and popularize scientific knowledge, also, in no small measure, contributes to the unfortunate demise of its citizens. This critical 'knowledge gap' results in the African populace being left vulnerable in profound ignorance and lacking the basic scientific information and understandings, that would enable them to make the empowering informed choices that would improve their health, resilience in the face of opportunistic infections, especially newly Emerging Infectious Diseases (EID), well-being and quality of life.

Africa's scientists need to engage with society routinely, during periods of calm, not just during crises. This would boost their credibility so that, during crises, there is already a foundation of trust with which to engage, empower and upscale public knowledge, enrollment and understanding (Oni 2016).

African Gong, in line with current research good practices, advocates for a 'societal literacy' approach to public engagement in science in Africa. This should ideally follow a two-way dynamic that highlights the role of scientists. Furthermore, for African scientists and researchers, routine engagement with society can also

E. Rasekoala (✉) · African Gong
African Gong, Capetown, South Africa

 
G. B. Tangwa et al. (eds.), *Socio-cultural Dimensions of Emerging Infectious Diseases in Africa*, https://doi.org/10.1007/978-3-030-17474-3_7

create a more critically engaged public, necessary for navigating science advice in a 'post-normal science' era. In addition, if we want science to be credible to the public and engender the 'common good' of societal transformation and equity, we need to fundamentally reimagine how science communication in Africa can operate, within an ethos of social justice (Oni 2016).

The imperative for Africa's scientists, researchers and experts to adopt this 'societal literacy' approach is of critical importance given the challenging contexts of the weak state of education systems at Primary, Secondary and Tertiary levels, in many countries, in general, and the parlous state of science education at all these levels, in particular. The resultant legacy is an African populace that is generally lacking the most basic scientific knowledge, leaving them susceptible to the predatory approaches of 'quacks' and peddlers of superstitious beliefs, pseudo-religious mercenaries, posing as 'Pastors', and untrained and unscrupulous traditional healers.

Public Health emergencies and pandemics continue to impact disproportionately on the African populace, with the acute vulnerabilities of Africans in this regard, in no small measure directly attributable to the marginalised state of science communication and the public learning and understanding of science (PLUS), on the continent. This chapter outlines the challenges of science communication and PLUS in Africa, and the vision, mission and strategies of **African Gong**: the Pan-African Network for the Popularization of Science & Technology and Science Communication, in concert with African stakeholder partners such as **GET**, to deliver a transformed, multi-disciplinary, inclusive and empowering African–centric science communication, engagement and outreach platform, for the transformation of the quality of life and well-being of the continent's citizens.

## 7.2 Global Scenarios and Developments in Science Communication

Science communication and Public Understanding of Science (PUS) has been a growing and emerging international framework since the 1980's, particularly in the developed world. In these realms, it is 'mainstreamed' as a key plank of the Science, Technology and Innovation (STI) policy and outreach strategy for the advancement of society and entry into the economy of discovery.

A key driver of this development has been the growing recognition of the critical role of STI in the development trajectories of nations. This understanding, thus, drives the imperative to enhance the scientific knowledge base and capacity of citizens. Despite this, the African continent continues to lag behind in the domain of science communication and PUS.

The Post-2015 Global Sustainable Development agenda encapsulated in the Sustainable Development Goals (SDG's), have elaborated in much more detail than the Millennium Development Goal's (MDG's), the complex interlinkages between the multi-level development challenges across the globe. These challenges are profound, and nowhere more so than on the African continent. Science communication and the public understanding of science should help to overcome Africa's myriad and intractable development challenges by highlighting and promoting the pivotal role of science, through developing innovations and solutions. This is evident in the area of health where the very dismal levels of scientific literacy in African countries is a big challenge in addressing public health pandemics and pathologies, such as Ebola, HIV/AIDS, Tuberculosis, Malaria, high maternal and infant mortality rates and childhood vaccination programmes (Rasekoala 2015).

There is a strategic rationale for the development of science communication and public understanding of science capacity, expertise and innovative good practice in Africa, based on African-centred approaches. Despite major advances in the field of science communication and PUS in the global north, and in parts of the developing world such as Latin America, the Caribbean, India and some Asian countries, science communication and the popularization of science and technology on the African continent has woefully failed to take off and is very marginalized in the scientific landscape. That marginalization is due to certain factors, such as the lack of policy and institutionalization of the science communication and public understanding of science agenda by African governments, and science and technology institutions in Africa. There is thus, increasingly a growing understanding of the rationale for the strengthening of the science communication and PUS agenda within STI policies at African national levels, Regional Economic Communities (REC's) and within continental development frameworks such as the African Union's Agenda 2063 and the AU/NEPAD Science, Technology & Innovation Strategy for Africa (STISA) 2024.

### *7.2.1 African Contexts for Science Communication*

Here, the notion of Afrocentricity as a paradigm of transformation is critical. Asante (2007) defines Afrocentricity as: "*A consciousness, quality of thought, mode of analysis and an actionable perspective where Africans seek, from agency, to assert subject place within the context of African history*". Afrocentricity operates within African ways of knowing and existence and results in the implementation of principles, methods, concepts and ideas that are derived from our own African cultural experience. Afrocentricity derives from and enhances African agency and exhorts Africans to be agents rather than spectators of their development. Afrocentricity postulates that the African experience must guide and inform all inquiry and that the knowledge generated must be liberating (Asante 2007).

The science communication transformation agenda can also be enhanced by opening up discourse and practice, working with multiple and gendered perspectives and approaches, and incorporating communities of practice and epistemic frameworks from all parts of the world. In the African context, this would involve the mainstreaming of indigenous knowledge systems (IKSs) into ways of conceptualizing, delivering and practising science communication, so as to tap into local urban and rural communities and their traditional indigenous ways of knowing and understanding natural and scientific phenomena (Seleti 2013). The emphasis here is not on romanticizing or eulogizing IKSs, which, just as with any other knowledge systems, have their inherent flaws and challenges. The aim is to use IKSs to build foundations on which local communities can embark an evolving, empowering and progressive journey to own and include scientific notions in their everyday experience, so that they are better able to make informed choices and decisions that will improve the quality of their lives.

On the face of it, the problem of public learning and understanding of science, at the bottom, arises from either the inability/failure of scientists to communicate in a language accessible to the general public or from the inability/failure of ordinary people to comprehend scientific language. It may therefore seem that the solution to the problem lies in either scientists adopting ordinary language in communicating science or in the general public learning and using scientific language. But the disjunction is false if not taken in the inclusive sense, inasmuch as it can be demonstrated that both disjuncts are indispensable for achieving the aim of public learning and understanding of science, without which the fruits of science remain elusive for any community (Tangwa 2016).

Furthermore, for African scientists and researchers, routine engagement with society can also create a more critically engaged public, necessary for navigating science advice in a 'post-normal science' era where *"facts are uncertain, values in dispute, stakes high and decisions urgent"* (Oni 2016).

#### 7.2.1.1 The African Gong Story

African Gong is the Pan-African Network for the Popularization of Science & Technology, and Science Communication in Africa. It was formed as a result of side meetings between African delegates, senior representatives of Red-POP – The Latin American & Caribbean Science Communication Network and representatives of UNESCO-Latin America & the Caribbean Region, during the International 13th Public Communication of Science & Technology (PCST) Conference, held in Salvador, Bahia, Brazil, in May 2014. These discussions highlighted the driving imperative to address the marginalisation of science communication and the public learning and understanding of science (PLUS) on the African continent. In addition, the realisation of the need to enhance the capacity, visibility and collaborative partnerships among African practitioners, was amply demonstrated by the highly visible and systematic good practice of Red-POP, which has been in existence for over 20 years.

African Gong has thus, been developed with the strategic support of UNESCO, and aims to create a strategic platform from which Africa can contribute to global structures and institutional capacities for the advancement of science communication, science and society studies and the public learning and understanding of science (PLUS). It also contributes a uniquely relevant and inclusive African-centred paradigm and community of practice to the global development agenda and addresses the critical need for transformation in the science communication and the PLUS sector. This African-centred paradigm is reflected in the inclusion of an **L (for Learning)** into the international acronym of PUS – highlighting a key dimension of the challenges and imperatives for science communication on the continent, in the context of the weak state of education in general, and science education in particular. African Gong is encouraged by the support of partner pan-African networks such as GET, in adopting this African contextualised approach of PLUS rather than the international PUS. African Gong also facilitates and enables the strategic positioning of science and its applications at the heart of the African sustainable development framework.

In choosing the traditional African Gong instrument for its name and symbol, African Gong commits itself to the principles of its use in African societies, as an instrument to call folks together for debates, discussions and interactive engagement, on a communal basis, for the betterment of ***all***. Thus, in developing African Gong, there has been the envisioning of a network that is multi-disciplinary, inclusive, interactive and multi-level in its membership, constituencies and partnerships, for the purpose of the exchange of information, regional and continental co-operation, and including the African Diaspora. A critical component of this inclusive landscape is the commitment of African Gong to *Language Diversity*and thus**,** to work towards operating and delivering across the three main African working Languages of English, French and Portuguese, as well as Indigenous African Languages.

A critical goal is to encourage the creation, dissemination and utilisation of science and technology for addressing pressing developmental needs, such as public health epidemics and pandemics, on the African continent, in a sustainable manner. A pivotal role is envisaged for the harnessing of the Indigenous knowledge and participatory capacity of Africa's scientists and communicators, to enhance social inclusion, as well as cultural and political engagement. The membership of African Gong is both institutional and individual, including the following: Academics, Universities & Research Institutions, Media and Science Journalists, Science Academies (Senior & Junior), Civil Society Organisations (CSO's), Policy-makers, Researchers & Research Networks, Educators, Science & Technology Centres and Museums, and the Private sector across the African continent and the African Diaspora.

#### 7.2.1.2 African Gong: Strategic Aims and Objectives

**The Vision** To realise a scientifically literate African citizenry driven and powered by its ownership of scientific knowledge.

**The Mission** To embark and sustain African citizens and communities through science communication and the public learning and understanding of science (PLUS) on an evolving, empowering and progressive journey to own and include scientific notions in their everyday experience, so that they are better able to make informed choices and decisions that will improve the quality of their lives.

To support and advance science communication and the public learning and understanding of science (PLUS) in a strategic framework encompassing the key parameters of:

**Policy Development** The agenda is to strive for the 'mainstreaming' of science communication and the public learning and understanding of science (PLUS) within Science, Technology and Innovation (STI) policies at African national levels, Regional Economic Communities (REC's) and within continental development frameworks such as the African Union's Agenda 2063 and the AU/NEPAD Science, Technology & Innovation Strategy for Africa (STISA) 2024. To this end, African Gong contributes to the provision of advisory support, training and expertise to African Member states and REC's for the delivery of innovative policy and programme development for science communication, science and society and the PLUS.

**Practice and Programme Development** The Agenda is to work across diverse stakeholders and partnerships to develop, conceptualise, embed, identify, showcase and highlight good practice initiatives, programmes, approaches, tools, methodologies, strategies, partnerships, etc., in the innovative delivery of science communication and the public learning and understanding of science (PLUS) in Africa and in the African Diaspora.

**Capacity Development** To support African universities and research institutions in growing the human capital for the continent's science communication and the PLUS outreach and programme delivery, through contributing to the development of innovative training modules, transformative and African-centric curricula development, science and society studies, promotion of international student exchanges, international research collaborations, and the involvement of the private sector operating on the African continent, and in the African Diaspora.

#### 7.2.1.3 African Gong: Framing the Science Communication & PLUS Agenda in Africa

African Gong is ambitious in aiming to achieve a re-imagined and re-fashioned landscape of transformative science communication and the public learning and understanding of science (PLUS) for sustainable development in Africa. Key parameters of the hallmarks of this innovative landscape include the following:

***Citizen-centred approaches*** that prioritize gendered, social and cultural paradigms to transform the Eurocentric and masculine-biased programmes that currently dominate (Rasekoala 2014). These also involve the mainstreaming of indigenous knowledge systems (IKS) into ways of conceptualizing, delivering and practising science communication and PLUS, so as to tap into local, urban and rural communities and their traditional indigenous ways of knowing and understanding natural and scientific phenomena. There is also the need to address language diversity so that science communication and PLUS materials, resources and engagements can be produced, disseminated and interacted in diverse local African languages and incorporated as early learning tools in school curricula. This would deliver enhanced reach, sustainable impact and empower local communities and the youth.

The active ***involvement of social scientists*** to help address sociocultural contexts. There is a growing acknowledgement that multidisciplinary scientific endeavour is critical to enabling societies to overcome multiple development challenges. The imperative of multi-disciplinarity should thus, also apply in the ways that science is communicated—the what, the how, the where, the tools, the methodologies and so on. Science communication and PLUS initiatives should then be co-designed in transdisciplinary, trans-science contexts to address multifaceted development challenges and engender mutual and transformational learning. Integrating social science and co-framing and co-producing the science communication and PLUS agenda will stimulate and support innovation and enhance inclusion (ISSC 2012).

Effective ***joint leadership and control*** by local actors (governments, civil society and community-based organizations) as well as international groups. The utilisation of participatory approaches to determining and achieving alternative, empowering and inclusive visions of a scientifically literate society. Building consensus on directions and mechanisms of progress and development in ways that include marginalized and non-scientific views and voices is a key challenge. Science communication and science and society strategies that are based on good-quality and appropriate community engagement are the key to achieving development goals.

An ***emphasis on the long-term sustainability of initiatives***, such as training a new generation of multidisciplinary science communicators, public health practitioners, community leadership advocates and journalists, to work with their fellow citizens to communicate the pivotal role of science in sustainable development and the transformation of societies, in inclusive and empowering approaches. One area where this is needed is in incorporating engagement skills into scientific education and training, particularly in tertiary institutions at the undergraduate and postgraduate levels. Not all scientists feel naturally inclined to interact with society beyond academic spaces, but many can be equipped to do so if teaching the relevant skills becomes a higher priority within the education and training system – through the integration of science communication skills/expertise into course curricula, modules and research frameworks (Oni, 2016).

### 7.2.2 African Gong and GET: Partnership for Change

African Gong is strategically committed to working in partnership with Africa-based and international institutions, organisations and entities in the delivery of its laudable goals, vision and mission. This is a manifestation of its core strategy of the capacity-building of African agents, drivers and innovators to deliver sustainable change and impact. There is a need for new ways of approaching the craft and delivery mechanisms of science communication and PLUS, in order to maximize impact and enhance development gains in Africa.

In this regard, African Gong has partnered with GET to engage in engendering the 'mainstreaming' of the science communication agenda in the pan-African framework for the prevention, mitigation and containment of Emerging Infectious Disease (EID) and Bio-Security, through co-convening and leading the *Science Communication &PLUS Faculty* of the *2nd African Conference on EID and Biosecurity, which tookplace in Lagos, Nigeria, in July 2016***.**The strategic and far-reaching outcomes of this partnership, which will have substantial impact on policy, practice and the capacity development foot-print for science communication and PLUS in Africa, are as follows:

- Provide a networking platform to shape the future of Science Communication and PLUS Policy, Practice and Capacity-building in Africa.
- Raise awareness and prompt action in the promotion of Science Communication and PLUS Policy, Practice and Capacity-building in Africa.
- Contribute to the principles of sustainable development and the role of Science Communication and PLUS in the prevention, containment and management of EID's in Africa.
- Engender and grow the pan-African network and interest group in Science Communication and PLUS which will facilitate the transfer and sharing of knowledge and good practice amongst practitioners.

The Science Communication and PLUS Faculty was predicated on transformative and inclusive Multi-disciplinary and Trans-disciplinary discourses, deliberations and contributions. In this regard, it welcomed contributions from across all the science disciplines (Natural, Life and Physical), the Humanities, Social Sciences, Anthropology, etc.

These outcomes were achieved through engaging on the following themes:

#### 7.2.2.1 Science Communication & PLUS in Africa: Policy Development Challenges and Opportunities

This theme focused on the policy landscape for science communication and PLUS on the African continent, and assessed the policy space in terms of available frameworks, interventions and gaps at national levels, Regional Economic Communities (REC's) and the continental level. It also focused on the knowledge gaps for policy development as regards levels of awareness, sensitization and understanding amongst African policy-makers. These discussions were further fully elaborated in the two sub-themes as follows:

- Science communication & PLUS in Africa: Defining the Agenda and knowledge development processes
- Science communication & PLUS in Africa: Policy sensitization strategies

#### 7.2.2.2 Good Practice Programmes and Projects Implementation – African Models for Science Communication and PLUS as a Containment Strategy for EID

This theme focused on the skills and capacity-building landscape for science communication and PLUS on the continent, and addressed the challenges inherent in delivering this capacity. It also focused on identifying, showcasing and highlighting good practice initiatives in science communication and PLUS across diverse stakeholders and practitioners, particularly regarding the development of innovative African models for Science Communication/PLUS and its role in preventing and curtailing public health crises emanating from EID's. These issues were further fully elaborated via the two sub-themes as follows:

- Capacity and skills development for science communication & PLUS
- Outputs on successes, challenges and opportunities for Science Communication/PLUS and EID prevention

#### 7.2.2.3 Strengthen Evidence Base Through Sharing of Research, Information and Capacity-Building

This theme focused on the research and development landscape for informing on policy development and good practice on science communication and PLUS. It also addressed the challenges of bridging the research/researcher-policy divide and the effective and cohesive networking of African practitioners in science communication and PLUS, in order to engender enhanced partnership working, increased programmatic delivery and innovative good practice development. These issues were further fully further elaborated in the two sub-themes as follows:

- Strengthening partnerships for Science Communication & PLUS – Policy interfaces
- Strengthening partnerships and networks amongst practitioners: Inclusion & Innovation

To further set the stage for deliberations and enrich the discussions on the above themes and sub-themes, presentations were made by delegates who had submitted Abstracts for Oral presentation at the Conference.

## 7.3 Science Communication & PLUS Resolutions

The resolutions to the above discussions, deliberations and discourses, highlighted the importance of effective science communication and public learning and understanding of science, in Africa. Specifically, how African populations can interact with scientific information in a language they can relate to. There was a general agreement to the effect that this has profound implications for health research in

Africa, and the overall welfare of African populations. The following resolutions were reached at the end of the sessions:

- African scientists, researchers and academics were encouraged to learn to communicate their research findings to the public in a language that is easy to understand. This would enhance more effective community engagement practices in research, and the promotion of public understanding of the sciences. It may also facilitate public debate on issues relating to science and technology.
- In communicating science to African populations, scientists need to take into consideration relevant cultural norms, beliefs and practices.
- There is need for communication between researchers, policymakers and community leaders. This would enhance policymakers' understanding of science and technology matters that are relevant for effective policymaking and development. It would further enhance greater communication between scientists, policymakers and society as a whole.
- Scientists need to engage investors and diverse stakeholders' in a sustained conversation, thereby encouraging them to invest in science and technology related activities in Africa. Such conversations are only possible if both sectors can learn the art and practice of science communication, through empowering capacity-building, knowledge sharing and engagement platforms.
- There is an increasing demand for African professionals with skills in the public communication of science and technology.
- Networking among researchers and academics of varying specializations and professionals in the scientific industry, is key in promoting science communication and PLUS in Africa.

At the end of these discussions, the following areas of **interventions** were proposed:

- There is a need to support and advocate for policy development for science communication and PLUS in Africa, given the dearth of policies, programmes and capacities on the continent;
- Practice and Program development for science communication and PLUS should be encouraged in Africa;
- The pressing need to strengthen human and institutional capacity for Science Communication and PLUS in Africa and the importance of fostering networking on Science communication at the continental level – perhaps taking the form of sub-regional and national chapters;
- Science communication should be mainstreamed in all aspects of the other Conference thematics on emerging and infectious diseases;
- Monitoring and Evaluation (M&E) frameworks should be developed for all science communication and PLUS activities to assess, enhance and sustain impact and good practice;
- The importance of building and/or strengthening the researcher-policymaker relationship for the advancement of science communication and PLUS in Africa;

- African governments should promote the development/strengthening of science communication and PLUS in their national Science, Technology and Innovation (STI) policy frameworks;
- The need for the training of communicators in Science; science journalism, and the mass media, and the strengthening of communication links between scientists and the general public;
- The establishment of science communication/PLUS Scientific Awards in Africa with different focus on youth, women, etc. Themes can be selected based on current and emerging issues (e.g. Ebola research, climate change, food security, etc.);
- The establishment of African Research Grants' programmes targeting science communication and PLUS research initiatives;
- The establishment and promotion of Science Centres, Science Museums, and Libraries (e.g. the Library of Alexandria), in African countries, with special targets for children and youth.
- The establishment of a Public Lecture Series to be delivered by renowned African scientists who can act as role models for African youth, raise the profile of science on the continent, and generate interest in science communication and PLUS;
- Promoting STEM education at all levels, with specific emphasis on girls and women;
- Promote alternative funding mechanisms for science communication and PLUS programmes, particularly focusing on domestic (mostly African funds);
- A consensus statement and *Call to Action document* should be established on the PLUS Faculty's Communiqué, and once finalized, should be widely disseminated to all stakeholders and relevant institutions, at national, sub-regional, regional and international levels.

## 7.4 Africa's Road-Map for Science Communication and PLUS Development

The Science Communication & PLUS Faculty Consensus statement and a key outcome document from the 2nd African Conference on EID and Biosecurity, which took place in Lagos, Nigeria, in July 2016, has been the **Lagos Declaration and Call to Action on Science Communication and PLUS in Africa**. This seminal and ground-breaking document, and the first of its kind in Africa, is a strategic, inclusive and empowering exhortation to all African scientists, researchers, academics and policy-makers, in Universities, Research Institutions, public and private sectors, and in the African Diaspora, to mobilise action, resources, policy development, programmes and capacity-building for the delivery of innovative, African-centric, culturally and locally relevant and contextualised science communication and the public learning and understanding of science (PLUS) for African publics.

### 7.4.1 Lagos Declaration and Call to Action on Science Communication and the Public Learning and Understanding of Science (PLUS) in Africa

We, African scientists, medical practitioners, science communicators', science journalists', health researchers, experts in Bio-safety, Bio-security and Bio-ethics, leaders, decision-makers, civil society activists, Representatives of Health Ministries in the ECOWAS Region, Representatives of the New Partnership for Africa's Development (NEPAD Agency), Representatives of the African Union Commission, UN Agencies and other bilateral and Multi-lateral international development partners, meeting at the 2nd African Conference on Emerging Infectious Diseases (EID)& Bio-security 2016, held from 27–29 July 2016 in Lagos, Nigeria.

**Recognising**, the unique developments at this second Conference, following on from the first, in 2015 (Dakar, Senegal), in the strengthening and expansion of the platform, debate and knowledge development, to address the pertinent critical relevance of Science Communication and the Public Learning and Understanding of Science (PLUS) as crucial to the prevention, mitigation, and containment of Emerging Infectious Diseases (EID) in Africa, in line with global recognitions and developments.

**Noting,** with concern that, despite progressive developments in the global north and many parts of the global south, science communication and PLUS in Africa, continues to lag behind, in spite of the international recognition of the fundamental role that it plays in the prevention, mitigation and containment of Emerging Infectious Diseases, good health, and the wellbeing of citizens.

**Acknowledging,** the progress made in the adoption of the African Union's ten year Science, Technology and Innovation Strategy for Africa (STISA-2024), by African Heads of State in 2014, and the adoption of its Implementation Plan, with the Priority 3 – Theme on Communication (Physical & Intellectual Mobility).

**Recognising,** the transformative vision of the African Union's Agenda 2063 for Africa's development, '*The Africa we want*', and the imperatives of the UN's Sustainable Development Goals (SDG's) for the global development agenda, and affirm that science communication and PLUS are key parameters for the pro-active delivery of these laudable development paradigms in Africa.

**Further Recognising**, the urgent need for the popularization of science and technology in Africa, so that citizens can learn and understand science, thereby making informed choices that will improve their health, resilience in the face of EID's, well-being and quality of life; the need for African scientists, researchers and academics to learn to communicate to their unscientific audiences and publics in a language they understand, in order for scientific knowledge to be shared, particularly in rural areas; the need for communication between researchers and policy-makers and to build the interface between researchers and the users of scientific results and technology; Knowledge is power, and in order to appreciate and benefit from scientific achievements, Africans need to learn science and to popularize scientific knowledge.

We, therefore elaborate a Call to Action as follows:

1. African Member states, Regional Economic Communities' (RECs), African Union Commission (AUC), New Economic Partnership for Africa's Development (NEPAD Agency) and the relevant partners, to strengthen the **STISA 2024 Priority 3 on Communication (Physical & Intellectual Mobility)**, so that it comprehensively addresses the critical relevance of science communication and PLUS in Africa's STI framework, in line with international developments in this strategic area.
2. RECs, the relevant partners and African national governments to domesticate the STISA 2024 within the overall people-centred African Union (AU) Agenda 2063 in their national STI policy frameworks, and advance the development of inclusive policies, programmes and capacity-building initiatives on the popularization of science and technology, science communication and PLUS.
3. AUC and NEPAD to put in place a cluster on science communication to support the implementation of STISA 2024, particularly, *Priority 3*, through the popularization of science and technology, science communication and PLUS.
4. African national governments and Ministries of Education to:

    (a) Advance, progress and implement good practice initiatives to develop enhanced Science, Technology, Engineering and Mathematics (STEM) education at all levels, on the African continent, particularly for girls and women, as a foundational strength for the Public Learning and Understanding of Science by citizens.
    (b) Promote the development of science centres, science museums, and libraries (such as the Library of Alexandria, in Egypt) within an empowering and affirming Africa-centred institutional and knowledge framework, as a strategic mechanism with which to enhance the popularization of science and technology, science communication and PLUS on the continent, in line with international good practice. This is in line with UNESCO having designated the World Science Day for Peace and Development on November 10, 2016, as the International Science Centre and Science Museum Day (ISCSMD), to highlight the contribution of science centres and science museums to the delivery of the SDG's globally.

5. Regional Economic Communities (REC's) to provide leadership, support and capacity-building to member states in their regions for the advancement of science communication and PLUS, in policies, programmes and development frameworks.
6. African scientific societies, academies, institutions and expert associations to provide:

    (a) Leadership, support and drive for the advancement of science communication and PLUS on the continent, at all levels of operation, to address the need to close the major knowledge gaps that impact profoundly on the scientific literacy, learning and understanding of science of African citizens, making them vulnerable to opportunistic infections especially new emerging infectious diseases and general poor health.

(b) Training, support and partnership networking programmes with African mass media organisations, in newsprint, television, radio, online, social media, etc., to enhance the capacity-building and knowledge-base of science journalists and generic journalists, in their delivery of science-based and science-related news, articles, stories and communications, so as to make them more effective partners in the delivery of the popularization of science and technology, science communication and PLUS on the continent.

7. International development partners, bilateral and multilateral international partners to support African governments and African scientific institutions in the advancement of Science Communication and PLUS on the African continent, for the betterment of the education, health, and well-being of citizens.

The **Lagos Declaration and Call to Action on Science Communication and PLUS in Africa,** as elaborated above, has been conceptualised and realised as a uniquely game-changing platform for the advancement of science communication and the public learning and understanding of science policy, practice and programme development, capacity-building, and thecontainment of EID's, in Africa. It is highly opportune that this document has been initialised by the **2nd Conference on EID and Biosecurity**, which tookplace in Lagos, Nigeria, in July 2016, in the context of Africa's challenges in the containment of EID's.

The challenges to the delivery of innovative, inclusive and empowering science communication and PLUS in Africa are many and severe, and are often different to the contexts, conditions and scenarios found in other global regions. The implementation of this **Call to Action** is thus, an opportunity not only to strengthen the skills, capabilities, knowledge-base, networks and strategies of practitioners in the sector, but also to accelerate the promotion of evidence-based practices that have the potential to influence policy and deliver systematic change in Africa's development framework, and how it prevents, mitigates and contains Public Health Emergencies and Pandemics.

## 7.5 Summary

International studies, research and good practice developed since the 1980's, have demonstrated that science communication and the public learning and understanding of science and technology (PLUS), have a pivotal role in advancing the systematic footprint of science in the development trajectory of nations. Innovative, interactive and inclusive science communication and PLUS frameworks, have been shown to deliver substantial gains for societies, in terms of enhanced science education outcomes, skills development profiles, professional development, and importantly, enhancing the scientific literacy of the general population, leading to direct impact and benefits on health, quality of life indicators, and other socio-economic parameters.

The profoundly challenging socio-economic conditions for many communities on the African continent, require a dynamic step change in the response of Africa's scientists, researchers and academics, and policy-makers, in order to deliver transformative and empowering 'societal scientific literacy', community engagement and scientific outreach. This should be undertaken with the critical aim of reducing 'knowledge gaps' at the individual, policy, institution, government levels and at socio-economic (gender, social class, age, etc.) levels, and the knowledge gaps in legislation and implementation (Rasekoala 2015).

**African Gong** has created a strategic and enabling pan-African leadership and practitioner platform and thus, calls on Africa's scientists, researchers, academics and STEM professionals, on the continent and in the Diaspora, to come on board, and empower Africa's citizens with the scientific knowledge which will transform their lives and well-being, and radically transform the development trajectory of the continent. These progressive developments will only yield sustainable impacts if enacted upon by the diverse stakeholders (policy-makers and governments, scientists/researchers, and health professionals, etc.) required to achieve sustainable change in the prevention, mitigation and containment of Public Health Emergencies and Pandemics, and their devastating impact on the quality of life and well-being of African citizens.

In this regard, African Gong makes the following **recommendations** as the way forward for the various actors and stakeholders on the continent and internationally:

### *7.5.1 Science Communication & PLUS for African Development on Public Health Emergencies: Policy Frameworks*

The systematic mainstreaming, adoption and synergising of science communication and the PLUS in the African Science, Technology and Innovation (STI) Policy arena needs to be driven and framed at the following levels:

- National STI & Health Policies
- Sub-Regional (REC's) STI & Health Policies
- Regional & Continental Frameworks: Agenda 2063
- Regional & Continental STI Policies: STISA 2024
- African implementation of Global Development Frameworks such as the SDG's

### 7.5.2 Science Communication & PLUS for African Development on Public Health Emergencies: Practice and Programme Frameworks

The proliferation and extensive foot-print of Science Communication and PLUS practices and programmes and which encompass a wide and diverse range of activities, methodologies and approaches, such as:

- Community engagement through outreach communication via communication platforms such as Radio, Television, social media, etc. driven in partnership with science journalists and media experts;
- Scientific infrastructure based programmes such as science centres and science museums, which provide the public with interactive, hands-on engagement and experiences with science and technology kits, games, gadgets, displays, exhibitions, etc.;
- National Science Weeks' and Scientific outreach and curriculum (teaching and learning) enrichment programmes with schools, utilising science kits for pupils and including professional development good practice for science teachers, etc.;
- Science Fairs, Science Festivals, and other 'fun' science outdoor activities in local Parks, Theatres, and community halls, for the 'edutainment' of adults, youth and children, etc.

### 7.5.3 Science Communication & PLUS for African Development on Public Health Emergencies: Capacity-Building Frameworks

The proliferation and extensive foot-print of Science Communication and PLUS Capacity-building programmes, such as:

- University Courses on Science Communication and PLUS at undergraduate and post-graduate levels;
- Science Journalism courses at Undergraduate and Post-graduate levels;
- Customised training programmes for science communicators, scientists, and science journalists in diverse institutions and multi-disciplinary formats;
- Science Communication Competitions and Awards for African scientists, science communicators and science journalists, and Public Health professionals.

## References

Asante, M. K. (2007). *An Afrocentric manifesto: Toward an African renaissance*. Cambridge: Polity Press.

International Social Science Council. (2012). *Transformative cornerstones of social science research for global change*. Paris: International Social Science Council. www.worldsocialscience.org.

Oni, T. (2016). *Don't wait for crises to reach public with science*. SciDev.net, www.scidev.net/global/cooperation/opinion/crises-science-public-engagement-sdgs.html. Accessed 12 Dec 2017.

Rasekoala, E. (2014). *Science must evolve or risk being marginalised. SciDev.net*, www.scidev.net/global/technology/opinion/science-must-evolve-or-risk-being-marginalised.html. Accessed 12 Dec 2017.

Rasekoala, E. (2015). Science communication in a post-2015 world: the nexus of transnational, multidisciplinary and sociocultural contexts. In B. Schiele, J. Le Marec, & P. Baranger (Eds.), *Science Communication Today – 2015: Current strategies and means of action* (pp. 39–45). De Lorraine: Universitaires De Lorraine.

Seleti, Y. (2013). The value of indigenous knowledge systems in the 21st century. In J. Gilbert & S. Stocklmayer (Eds.), *Communication and engagement with science and technology—Issues and dilemmas* (pp. 261–272). New York: Routledge.

Tangwa, G. B. (2016). *'Scientifying' villagers or 'Villageising' Scientists: A false disjunctive dichotomy in the communication conundrum*. 2nd African Conference on Emerging Infectious Diseases and Biosecurity, Lagos, Nigeria, 27–29 July 2016.

**Dr Elizabeth Rasekoala** is the President of African Gong – the pan-African Network for the Popularization of Science & Technology and Science Communication, which aims to advance the Public Learning and Understanding of Science (PLUS), scientific outreach and scientific literacy on the African continent (www.africangong.org). She is a member of the African Union Commission (AUC) Monitoring and Evaluation (M&E) Committee for the 'Science, Technology and Innovation Strategy for Africa' (STISA-2024).
Dr. Rasekoala with a professional background in Chemical Engineering and industry internationally, has championed, advocated, researched, presented and written widely on public innovation and transformative development through advancing diversity, sociocultural inclusion and race and gender equality issues in science communication and science, technology, engineering and mathematics (STEM) education and skills development. She has provided extensive advisory and consultancy expertise to governments and multilateral international organisations over the past 15 years, including the European Commission, the UN Commission on Human Rights, the UN Economic Commission for Africa, UNESCO, the African Union Commission and the African Development Bank.

**The African Gong** Executive Committee is comprised of the following members: Dr. Elizabeth Rasekoala (Nigeria/South Africa); Dr. Judith Gbenoudon (Benin); Prof. Aziz Bensalah (Morocco); Mr. Rodrick Sambakunsi (Malawi); Ms. Funmi Eyeoyibo (Nigeria); Dr. Bernard Appiah (Ghana/USA); Dr. Chux Daniels (Nigeria/UK); Mr. David Mbulumi (Tanzania); Mr. Joao Cossa (Mozambique); and Ms. Deborah Nyirenda (Malawi).

# Chapter 8
# Ebola and the Reimagining of Health Communication in Liberia

**Sally Deffor**

## 8.1 Introduction

The Ebola Virus Disease (EVD) outbreak devastated many communities in the key countries of Sierra Leone, Guinea, and Liberia. Now thought to have originated from a village in Guinea in December 2013, it tested the health systems of not only these countries but also the global responsible body, the World Health Organisation (WHO). These three countries, including others in the sub-region where the virus was detected – Nigeria, Senegal, and Mali – each employed its own means of tackling the disease using health communications techniques. Health communication, sometimes used interchangeably with social marketing, has been defined as the use of communications strategies and tools to influence changed behaviors and attitudes with respect to health (Munodawafa 2008). Through a thorough case study analysis, this chapter attempts to understand some of the edutainment approaches employed in Liberia specifically, towards these health communications goals. Edutainment, which has been defined as the use of a combination of entertainment and education in one piece or process (Colace et al. 2006), has featured consistentlyin health communication initiatives on the continent. One of the very earliest definitions noted it as a "process of purposely designing and implementing a media message to both entertain and educate, in order to increase knowledge about an issue, create favorable attitudes and change overt behavior" (Singhal and Rogers 1999, p. 229). The implementation of health communication using edutainment approaches, is still nascent in much ofsub-Saharan Africa, especially in Liberia, where there is very little evidence to suggest its prevalence. Govender 2013 (p. 7) noted "Edutainment interventions and programs were evident in several African countries, however many were often under-researched or undocumented and did not employ a purposive entertainment education strategy as suggested by the definition."

S. Deffor (✉)
Internews Network, Washington, DC, USA
e-mail: sdeffor@internews.org



G. B. Tangwa et al. (eds.), *Socio-cultural Dimensions of Emerging Infectious Diseases in Africa*, https://doi.org/10.1007/978-3-030-17474-3_8

Researchers have traced the genesis of edutainment in health communication back to the highly popular and highly successful BBC radio drama series named *The Archers* set in 1950s Britain (Soul City Institute 2013). A review of edutainment approaches in Africa, captured in Govender 2013 however revealed a large concentration of such initiatives in southern Africa, with the only ones from West Africa making the cut being from Ghana. It was noted, "The application of EE in West Africa seems to be scarce with only evidence of purposive EE interventions in Ghana through MARCH and Stop AIDS, loveLife interventions", (Govender 2013, p. 13). The most high profile one on the continent was the *Soul City* radio and tele-drama series employed inSouth Africa, which later expanded to other countries in the sub-region, to combat HIV/AIDS.[1] In Liberia however, it appears that health communication was dominated by traditional approaches removed from edutainment.

Overall, edutainment is well regarded as an effective tool in achieving the objectives of health communication. Both goal and process oriented definitions of health communication are therefore important considerations for this analysis. According to Munodawafa (2008), the goal of health communication is to seek to increase knowledge gain, and as such, those who initiate these initiatives have to have an understanding of how it can lead to the intended outcomes. A process element of this definition further outlined by Munodawafa (2008) requires first of all an awareness of the desired outcomes, a determination of the environment in reference to the intended audiences, and selecting the right tools and channels. A widely-accepted set of criteria for what constitutes effective health communication has been put forward by the *Office of Disease Prevention and Health Promotion* (2010). These include accuracy, accessibility, and consistency of the message being conveyed, cultural competence (awareness) in relation to the community being targeted, as well as incorporating evidence-based facts and utilizing reliable sources, and finally ensuring a wide reach and repetitiveness of the message so that it gets to all intended targets. Contemporary perspectives, for example, from Brown et al. (2015) hold that it needs to engage media and technology, but most importantly must embrace popular culture. This will be an overarching consideration that informs the analysis of the health communication activities that unfolded in Liberia during and after the epidemic. These different strands of thinking will be explored using how the Ebola story unfolded in West Africa generally, and Liberia specifically.

## 8.2 The Ebola Story

The Ebola outbreak was a lengthy episode of pain, helplessness, and untold suffering on victims and their families. The epidemic also provoked frantic efforts on the parts of the health and humanitarian community to provide a structured response and find solutions. It prompted governments all over the world to attempt to restrict

[1] http://www.who.int/bulletin/volumes/87/8/09-050809/en/

the geographical movement of persons, and invariably the spread of the disease. Towards the end of the crises however, the stories that subsequently emerged were those of hopefulness – resilience on the part of local communities, the dedication of local health and aid workers, and of course the determination on the part of the survivors and their families to overcome the disease.

Many different media organizations, both national and international, made us privy to these stories. However, their respective narrative stances have been contested and debated on many platforms and in different research outputs. For example, Kummervold et al. (2017) revealed from their analysis of news covering the Ebola Vaccine Trial in Ghana that the said media coverage was characterized by rumour mongering developed from deep-seated historical norms within the Ghanaian political context. Meanwhile Sastry and Dutta (2017) discovered a culture of disregarding local agency of the affected communities, which did not augur well for the crisis response. They therefore sought to get us thinking about these crucial questions:

> Ebola emerges as a site of storytelling, punctuating stories of death amid a globally circulating network of affect. What particular stories of disease are narrated on a global map? What are the imaginaries anchored in stories for addressing epidemics such as Ebola? (pg. 10)

They concluded that these media narratives related the Ebola outbreak to a particular place – that is among the West African people, and spurred by cultural dynamics. Thus, most of these narratives were generally regarded as faulty at best. They mostly attributed the spread of the disease to cultural dynamics and practices such as funeral and burial rites. These ignored the wider interplay of factors such as language barriers, distrust of foreign aid workers, and corruption in local and national health systems and institutions.

It is therefore of prime importance to explore the approaches that incorporated those same cultural dynamics and practices as more effective alternatives to help curb the spread of the disease in the future.

Roberts et al. (2017) analysed thousands of online stories on the Ebola crisis. Their study revealed a prevalence ofmisinformation, amply aided by the medium of the internet. This fuelled rumours and subsequent stigmatization of affected persons and countries. However, Abramowitz et al. (2017) found from a study on Liberia's information sharing norms at the height of the crises, a rather positive public awareness about the disease and its causes and modes of spread.

Roberts et al. (2017), also tackled the issue of the digital (technology) aspect of the Ebola response. Their big data analyses of Ebola related information and news on the internet led to the conclusion that there was some elements of the prevailing networked society that shaped the discourses, and hence the public responses to the crises. It is however important to note that this study focused only on US-based information sources. They also discovered a tendency for these media content to feature scientific arguments and to reference expert sources such as the Centers for Disease Control and Prevention (CDC) and WHO, in contrast to the news and information reported on the outbreak in the West African region.

These sorts of insights are important for researchers and health communications experts. It gives them an understanding of what will work in each case should the opportunity for undertaking large scale health communications arise in the event of a similar crisis or epidemic. Storey et al. (2017) explored the effects of community engagement on the Ebola crises. They concluded that international responders did not at the start of the outbreak seek to understand the community's culture in order to identify the most feasible communications method to use in tackling the disease. They therefore advocated the use of tried and tested communications models and frameworks, however to be foregrounded by local knowledge and community-led approaches. The next sub-section explores the extent to which these recommendations were evidenced in the case of the Liberian response.

## 8.3 When the Crisis Hit: Making the Case for Edutainment

In the event of a devastating disease outbreak, like Ebola, the last thing anyone, much less seasoned health communicators, would be considering is how to provide entertainment. In Liberia, this need arose from March 2014 when the disease was first reported from some areas in Lofa County (Nyenswah et al. 2014/2015). Though traditionally, some health campaigns will incorporate an entertainment element in order to make the audience more receptive to the educational or informational messages, in the case of the Liberia, there were further incentives. These included keeping Liberians hopeful by diverting their attention from the devastating effects of Ebola through films and music. This further encouraged people to stay at home or indoors, enabling the containment of the spread of the disease.

The case studies considered here are underpinned by the philosophy of edutainment, as pioneered by Miguel Sabido in the 1970s.The film executive sought ways to use the platform of serialized film or radio content to change lives in his native country of Mexico. Since then, the edutainment approach has been used in many places all over the world, albeit to a limited extent in Liberia. It has been used with various social change projects – from uniting communities in conflict to fighting climate change. Edutainment is defined simply in layman's terms as any form of entertainment that seeks to educate. Many communicative pieces can fit this bill – from comics, to community theatre, to poetry recitals – as long as they seek to incorporate both the elements of education and entertainment. The Sabido Methodology[2] requires an approach to mid and long-term goals of changing behaviours. It requires harnessing popular culture – in whatever form it may exist in each locality – and using it as a force for social change. In one such health related success story, it was used in the *Soul City* of South Africa (in this case radio and teledramas) in the fight against HIV/AIDS.[3] So, it is not out of place that the approach to fighting Ebola will bean appropriate platform to employfilm and song as tactics for behaviour

[2] http://www.comminit.com/content/sabido-methodology

[3] http://www.who.int/bulletin/volumes/87/8/09-050809/en/

change. Even though not exactly labelled as edutainment, Liberia's creative industry outputs during those turbulent months were geared towards achieving goals akin to that of social change. Even though in principle, edutainment works more effectively through a more long-term series of creative products, e.g. serial drama (Soul City Institute 2013), I will argue that the films and songs used during the Ebola crises in Liberia were simply a rewriting of the script, as they were better suited to the times, and nonetheless achieved the same results.

Other scholars also sought to advance some of these alternative approaches. Sastry and Dutta (2017) explored the critical role that the Culture Centered Approach (CCA) could play in theorizing and implementing a more effective health communication in the wake of epidemics such as the Ebola crises. However, it can be concluded from a cursory look into some of health communication campaigns in Liberia over the period that the approach still very much reverted to the status quo. This was characterised by the use of persuasive messaging by external actors with the intention to change behaviors with the inadequate involvement of local communities and voices – a contrast to the approach Dutta et al. (2014) so strongly advocated for. I will argue that the artistes involved in the three case studies were professional performers after all, bringing some element of professionalism by way of storytelling and scripting messages that have both educational and entertaining features. One may rightly argue, that these actors nonetheless embody a certain understanding of the Liberian local community, and thus can be seen as representing the voice of the community.

That is not to say that other channels for conveying health messages beyond entertainment media, in particular direct marketing and interpersonal communications were not also in use during the campaign in the various country settings. They were indeed, and plentifully so. Mention can be made of the most high profile one, which was the Halt Ebola campaign of Nigeria (which was locally driven). Nabarro (2017) attempted to identify the best practices with health communications approaches in the height of the Ebola crises. He also noted the engagement and inclusion of local people in the response, though did not go as far as specifying what these could look like in specific contacts. However, he looked at this from the lenses of policymakers (the United Nations (UN) in particular), which made his views particularly insightful. His articulation of the view of the various researchers who have delved into the issue of the role of community based engagement, seems to point to the fact that no matter the channels used, it is the one that incorporates local voices to the largest extent possible that can be considered as best practice. Noting for example:

> They propose, for example, that communities be regarded as experts in their own culture and as sources of solutions and innovation. They maintain that communication is most effective when information is conveyed by individuals who are known and trusted by communities and when communication channels encourage participatory dialogue. They suggest that care is taken to appreciate the impact of social media and new communication technologies— and to use these means sensitively. They indicate the ways in which efforts to reach marginalized or out-of-reach communities (whether due to economic, political, geographic, or social factors) should take their literacy, language, and access to technology into account. (pg 2).

Regarding the incorporation of the platform of entertainment media specifically, it is important to note that this approach is certainly not new. Large humanitarian and health organizations such as the United Nations Children's Fund (UNICEF), CDC and WHO have generally experimented with this approach in different forms all over the world and on various projects. However, it is usual of longer-term health responses such as required for HIV/AIDS and cancer. Applying this same approach to highly infectious diseases such as Ebola was quite a bold move. Rivera (2017) carefully dissected how two such Ebola songs showed the Non-governmental Organization (NGO) and creative communities working together, not just to educate but also to sort of contextualize the crisis response within the Liberian community. Similarly, Nyenswah et al. (2014–2015) explored how different novel health communications approaches were adopted – from public campaigns to incorporating the voices of local traditional leaders.

## *8.3.1 Film and Music in the Times of Ebola*

Below, I explore further what each film and music project brought to the table, in those times of Ebola at the height of the crises.

### 8.3.1.1 Film in Ebolawood

Much like any other ordinary time in Liberia, music and film was in plentiful supply during the crises. In many ways, this alluded to a sense of normality, though this was not in fact the case. That in itself is telling, of a people who were determined to achieve some semblance of normality in order to escape the horror of the outbreak. A total of 11,315[4] persons were reported to have died from the virus, many families were torn apart by death, and many kids were left orphans.

In the midst of these, Ebolawood emerged. It is exactly what it appears to be – a movie industry much like Hollywood or Bollywood. This moniker does not point to a geographic location, but rather strangely a hopefully fleeting disease. It was the brainchild of Filmmaker and Producer Richard Dwumoh. The production in question which heralded the industry was given the witty title 'Killer Bean and Falcao'. He admitted that the film was not intended to be a 'blockbuster", nor was it going to break the box office. Yet, it was sufficient to serve a purpose – to provide some much needed relief from the pain, and get some key messages across.[5] Liberia has always had a long history with the creative arts especially film and music. Like many cities across West Africa, it hosted cinemas decades go which has since fallen into some sort of disrepair, and the resurrection through the likes of Silverbird cinemas in neighboring Accra and Lagos haven't quite made its way here. Hence, these movies

[4] https://www.bbc.com/news/world-africa-28755033

[5] http://edition.cnn.com/interactive/2017/08/world/ebola-lollywood-liberia-film/

were expected to be distributed on DVDs, to be watched at home, well away from crowds who may well be harboring the dangerous virus. This was an approach well suited for the particular environment and the objective of curbing the spread of the virus.

These movies were pure comedy with hilarious scripts built around the comical central character Killer Bean. They were devoid of any educational aspects that can be directly linked to Ebola. However, the motivations of its creators is key here to considering them within the remit of edutainment-focused health communication products.

To producer Dwumoh, it was an enterprise that was well worth the effort and risk it took. Some credit these Ebola productions for raising the profile of the film industry in Liberia. Although his production company had been operational for close to a decade, it was this Ebola production that brought him on the radar of international media like the BBC. However, as noted, the films itself were no Oscar-winners. They were very simply structured. However, like any good old script, it borrowed storylines and plots from Hollywood – the tension, suspense, and eventual miracle. However, it filled a much-needed gap – that of the lack of DVDs due to the closure of borders, a popular medium of entertianment which most Liberian city dwellers depend on. The state of emergency (or curfew) instituted during the period also curtailed all possible movements in search of other forms of entertainment. Actors such as Abdul Jah and Director Abdul-Karim Sheriff were all local, home-grown products. Together, they both entertained and captivated hundreds of homebound Liberians in the midst of the crises. An added motivation for these actors, was to relieve the tension that was ever-present, as many hundreds of new cases were reported each day, and quarantines (often forcefully enforced) were undertaken by a mix of security forces and health workers. Threats of infections among the crew and cast, made the experience even more daunting for all those involved. Yet, they prevailed motivated by the quest to provide some respite to Liberians, from the disease.

Though movies in Ebolawood were most often comedy, contextualised to appeal to local audiences in Liberia, there was a significant unintended consequence. It also provided an opportunity to educate people beyond the shores of Liberia about Liberia and its people – their creativity, hopes, and dreams amidst the crises.

#### 8.3.1.2 Music: Ebola in Town

Liberian rapper and producer Samuel "Shadow" Morgan, collaborated with fellow Liberian artistes Edwin "D-12" Tweh and Kuzzy of 2-Kings to put out the music track titled *Ebola in Town* at the height of the crises in 2014. It was ironically described as an infectious song by some, and has been credited as Liberia's first Ebola song.[6] Though these three were all of Liberian origin, they had honed their

[6] http://www.npr.org/sections/goatsandsoda/2014/08/19/341412011/shadow-and-d-12-sing-an-infectious-song-about-ebola

craft in the West African country of Ghana. Like Dwomoh and his crew, they were looking for a way to still earn a living from their craft, as curfews imposed on many towns across the country meant there was no longer an opportunity to perform for large gatherings.

But, this hit song was also inspired by a need to educate. They had dabbled in social messaging before – notably issues of poor sanitation and irresponsible parenthood. The latter established some striking parallels between these and their Ebola song. Shadow maintained the view that the song opened up the world to the possibility of Liberian music.[7] It certainly garnered him some international media attention. For an artiste who was used to the backing of so-called donors, he went this one alone. In fact, the first major project of his entertainment company was a collaboration with Canada's University of Alberta, to highlight the plight of child refugees based in Ghana who had fled the Liberian war.[8] *Ebola in Town* itself, could pass for any other local song common to the sub-region, danceable tunes and funk beats. But, the lyrics are all educational, written completely in English (including Pidgin), with simple rhythms and sentences. It notes the actions that can lead to the spread of the virus and urged listeners to desist from these actions. There is the inevitable allusion to God (Liberia, just like much of West Africa, is thought to be very religious) – requesting the intervention of God to save them from the disease.

However, the extent to which it went further to influence changed behaviors in affected communities across the country is not immediately clear. Nonetheless, its impact in lifting the spirits of affected victims of the disease, dispelling tensions, and changing the narrative of the Liberian among western audiences was evident, much like Ebolawood discussed above.

#### 8.3.1.3 Ebola Song

The last set of artistic pieces to be considered are those funded by UNICEF, which is a sharp contrast to the independent productions from Dwomoh and Shadow, discussed in the preceding two sub-sections. These however fit squarely in the domain of health communications – going by the Office of Disease Prevention and Health Promotion (2010) set of prescribed criteria as discussed above. They saw collaborations from local artistes, international NGOs and government agencies including Crusaders for Peace, Hott FM Radio, and the Ministry of Health. The two songs developed as part of the project were simply titled *Crusaders for Peace Ebola Song* and *Hottfm Ebola Song* respectively, and they had none of the frills associated with an independently-produced music piece for purely entertainment purposes. Also produced in 2014 at the height of the Ebola elimination campaign, one had a description tag that said "…inform people about how to protect themselves from this deadly disease, and we won't stop until #Ebola is history!" The accompanying promotional images were also a contrast to those seen from the self-initiated content discussed

[7] http://www.okayafrica.com/shadow-liberian-mc-producer-killing-me/

[8] http://www.globaled.ualberta.ca/en/OutreachandInitiatives/BuduburamCDProject.aspx

in the preceeding two sub-sections They did not feature the photos of the artistes, but rather, educational flyers displaying the Dos and Don'ts in relation to avoiding the spread of the virus, and what to do in the event of contracting the virus. The artistes behind these creations Deng, SoulFresh and FA were not personally named either.[9] The songs' respective pages on SoundCloud garnered 4750[10] and 18.6 k[11] views as at the time of this research. They nonetheless also embodied the cultural identity of the Liberian people. They were however widely distributed on CDs, to all radio stations across the country, and due to the backing of donor funds, received substantial airplay, reaching as many audiences as possible.

The lyrics were also more comprehensive comparatively, with long narrations dedicated to outlining the scientific facts associated with Ebola. One featured a list of the possible ways to prevent contracting the virus, as well as the symptoms of the virus. From a health communications perspective, it was certainly more direct and streamlined – messages and key takeaways well apportioned in each verse. It had all the hallmarks of a professional health communications touch, including accuracy, accessibility, and consistency of message, as well as use of evidence-based information and reliable sources. While it was also done in a mix of English and pidgin, both well-spoken in Liberia, the tune could indeed pass for any contemporary pop song emerging from the sub-region. The educational elements were certainly stronger than the artistic elements, which made it very obvious what the aim was first and foremost educational. After all, they end with an acknowledgement that this is in fact a message from the Ministry of Health and Social Welfare and partners. Nonetheless, the latter of the two songs had a catchy tune that was sure to appeal to the large swaths of Liberians who had to listen to the song over and over again over the period. No wonder it garnered the most views. Anecdotal accounts seem to support the view that the tunes were perceived by locals to be filled with hope.

## 8.4 Health Communications from the Margins

While it is important to consider overarching frameworks of health communications in investigations such as this one, it is obvious that no two health communication projects are the same. More importantly no two similar health messages transmitted via entertainment media are motivated by the same goals.

The presented case studies are indeed three very different film and music projects with varying motivations, structures, and approaches. But to what extent do they lead us to question, whether they fit within the realm of "traditional" health communication? Relatedly, it is worth questioning if these approaches are any more effective in creating awareness of the disease taking the economic and cultural context of Liberia into account. Many a researcher has identified the shortfall that the

[9] https://www.UNICEF.org/liberia/media_8291.html

[10] https://soundcloud.com/UNICEF-liberia/crusaders-for-peace-ebola-song

[11] https://soundcloud.com/UNICEF-liberia/hott-fm-ebola-song-liberia

economic disadvantages of countries in the global South (such as Liberia, Guinea, and Sierra Leone) present when attempting to combat such epidemics within their borders. However, it is important to understand that collectively, edutainment projects such as the ones being profiled here come at a cost, and can be taxing on any community, especially one that has taken a beating economically such as Liberia did. These production pieces cost a great amount of money to assemble, and to air these on radio and television requires quite an investment, which may well be beyond the capacities of local governments, even though most do get the support of donor communities. As such, the contribution of private sector actors (like Dwomoh and Shadow) should be considered, their outputs evaluated as health communications content, and their overall impact in contributing to health communications goals well-articulated.

Though the differences in these three case studies have been outlined, it is also important to showcase the instances when they mirror each other. Interestingly, this is mostly in the domain of the incorporation of cultural dynamics peculiar to the locality, which many scholars and practitioners have touted as key considerations in building health communications approaches that more effectively speak to the needs of the intended target communities. The same cultural norms that made their way into these artistic pieces, though depicted as villains in the media and scientific publications as far as the transmission of the Ebola virus is concerned – such as indiscriminate touching, and the love for the consumption of bush meat – received a funny treatment in the songs. By projecting these norms through the medium of music and film, these actors are all considering the vital role of popular culture in tackling the disease.

Though the increasing relevance of digital technology has been advanced as one of the defining elements of effective science and health communication in the present time, it is obvious from the distribution of these media content on DVDs and CDs that traditional mediums still served as the main channels in countries such as Liberia. It is evident that contextual socio-economic and cultural factors are more integral in shaping the types of approaches and channels adopted to do health communications in each locality, and the degree of effectiveness depends on these. There is also the element of the role of citizens as producers or actors in the development of health or science communication content, which is increasingly gaining popularity in many parts of the western world. Strictly considered, not all of the actors identified from the case studies discussed above fit this bill, and certainly not the donor organizations that sponsored some of these productions. The solutions presented by these cases studies were indeed a marriage of actors and approaches – donors (western), production teams (both local and foreign), and artistes (mostly local).

Finally and more importantly, there are considerations to do with the motivations behind these media productions. Of all the three case studies, only the case of the *Ebola Songs* produced in partnership with UNICEF was intended to be health communications from the most complete understanding of the term, referencing Office of Disease Prevention and Health Promotion (2010) guidelines. The aim of the project was primarily to provide information (through songs) for audiences to change their behaviours and ultimately contribute to curbing the spread of the virus, and also reducing the fatality rates from the infection. Shadow and his collaborators, though seeking to educate fellow Liberians with the content of their songs were nonetheless also motivated by a mix of factors including earning an income from their trade due to the inability to perform for large gatherings, and a desire to expand the reach of their content considering the fact that Ebola had offered a global platform as awareness about the virus increased worldwide.

Finally, *Ebolawood* can be considered as the production space where the creators had the least motivation for engaging in any form of health communication. Dwomoh and the rest of his team had no intention of undertaking a health communications campaign in the strictest sense. They were merely taking advantage of the situation to do a number of things, namely capitalize on the shutdown of borders and movements to churn out home-grown DVDs and to earn an income through these, and not unlike Shadow and his team, put Liberian media content (in this case film) on the map, at least within the sub region. However, they both inadvertently achieved some of the ultimate goals of health communication in Liberia that the relevant stakeholders – government, donors, international NGOs – would have sought to achieve at that time, i.e. keeping spirits up, and people indoors and away from crowds.

## 8.5 Conclusions: Presenting a Blueprint for Future Outbreaks

In this chapter, I have attempted to use a case study of some media content put out during the Ebola outbreak in Liberia, to contest the idea that only content that satisfy the notion of traditional health communications can be considered as such. The investigations considered a number of factors; the approaches of these pieces, the messages within the content, the channels used, and the impact that they made. These were used to conclude that they can indeed be considered to be health communications products that ultimately contributed to the Ebola campaign in Liberia.

However, what sets them apart from each other is the motivations behind these projects. While the totality of the examination undertaken here does not in any way assist us in developing a sure blueprint for undertaking effective health communications interventions in the event of a future outbreak of a similar nature, it does put us firmly on the path of doing so. While the remit of this chapter is limited to posing salient questions about what qualifies as health communications, it can however make the recommendations through the main findings for future scholarly research, and for practitioners to consider in the design of future interventions. Firstly, there is a need to cast the net wide as far as labeling what constitutes a health communications intervention is concerned. Dwomoh and Shadow's respective projects fall at the periphery of traditional interventions. However, their collective contributions towards achieving health communications goals are remarkable. Practitioners and scholars should therefore consider evaluating their impact in terms of overall effectiveness in order to identify what approaches are best suited to achieving results taking the contextual norms of Liberia into consideration. However, while these cases studies and resulting conclusions and recommendations are specific to Liberia, it is important to note that any examination of other affected areas (for example Guinea or Sierra Leone) and their respective interventions as far as edutainment approaches in health communications is concerned, are likely to yield similar results, hence making these recommendations applicable across the board.

While we know more now about how to possibly contain the disease than we did then, it appears that whatever interventions are in place as far as raising awareness or curbing the spread of the disease is concerned need not necessarily follow a particular theory or approach of health communication. However, we do emphasize that how the story or messages are packaged and disseminated in each instance is indeed a marker of how the epidemic would end and the number of fatalities when it does. As the potential for more outbreaks of infectious diseases on the continent is sure, there is a need to emphasize among other things media literacy, on the part of the audience, circumspect actions on the part of journalists, writers, communications experts and media writers, and vigilance on the part of governments and global health bodies. This is more imperative now more than ever, especially in the age of Fake News. But, when an opportunity presents itself to cast the net wide to consider alternative forms of health communications messages, it is vital that these are taken.

What I have sought to do in this chapter, is to contest the idea that the approach should follow a particular path, and the actors must belong to a particular designated group that bears a formal responsibility for the health communications intervention. This is by no means the first or only publication that attempts to understand how the lessons learned from the Liberia response can be applied to other potential disease outbreaks. Bedford et al. (2017) believe that community focused engagements did lead to a change in behaviors, through increased knowledge levels. It is important to explore the impact that unintended health communications projects, such as Dwomoh's and Shadow's discussed above (which will certainly fall outside the radar of mainstream donor-funded evaluations), have had on changing behaviors and helping to curb the disease. This must certainly be an agenda for future research.

## References

Abramowitz, S., McKune, S. L., Fallah, M., Monger, J., Tehoungue, K., & Omidian, P. (2017). The opposite of denial: Social learning at the onset of the Ebola emergency in Liberia. *Journal of Health Communication, 22*, 59–65.

Bedford, J., Chitnis, K., Webber, N., Dixon, P., Limwame, K., Elessawi, R., & Obregon, R. (2017). Community engagement in Liberia: Routine immunization post-Ebola. *Journal of Health Communication, 22*(1), 81–90. https://doi.org/10.1080/10810730.2016.1253122.

Brown, B., Nasiruddin, M., Dao, A., & Halabi, M. (2015). Responsible use of pop culture and communication in the face of Ebola virus. In O. B. Akogun (Ed.), *PLoS Neglected Tropical Diseases, 9*(8), e0003890. *PMC*.

Colace, F., De Santo, M., & Pietrosanto, A. (2006). *Work in progress: Bayesian networks for edutainment*. 36th ASEE/IEEE Frontiers in Education Conference, https://doi.org/10.1109/FIE.2006.322573

Dutta, M. J., Anaele, A., & Jones, C. (2014). A culture-centered approach to listening: Voices of social change. *International Journal of Listening, 28*(2), 67–81. https://doi.org/10.1080/10904018.2014.876266.

Govender, E. (2013). Working in the Greyzone: Exploring education-entertainment in Africa. *African Communication Research, 6*(1), 5–32.

Kummervold, P. E., Schulz, W. S., Smout, E., Fernandez-Luque, L., & Larson, H. J. (2017). Controversial Ebola vaccine trials in Ghana: A thematic analysis of critiques and rebuttals in digital news. *BMC Public Health, 17*, 642. https://doi.org/10.1186/s12889-017-4618-8.

Munodawafa, D. (2008). Communication: Concepts, practice and challenges. *Health Education Research, 23*(3), 369–370. https://doi.org/10.1093/her/cyn024.

Nabarro, D. (2017). Including communities in public health action: Harnessing best practices. *Journal of Health Communication, 22*(1), 1–1. https://doi.org/10.1080/10810730.2017.1283203.

Nyenswah, T., Kateh, F., Bawo, L., Massaquoi, M., Gbanyan, M., & Fallah, M.. (2014–2015). Ebola and its control in Liberia. *Emerging Infectious Diseases*, *22*(2), 169–177. https://doi.org/10.3201/eid2202.151456.

Office of Disease Prevention and Health Promotion. (2010). *Health Communication*. https://ecdc.europa.eu/en/health-communication/facts

Rivera, M. (2017). Music, media, and the ethnopoetics of two Ebola songs in Liberia. *Africa Today, 63*(3), 63–76. https://doi.org/10.2979/africatoday.63.3.05.

Roberts, H. B. S., Alden Fish, S., II, Robinson, E., & Zuckerman, E. (2017). Digital health communication and global public influence: A study of the Ebola epidemic. *Journal of Health Communication, 22*(1), 51–58. https://doi.org/10.1080/10810730.2016.1209598.

Sastry, S., & Dutta, M. J. (2017). Health communication in the time of Ebola: A culture-centered interrogation. *Journal of Health Communication, 22*(1), 10–14. https://doi.org/10.1080/10810730.2016.1216205.

Singhal, A. And Rogers, E.M. 1999. Lessons learned about entertainment education. In A. Singhal and E.M. Rogers (Eds.), Entertainment education: A communication strategy for social change (pp. 205–227). Mahwah: Lawrence Erlbaum Associates.

Soul City Institute. (2013). *Edutainment: Using stories and media for social action and behavior change*. https://www.soulcity.org.za/research/published-articles/edutainment-using-stories-and-media-for-social-action-and-behaviour-change/download

Storey, J. D., Chitnis, K., Obregon, R., & Garrison, K. (2017). Community engagements and the communication response to Ebola. *Journal of Health Communication, 22*(1), 2–4. https://doi.org/10.1080/10810730.2017.1283200.

# Part III
# Global Health and Governance

# Chapter 9
# A Political Conception of Pandemics and Epidemics in Africa

**Frank Aragbonfoh Abumere**

## 9.1 Introduction

This chapter is dealing with health. Nevertheless, the framework of the chapter is neither biological nor medical, but political. This is what is referred to in the chapter as a *political conception* of pandemics and epidemics. In this political conception, I contend that the interactional and institutional failure to conform to the communal basic structure of society (assuming the communal basic structure is itself just and not unjust) causes, enables or contributes to pandemics and epidemics in Africa. Pandemics are diseases that are prevalent over a sizable geographical area such as a country, sub-region, continent or the entire world. While epidemics mean widespread occurrences of infectious diseases in a particular community and at a particular time. Pandemics and epidemics include cholera, Ebola, yellow fever, etc.

Specifically, the concern of the chapter is with the individual's morally unjust actions and inactions that may cause, enable or contribute to pandemics and epidemics in Africa. I consider the actions and inactions to be moral injustice because of the resultant pandemics and epidemics. *Prima facie*, this argument is a consequentialist one. However, the arguments in this paper will be based on deontological grounds where as a moral agent and member of society, the individual has certain duties or obligations, and these obligations are formalised in terms of norms or rules. Whether the consequences of her actions and inactions are positive or negative do not determine their moral rightness or wrongness. What determines the moral rightness or wrongness of her actions and inactions is whether she acts or fails to act in accordance with her duty or duties.

F. A. Abumere (✉)
Department of Philosophy, The Arctic University of Norway, Tromso, Norway
e-mail: frank.a.abumere@uit.no; frank.abumere@area.ox.ac.uk



G. B. Tangwa et al. (eds.), *Socio-cultural Dimensions of Emerging Infectious Diseases in Africa*, https://doi.org/10.1007/978-3-030-17474-3_9

### 9.1.1 *The Structure of the Chapter*

I will focus on cholera in Nigeria. There have been many cholera outbreaks in Nigeria. The most recent outbreak was in 2017 (WHO 2012). Cholera is an infectious and fatal bacterial disease of the small intestine which causes severe vomiting and diarrhoea. Since cholera is typically contracted from infected water supplies, cholera outbreak implies the failure to provide healthy water supplies. If we are to successfully prevent cholera outbreaks in Nigeria, quickly eradicate them when and where they have already occurred, and to shield victims and families of victims from suffering the after-effect when and where outbreaks have already been eradicated, then we must pay attention to how members of society can have a causal, enabling or contributory roles in cholera outbreaks.

In the above regard, we must pay attention to all agents, both the more important and the less important, and both the more powerful and the less powerful. However, because individuals are less powerful and less important in terms of how agents affect cholera outbreaks in Nigeria, the causal, enabling and contributory roles of individuals do not receive adequate attention. Therefore, the focus of this chapter is on individuals. The chapter engages in both the descriptive and prescriptive analyses of the failure to conform to the communal basic structure of society which in turn causes, enables or contributes to cholera outbreaks. The descriptive analysis shows us what the actions and inactions of members of society are. While, relying on the descriptive analysis, the prescriptive analysis tells us what the duties or responsibilities of the members of society ought to be.

The chapter is divided in to six sections. The first section is this introductory and structural section. In the second section, I present my conception of communal basic structure. In the third section, I present a descriptive analysis of how members of society have causal, enabling or contributory roles in cholera outbreaks in Nigeria. In the fourth section, I explain the systemic nature of the individual's actions and inactions. In the fifth section, I explain, within the context of our subject matter, the relationship between causal responsibility (actions or inactions) and the corresponding moral responsibility (the consequences generated by the actions or inactions). Finally, in the concluding section, I reiterate my conception of responsibility – throughout the chapter, it is this conception that allows us to see the culpability of agents in pandemics and epidemics.

## 9.2 Communal Basic Structure

The fundamental concept of this chapter is "communal basic structure." By "communal basic structure," I mean the basic structure of a moderate communitarian society in which the explicit focus on the rights of the community and the duties of individuals is complemented by an implicit focus on the duties of the community and the rights of individuals. In other words, on the one hand, even when and where the society emphasizes the rights of the community, it does not negate the rights of individuals. On the other hand, even when and where the society emphasizes the duties of individuals, it does not negate the duties of the community.

The concept is a derivative of John Rawls' (1999) 'basic structure' and Kwame Gyekye's (1997) 'moderate communitarianism.' According to Rawls (1999), "the primary subject of justice is the basic structure of society…the way in which the major social institutions distribute fundamental rights and duties and determine the division of advantages from social cooperation" (6). While for Gyekye (1997), in moderate communitarianism, the rights of the individual and the individual's obligations to society are given equal weight (52). By virtue of the equal weight given to both the individual's rights and her obligations to society, Robert Nozick's (1974) libertarian assertion that "Individuals have rights and there are things you cannot do to them without violating their rights" (IX) will not be allowed to stand alone in a moderate communitarian society. It must be balanced with a counter assertion that communities and societies have rights and there are things individuals cannot do to them without violating their rights.

In spite of the above counter assertion, a moderate communitarian society – unlike a non-moderate communitarian society – does not negate the individual's rights while affirming the society's rights. In other words, it does not deem the individual to only be a communal being whose existence and essence can only be defined in terms of the obligations she owes the society. Therefore, a moderate communitarian society avoids the danger of a non-moderate communitarian society. The danger of a non-moderate communitarian society is that, like utilitarianism, it does not respect the separateness of persons. It does not recognize that:

> Each person possesses an inviolability founded on justice that even the welfare of society as a whole cannot override….justice denies that the loss of freedom for some is made right by a greater good shared by others. It does not allow that the sacrifices imposed on a few are outweighed by the larger sum of advantages enjoyed by many….the rights secured by justice are not subject to…the calculus of social interests (Rawls 1999, 3–4).

In a moderate communitarian society, while the individual is seen as a communal being with obligations, she is also seen as an autonomous being with rights. According to Gyekye (1997), "The capacity for self-assertion that the individual can exercise presupposes, and in fact derives from, the autonomous nature of the person. By autonomy, I do not mean self-completeness buthaving of a will, a rational will of one's own, that enables one to determine at least some of one's own goals and to pursue them, and to control one's destiny" (54). Consequently, the autonomous nature of the individual entails that "the communitarian self cannot be as a cramped or shackled self, responding robotically to the ways and demands of the communal structure. The structure is never to be conceived as reducing a person to intellectual or rational inactivity, servility and docility" (55–56).

Within a moderate communitarian society, there are two normative relationships, namely the vertical and the horizontal, and the communal basic structure is the hub which these special relationships revolve around. On the one hand, the vertical relationship is the relationship that exists between the society and individuals. On the other hand, the horizontal relationship is the relationship that exists among the individuals. Combining both relationships, the communal basic structure forms and shapes, and guards and guides the life of the society. For this reason, to know whether the society is structurally just or unjust, or to know to what extent the society is structurally just or unjust, we only need to look at how far away or close the interactions and institutions within the society are from or to the communal basic structure. My contention is that actions and inactions that fail to conform to the communal basic structure of society can cause, enable or contribute to pandemics and epidemics.[1]

## 9.3 The Role of the Individual in Cholera Outbreaks in Nigeria

The individual can be said to contribute to causing or enabling cholera in Nigeria due to certain actions or inactions For instance, the unavailability of water supply from a water board or ministry of water resource usually forces people to have alternative water supplies. While some alternative water supplies are clean, many are contaminated. In this case, if there is a cholera outbreak due to the usage of contaminated water, the individuals who are responsible for water supply at the water boards or ministries of water resource are morally responsible for the cholera outbreak. Further instances include the supply of contaminated water for consumption, pollution of water bodies, etc. While the aforementioned instances directly result in outbreaks, instances such as non-enforcement of laws, non-implementation of policies, non-prosecution of offenders, making of bad laws and policies, lobbying, etc. can indirectly cause or enable outbreaks.

The aforementioned actions and inactions of individuals can affect cholera outbreaks at one, two or three of the following stages; pre-outbreak, outbreak and post-outbreak. At the pre-outbreak stage, individuals are said to have a causal or contributory role in an outbreak if or when their actions or inactions pre-outbreak (that is before the actual occurrence of the outbreak) are responsible for the *fact, condition or situation* that the outbreak could not be prevented. At the outbreak stage, individuals are said to have an enabling or contributory role in an outbreak if or when their actions or inactions during an outbreak are responsible for the *fact, condition or situation* that the outbreak was allowed to spread or could not be eradicated, or at least could not be eradicated as quick as possible.

At the post-outbreak stage, unlike the pre-outbreak and outbreak stages, when I say individuals are responsible for an outbreak, I do not mean that they caused or contributed to the failure to prevent the outbreak (as inthe pre-outbreak stage).

[1] Throughout this chapter, I am dealing with political agents, rather than biological and medical agents. In other words, I am not dealing with fungi, bacteria, viruses, environmental conditions, natural elements, etc., but with individual agents (human beings or persons) who are part and parcel of the communal basic structure of society.

Neither do I mean that they contributed to the spread or the failure to eradicate the outbreak (as in the outbreak stage). But what I mean is that the actions and inactions of these individuals caused or contributed to the *fact, condition or situation* that those affected by the outbreak are allowed to suffer the after-effect of the outbreak.

The actions and inactions of individuals, in the above instances and stages fail to conform to the communal basic structure of society in two senses. In the first sense, the individual fails to conform to the communal basic structure of society by failing to performing her duty to society or by not refraining from performing acts which violate the rights of society. For instance, when individuals pollute common water bodies, they violate the right of the community to clean water and fail in their own duty to refrain from such violation. In the second sense, the individual fails to conform to the communal basic structure of society because by failing in her duty to society she consequently violates the rights of other members of society. In other words, the individual's failure in her duty to society mitigates the ultimate end of society which is the creation and sustenance of a just and fair society for the wellbeing of the entire membership. Ultimately, in the context of our discussion, this is what causes, enables or contributes to a condition or situation whereby cholera outbreaks: (i) are not prevented; (ii) are either not eradicated or not quickly eradicated, and; (iii) victims and family members of victims are allowed to suffer the after-effect.

## 9.4 The Systemic Nature of the Individual's Actions and Inactions

When isolated as singular actions and inactions, individuals' actions and inactions that are held responsible for cholera outbreaks in Nigeria may neither be necessary nor sufficient conditions for the outbreaks. Nevertheless, when all the actions and inactionsare not seen in isolation, but are seen holistically, then we can see how together they cause outbreaks. In other words, outbreaks are 'up to the actions and inactions' collectively, therefore the actions and inactions "have a collective *causal* responsibility for" (Pogge 1989, 276) outbreaks. What this means in terms of cholera outbreaks in Nigeria is that many outbreaks could have been prevented, many could have been eradicated quickly, and many victims and families of victims could have been shielded from the after-effect of such outbreaks if not for the actions and inactions of certain individuals who do not respect the communal basic structure of society. In view of the grave consequences of such actions and inactions, it is apt to conclude that such individuals have no value for human life or at least they do not care about human suffering.

But how can an individual be said to have caused cholera outbreakswhen her actions and inactions are not causality if causality is understood as a necessary and sufficient condition for an effect? Before answering the question, I will briefly explain what I mean by 'necessary and sufficient condition' in the context of cholera outbreak. In the context of cholera outbreak, just like in ordinary language sense, an individual's action or inaction is necessary and sufficient for an outbreak if: (i) the outbreak will not occur except the action or inaction has already taken place; (ii) the action or inaction must precede the outbreak and the outbreak must follow the action or inaction. In my argument, the individual's actions and inactions are not a necessary and sufficient condition for cholera outbreaks. Other than the individual and her actions or inactions, other agents and factors can be responsible for the outbreaks; in this sense, the individual's actions or inactions are not *necessary* for an outbreak. In spite of the individual's actions or inactions, there may not be an outbreak; in this sense, the individual's actions or inactions may not be *sufficient* for an outbreak. However, while the individual's actions and inactions may not be *the cause* of an outbreak, such actions or inactions may be *part of the cause* of an outbreak.

The above explanation shows that while the individual's actions or inaction may be inconsequential when viewed in isolation, it may be consequential when view in relation to other enabling actions. In this sense, the nature of the combined actions or inactions is systemic, and the individual's action or inaction is accurately understood when it is viewed as part of a system. To see the individual's role as part of a systemic one, an explanation of systemic causation will suffice. According to George Lakoff (2012):

> Systemic causation, because it is less obvious, is more important to understand. A systemic cause may be one of a number of multiple causes. It may require some special conditions. It may be indirect, working through a network of more direct causes. It may be probabilistic, occurring with a significantly high probability. It may require a feedback mechanism. In general, causation in ecosystems, biological systems, economic systems, and social systems tends not to be direct, but is no less causal. And because it is not direct causation, it requires all the greater attention if it is to be understood and its negative effects controlled. Above all, it requires a name: systemic causation.

Moreover, as Thomas Pogge (1989) says, "injustice can be systemic, can exist without being traceable to any manifestly unjust actions by individuals or groups. Our causal contribution to suffering is extremely indirect and intermixed with the causal contributions of others" (11–12). In this case, although we may not be able to trace an outbreak to any manifestly unjust actions and inactions of an individual, yet their causal and constitutive contributions are indirect and intermixed, hence systemic.

A brief description of the enabling conditions of the 1996 Cholera Outbreak in Niger State, Nigeria suffices to illustrate the systemic nature of the individual's actions or inactions. No particular source was identified as the source of the outbreak and no specific persons were identified as being responsible for the outbreak. In the absence of pipe borne water, in some parts of the State people were dependent on certain sources of water for their water supply although such sources were reported to be contaminated. The sources included River Guarara, private wells and public wells.

The state had ministry of water resource and water boards that were responsible for the supply of clean water, yet there was no clean water for consumption in spite of the annual budgetary allocations for clean water supply. The politicians and civil servants who had the duty to provide clean water but failed in their duty are morally responsible for the cholera outbreak. Also morally responsible for the devastating effects of the outbreak are politicians and civil servants who were in charge of the ministry of health and medical practitioners and other health workers who were in charge of public health. These latter individuals were inefficient in their response to the outbreak hence the outbreak could not be quickly eradicated. Therefore, while no singular individual can be held morally responsible in isolation, collectively all the aforementioned individuals share responsibility for the outbreak.

Some arguments might be raised against my conclusion as reached above. For instance, it can be argued that in most of the scenarios above, if it were not a particular health worker, director of public health, commissioner of water resource or minister of environment, some other health workers, directors of public health, commissioners of water resource or ministers of environment would have taken their places and done the same immoral deeds because the structures, system or institutions are such that there will always be some actors to do the exact deeds. However, this does not negate the fact that the actors that actually did the deeds are blameworthy. What it shows is that the structures, systems or institutions are also blameworthy. When someone has committed a crime or moral wrong, we do not say that the person is not to blame because others would have done that crime or moral wrong. For instance, when there is a vicious and violent xenophobia in a community, the targets will be prone to crimes being committed against them and moral wrongs being done to them. But we do not exonerate a xenophobe from her morally wrong act or crime of killing someone because if she did not do it someone else would have done it.

Perhaps a stronger argument against my conclusion regarding the particular health worker, public health director, commissioner of health or minister of environment will say that rather than acting or failing to act on their own, such individual merely acted or failed to act as an agent of the government. Hence it is the government that should be held morally responsible rather than the individual. Nevertheless, holding the individual morally responsible does not negate holding the government she represents morally responsible. Ultimately, the government is responsible for the actions and inactions performed on its behalf with its approval. But as a moral agent, the individual is morally responsible for her part in the actions and inactions.

In summary, in the context of our discussion, the health worker, civil servant or politician faces a two-count moral charge namely action and inaction. On the one hand, *when she acts*, for instance, when she uses her executive power to make harmful public policies, she is guilty of causing, enabling or contributing to a condition or situation whereby cholera outbreaks: (i) are not prevented; (ii) are either not eradicated or not quickly eradicated; (iii) victims and family members of victims are allowed to suffer the after-effect. On the other hand, *when she fails to act*, for instance, when she has the legislative power to stop the above harmful public policies but fails to do so, she is guilty of causing, enabling or contributing to a condition or situation resulting in the above.

## 9.5 Causal Responsibility and Corresponding Moral Responsibility

A moral agent can be causally responsible in action or in omission and yet can be said not to have any corresponding moral responsibility for the consequences of the action or omission. So also a moral agent can be said to have a moral responsibility for an event, condition or situation even if the agent has no causal responsibility for the event, condition or situation. Nevertheless, in this chapter, I am only concerned with the relationship between actions/inactions (causal responsibility) and the cholera outbreaks that result from the actions or inactions (corresponding moral responsibility).

The concept of responsibility is always difficult to define. This difficulty is usually resolved by proving that: first, a particular agent caused an undesirable incident or failed to prevent an undesirable incident; second, then the action or omission is shown to be against certain laws, rules, norms, codes or principles. When these two conditions of proof are met, then the agent is said to be responsible for the undesirable incident. This is usually the standard way of resolving the difficulty of defining responsibility in the context of the relationship between causal responsibility and the corresponding moral responsibility.

In the court of law, lawyers and judges have a constitution or legal code to serve as their frame of reference when proving the guilt of an accused. In moral philosophy, there is no canonical conception of moral responsibility. As Paul Ricoeur (2000) says, the concept of responsibility is "not really well-established within the philosophical tradition" (11). Nevertheless, there are standard conceptions of moral responsibility:

I. moral responsibility may refer to prospective responsibility whereby a moral agent has a certain moral role (Williams 2014), for instance a moral duty to care for or attend to a sick person during an epidemic and failure to perform this duty leads to blame or punishment;
II. moral responsibility may refer to retrospective responsibility which is a situation when the actions of a moral agent are judged to be morally wrong, and the moral agent thus deserves to be blamed or punished for the actions (Ibid.);
III. while theories of moral agency tend to regard an agent as either responsible or not, with no half-measures, our everyday language usually deploys the term 'responsible' in a more nuanced way….one way we do this is by weighing degrees of responsibility, both with regard to the sort of prospective responsibilities a person should bear and a person's liability to blame or penalties (Ibid.).

In summary, the three standard conceptions conceive of responsibility to be moral culpability for one's actions or inactions which cause moral harm. Having established the individual's causal and constitutive (contributory) role in cholera outbreaks in the previous sections of this chapter, and in view of the standard conceptions of responsibility, the conclusion I will draw is that the individual can be morally responsible for cholera outbreak. But so also are the agencies they work for or the communities they belong to. Therefore, my conclusion is less emphatic, but it is nonetheless valid.

First and foremost, given that cholera outbreaksare 'up to all the agents' collectively, and therefore they "have a collective *causal* responsibility for" pandemics and epidemics, "this causal responsibility gives rise to a *moral* responsibility, which is a collective responsibility for [their] collective role in" (Pogge 1989, 276) the outbreaks. Second, but of equal importance as the first, contributory causal and constitutive role implies partial blameworthiness, which in turn implies partial responsibility. Linking contributory causal and constitutive role with partial responsibility suggests that the principle of commensurability is in application. It is with the help of the principle of commensurability that we are able to gauge the exact or approximate relationship between contributory causal and constitutive role and the corresponding partial responsibility.

Given the contributory causal and constitutive role the health worker, civil servant or politician plays in causing cholera outbreaks and given the principle of commensurability, it is only fair that she is *prima facie* morally responsible to the extent or degree that she is causally and constitutively responsible. In spite of the principle of commensurability, her moral responsibility, commensurate with her causal and constitutive role, should only be a *pro tanto* obligation. Because, as a member of society with a communal basic structure she may have a duty that goes beyond the extent of her role in an outbreak. Therefore, by seeing her responsibility as a *pro tanto* obligation, there will be enough room left for more demanding obligations. The nature of such obligations will depend on what the communal basic structure of her society stipulates.

To conclude this section, I admit that there are "cases of exception." By cases of exception, I mean there are cases whereby although a health worker, civil servant or politician has a role in a cholera outbreak, she may still be deemed not blameworthy because of certain circumstances. For instance, if a health worker has already done her fare share, she may not be expected to take up the slack when others refuse to do their own share. Furthermore, children who have not attained the age of reason, mentally disabled persons etc. cannot be held morally responsible for their actions even if such actions contribute to outbreaks.

## 9.6 Conclusion

In the above discussion, I contended that the interactional and institutional failure to conform with the communal basic structure of society (assuming the communal basic structure is itself just and not unjust) causes, enables or contributes to pandemics and epidemics. I contended that there are obligations the individual owes her society and failure to fulfil such obligations can lead to grave consequences such as the 1996 Cholera Outbreak in Niger State, Nigeria. In order to avoid situations of such grave consequences which result from the actions or inactions of individual members of society, a moderate communitarian society has a "communal basic structure" which explicitly focuses on the rights of the community and the duties of individuals, and implicitly focuses on the duties of the community and the rights of individuals. While the rights of individuals are not negated, the rights of the community are emphasized. And while the obligations of the community are not negated, the obligations of the individual are emphasised.

To summarise the crux of the discussion, individuals are morally responsible, albeit commensurately, for pandemics and epidemics. By implication, as already mentioned, they have *pro tanto* obligations which leave enough room for the possibility of more demanding obligations. The *pro tanto* obligations can be summed up into a negative and a positive duty. On the one hand, the individuals will have a negative duty *not to cause* harm and *not to act* in such ways that they will cause, enable or contribute to a condition or situation whereby: (i) pandemics and epidemics are not prevented; (ii) pandemics and epidemics are either not eradicated or not quickly eradicated, and; (iii) victims and family members of victims of pandemics and epidemics are allowed to suffer the after-effect of pandemics and epidemics. On the other hand, the individuals will have a positive duty *to make amends* for the harms they have already caused, and *to act* in such ways that they will cause, enable or contribute to a condition or situation whereby: (i) pandemics and epidemics are prevented; (ii) pandemics and epidemics are quickly eradicated, and; (iii) victims and family members of victims of pandemics and epidemics are shielded from the after-effect of pandemics and epidemics.

**Note**

I first worked on some of the ideas in my chapter – "A Political Conception of Pandemics and Epidemics in Africa" -in my PhD Dissertation. Some ideas have changed and some have remained the same. The conclusion I reached in the chapter is some ways different from, and in other ways similar to, the conclusion I reached in the PhD Dissertation. In other words, it is some ideas in the dissertation that metamorphosed into the chapter.

## References

Gyekye, K. (1997). *Tradition and modernity*. New York: Oxford University Press.

Lakoff, G. (2012). *Global warming systematically caused hurricane Sandy*. http://blogs.berkeley.edu/2012/11/05/global-warming-systemically-caused-hurricane-sandy/. Accessed 4 May 2013.

Nozick, R. (1974). *Anarchy, State and Utopia*. New York: Basic Books.

Pogge, T. (1989). *Realizing rawls*. Ithaca: Cornel University Press.

Rawls, J. (1999). *A theory of justice, rev*. Cambridge, MA: Harvard University Press.

Ricoeur, P. (2000). *The Just. Trans. D. Pellauer*. Chicago: The University of Chicago Press.

Williams, G. (2014). Responsibility. *Internet Encyclopedia of Philosophy*. http://www.iep.utm.edu/responsi/. Accessed 28 July 2014.

World Health Organization (WHO). (2012). Emergencies, Preparedness, Response: Cholera – Nigeria. *Disease Outbreak News*. http://www.who.int/csr/don/12-july-2017-cholera-nigeria/en/. Accessed 9 July 2018.

# Chapter 10
# Global Emerging Pathogens and the (Prescriptive) Role of the World Health Organization

**Godfrey B. Tangwa and Muhammed O. Afolabi**

## 10.1 Introduction

The WHO was created in 1948, the same year that the Universal Declaration of Human Rights (UDHR) was proclaimed by the United Nations General Assembly in Paris (10 December 1948, Resolution 217 A), as a common standard of fundamental human values binding on all and to be universally protected everywhere on earth. This came on the heels of the Nuremberg Code (1947), following the Nuremberg Trials consequent on the end of World War Two, which had been marked by indescribable atrocities, including the most wanton medical experimentations on human beings (Emanuel et al. 2003). The WHO is thus very well placed and equipped by its mission and very raison d'être to be the guardian of global health and the guarantor of ethics and good science practices in health-related research all over the world. This role is always severely put to test in emergency situations such as during the outbreak of a dangerous infectious epidemic. This was the case during the recent EVD outbreak in West Africa and the ZVD outbreak in South America.

G. B. Tangwa (✉)
Department of Philosophy, University of Yaounde 1, Yaounde, Cameroon

Cameroon Bioethics Initiative (CAMBIN), Yaounde, Cameroon

Global Emerging Pathogen Treatment Consortium (GET) Consortium, Lagos, Nigeria

M. O. Afolabi
Department of Clinical Research, London School of Hygiene & Tropical Medicine, London, UK



G. B. Tangwa et al. (eds.), *Socio-cultural Dimensions of Emerging Infectious Diseases in Africa*, https://doi.org/10.1007/978-3-030-17474-3_10

## 10.2 Ebola Epidemic in West Africa

The Ebola virus epidemic (EVE) erupted in December 2013 and started raging and "ravaging West Africa, with nearly 4000 deaths already as of October 2014, and threatening to migrate to other regions of the world. Shortly after the outbreak, the WHO convened a consultation meeting of ethicists, other experts and stakeholders, on 11 August 2014, to consider and assess the ethical implications for clinical decision-making of the potential use of unregistered interventions. On 12 August 2014, the WHO released a short statement detailing ethical considerations for the use of unregistered interventions to fight the Ebola epidemic, which generally was well received and appreciated around the world**.** The consultation panel had reached the consensus that, in the particular circumstances of this outbreak, and provided certain conditions are met, it is ethical to offer unproven interventions with as yet unknown efficacy and adverse effects, as potential treatment or prevention. This recommendation was justifiable by the fact and to the extent that the situation in question was clearly that of a deadly and highly infectious epidemic with no known, let alone available, cure. The context was a purely therapeutic one with all efforts directed at saving human lives in imminent danger of death."[1]

Later on, the WHO came out with another statement [http://www.who.int/immunization/diseases/ebola/WHO_consultation_ebola_sep2014/en/] **on phase 2 clinical trials for Ebola, "**being the result of 'an expert consultation to assess the state of the art work to test and eventually license candidate Ebola vaccines' in which 'more than 70 experts, including many from affected countries in West Africa... Ebola virus disease (experts), manufacturers, regulators from Africa, Europe and USA, those with expertise in vaccine science, clinical trials and clinical management of patients' took part. This panel considered and approved urgently carrying out clinical tests on humans of some candidate Ebola vaccines in the development pipeline, including Chimpanzee adenovirus serotype 3 (ChAd 3) by Glaxo Smith Kline and others and Recombinant vesicular stomatitis virus **(rVSV)** vaccine by a consortium involving Canadian Public Health plus others."[2]

In normal circumstances, a clinical trial of a biomedical product must pass through several phases focalized progressively on safety, efficacy, dosage, comparison with other standard interventions, monitoring of effectiveness as well as adverse effects associated with widespread use, over many years involving thousands of participants. But, in this case, given the urgency of the situation, it was decided to test the candidate molecule for safety and ability to generate appropriate antibodies in a few hundred volunteers and to proceed from there directly to use the intervention in the affected countries by January 2015. "This was a highly ambitious project, maybe consistent with the challenge at hand. But it was ethically highly controversial. The Ebola virus epidemic (EVE) as distinguished from the Ebola virus disease (EVD) as such was still raging unabated and threatening to migrate from its epicenter

[1] See www.gobata.com "Ebola Epidemic: the WHO gets it right, then wrong" October 09, 2014.

[2] See www.gobata.com "WHO DONE IT AGAIN!" September 07, 2015.

in West Africa to other regions of the world. All reports coming out from West Africa at the time described an overwhelmingly desperate and chaotic situation. How could anybody go there with an aim and intention, let alone with a clinical research project, whose immediate purpose was anything other than containing the spread of the epidemic and helping to save the lives of those in imminent danger of death? How could one go about asking for, let alone obtaining, the informed consent of participants in such a research project especially when extreme panic would predictably be the major driving force for participation?"[3]

If we recall the infamous TROVAN trial by Pfizer in Kano, Northern Nigeria, in 1996, the ethical issue was not that an experimental molecule should not have been tested on children but rather that Pfizer acted in an opportunistically exploitative manner while a meningitis epidemic was ravaging children and, more to that, without following proper informed consent and ethical approval procedures (Ezeome and Simon 2010).

In the case of the Ebola experimental intervention, "it is evident that, in that situation, any attempted testing of an investigative substance would be up against an insurmountable therapeutic misconception and illusion on the part of desperate parents and guardians. Besides, one of the proposed candidate Ebola vaccines to be tested belonged to a powerful pharmaceutical company with a reputation for controversial drug trials involving a legion of unethical practices. Also, no mention was made in the WHO statement of post-trial access to any successful vaccine or treatment that might eventually result from the trial, from which it could be deduced, in the light of past experience, that whatever vaccine or medicine resulted from the trials, it would be priced beyond the means of those who had helped to make it possible."[4]

With regard to using hopeful but unproven interventions in desperate attempt to save lives, the WHO was evidently on the side of the ethically defensible but, in the case of giving its approbation for clinically testing unproven substances during a deadly epidemic, it was as evidently threading on controversial grounds.

If clinical tests on any candidate vaccine or medicine for Ebola were to be carried out, after the epidemic had subsided or been brought under reasonable control, the following procedures at least would seem ethically recommendable:

1. Let the Phase 1 and 2 of such trials (expedited or not) be carried out on well-informed volunteers from amongst research scientists, members of ethics review committees, medical personnel including doctors, nurses, laboratory technicians etc., personnel of pharmaceutical companies, civil servants especially in the Ministries of Health and Scientific Research, University teachers, government ministers, members of parliament, experts in all domains. Such tests for the initial two phases of the trial could not hope to last less than 12–18 months. For, to take such a putative experimental substance which has previously only been tested in non-human animals requires appropriate caution. One cannot start

[3] ibid.

[4] ibid.

celebrating safety, let alone efficacy, only a couple of weeks after surviving the test and not contracting the Ebola virus whose incubation period is said to be 3 weeks. There is need to observe possible effects for at least a couple of months.
2. Phase 3 and 4 could then go "straight into very vulnerable people in African countries" as envisaged by the WHO and its expert consultants, while every effort is made to avoid exploiting the desperately poor, illiterate or ill who have been the guinea pigs of Allopathic medical research, the unacknowledged heroes/heroines of the great advancement of scientific Western medicine in the past century.[5]

By the end of July 2015, the very prestigious journal *The Lancet* (www.thelancent.com) made an exciting publication for all stakeholders of EVD. Entitled "Efficacy and effectiveness of an rVSV-vectored vaccine expressing Ebola surface glycoprotein: interim results from the Guinea ring vaccination cluster-randomised trial (Henao-Restrepo et al. 2015)", whose copyright was attributed to the WHO, this publication was announced and advertised in both the print and electronic media in exaggerated terms quite unusual within the scientific field. The results of the clinical study were described as: "spectacular", "first time ever", "100% effective", "game changer" (Farar 2015). In fact the "ring vaccination" design used in Guinea, whereby a network of people confirmed or suspected to have Ebola are administered the vaccine, has obvious limitations. Incidentally, this particular vaccine has recently caused a number of adverse events in phase 1 developed world participants, leading to suspension by the WHO of pre-qualification and licensing procedures until further safety trials are conducted.

"The "successful" molecule, hurriedly tested on Africans in Guinea, a country ravaged by civil war and epidemics, had originally not been developed or prepared against the Ebola virus but rather as an anti-bioterrorism product for North Americans, which had been subjected to non-human animal tests but not yet human tests. The following preliminary questions thus naturally arise:

1. Was the WHO statement on clinical trials for Ebola of September 2014 tailor-made to ensure tests in humans of this particular candidate vaccine?
2. Was this not an opportunistic trial reminiscent of the Trovan trials in northern Nigeria in 1996?
3. As an agency of the United Nations with oversight for global health, is it right for the WHO itself to engage directly in commercial drug discovery, development and clinical tests, while at the same time issuing guidelines and directives on how these should properly and ethically be done?
4. Is the spectacular success of any candidate vaccine a justification of any ethical lapses that might have occurred in the process of testing it?"[6]

Hindsight and retrospection would seem to render plausible the impression that the actions and releases of the WHO during the Ebola epidemic were anticipatory

[5] ibid.

[6] ibid.

and calculated to render inevitable the testing of the candidate Ebola vaccine that it ended up testing. The spectacular success of the test might becloud its essentially opportunistic and exploitative nature reminiscent of the 1996 TROVAN trials in northern Nigeria, but a good end can never justify ethically questionable means. By its very nature and global functions, it seems to us inadvisable for the WHO directly to be leading or taking part in commercial drug discovery. The WHO ought to stay above every possible suspicion.

## 10.3 The Zika Epidemic

Similar to the Ebola virus, the Zika virus is an emerging infectious disease. It takes its name from the Zika forest of Uganda where it was originally discovered in rhesus monkeys in 1947 (Bearcroft 1954) and later diagnosed in a young lady from Afikpo, South-eastern Nigeria in 1954 (Macnamara 1954). Ever since, sporadic outbreaks of Zika viral infection have occured in various parts of Africa and Asia. The current geographical spread of Zika outbreaks started in 2007 when it was reported in Pacific Island and Yap Island in 2013. Although Zika virus is known to share the similar epidemiology, clinical presentation and transmission route with chikungunya and dengue fever and vectored exactly in the same manner as yellow fever through the infected bite of an *Aedesaegypti* mosquito, Zika causes a milder illness.

In the first quarter of 2015, Zika virus was suspected to cause episodes of fever and rash in several parts of Brazil. By December 2015, Brazilian health authorities lost count of cases of Zika virus infection and the epidemic extended its tentacles to neighbouring countries and coast of Africa in Cape Verde and Guinea Bissau where more than 8000 suspected cases were reported. Posing considerable concern was the causal association of the Zika virus infection with microcephaly (a birth defect characterized by poor brain development) and other neurologic disorders in babies born to infected pregnant women.

Similar to delayed response experienced during the last Ebola outbreak in West Africa, it was not until after a year of continuous devastating effects of Zika outbreak, precisely on 1 February 2016, that an International Health Regulations (IHR 2005) Emergency Committee convened a meeting, and WHO declared Zika virus as a Public Health Emergency of International Concern. This declaration was quickly followed by a launch of global Strategic Response Framework and Joint Operations Plan to guide the international response to the cluster of microcephaly and other neurological complications that appeared to be linked to Zika virus infection. The strategy was underpinned by mobilization and coordination of partners to support affected and at-risk countries across three core areas: surveillance, response and research.

WHO's Regional Office for the Americas (AMRO)/Pan American Health Organization (PAHO) in conjunction with Global Outbreak Alert and Response Network (GOARN) supported Ministries of Health of affected countries to strengthen detection of Zika virus through rapid reporting and laboratory testing. The rescue team performed extensive assessment of the unprecedented number of microcephaly cases and their possible association with Zika virus infection and provided guidance on surveillance, disease control measures and epidemiological research to the health authorities. WHO subsequently published 16 guidance documents covering all aspects of the response and translated these documents into several relevant languages (http://www.who.int/csr/resources/publications/zika/en/). The global response, albeit tardy, succeeded in stemming the tide of the Zika virus infection and its associated complications.

Given the central role played by WHO in maintaining countries of the world in a state of optimal health, it is amazing to note that WHO response is usually very slow and comes very late when epidemic outbreaks would have claimed several lives which could have been saved by timely and prompt interventions. Prominent amongst reasons cited for the institutional slow response are gaps in funding (WHO 2016). This hampers the WHO efforts to play a leading role in facilitating the development of research agendas that address vital questions that must be answered to respond to an outbreak such as that of Zika virus. WHO usually utilizes its authority to convene meetings of large cohorts of experts in working groups to: produce guidance documents, set research priorities, and advice on surveillance and response strategies. As data are the basis for public health research and action, and rapid data sharing is critical during an unfolding health emergency, it takes a substantial amount of time to generate data which can be shared to allow open and early access to Zika-related research information that could shape the control of the outbreak (WHO 2016).

In view of the aforementioned challenges impeding WHO from rising promptly to respond appropriately to epidemic outbreaks, we suggest that standing committees (or working groups) on epidemic responses should be empowered to engage relevant stakeholders during the period when there is no outbreak to formulate appropriate policies that can be quickly implemented when epidemics rear their ugly heads. For example, vaccine manufacturers are usually discouraged investing funds in research and development for emerging infections such as Ebola and Zika viruses because they are convinced that they would not be able to re-coup their investments. No wonder, sporadic outbreaks of Ebola and Zika viruses have been occurring for decades without consideration for developing or evaluating vaccines that may effectively prevent or control the diseases. WHO may adopt ‘pull’ and ‘push’ method of incentives for research and development where “push” funding policies aim to incentivize industry by reducing industry’s costs during the conduct of research and development stages, whereas “pull” mechanisms create incentives for private sector engagement by creating viable market demand. Push mechanisms essentially pay for “effort” on the part of researchers, by underwriting the cost of that effort, while pull mechanisms pay for “results” (Cheri and Kyle 2009).

Similarly, ‘pull’ and ‘push’ model of human behaviour can be used in conjunction with community engagement processes to shape the research landscape such that communities are ‘pulled’ to genuinely support and participate in research involved in the evaluation of innovative tools such as vaccines during the time when there is no epidemic outbreaks; the outcomes of which can be rapidly deployed as control strategies when epidemic outbreaks occur.

## 10.4 Appraisal and Conclusion

Human well-being and flourishing are largely contingent on human health. The WHO, as the organization concerned with human health as a state of complete physical and mental well-being at the global level, is indisputably the foremost arm of the United Nations Organization, the only body in the world that can pretend to be charged with global governance. In our contemporary world, the rapid progress in medical science and medical technologies has been matched by the emergence and spread of deadly infectious diseases not experienced in the past. The WHO is thus frequently saddled with global health emergency situations requiring prompt appraisal, urgent advice and action. This is an extremely important role given that deadly emerging diseases can kill thousands of people within days and spread rapidly around the globe because of the efficiency and speed of human loco-motion around the world.

In this situation, our recommendations are that the WHO should stay focused and proactively prepared, remain clearly independent and objective in relation to all other stake holders, including national governments, pharmaceutical companies, academic researchers, patient organizations, etc., and refrain from itself conducting or sponsoring commercially valuable medical research. This would assure that it avoids conflict of interest or favouritism and can stand up robustly to the pressures of lobbyists, powerful stakeholders, and for-profit actors. It also needs to dilute as much as possible its understandably Eurocentric and Allopathic medicine perspectives with the genuine perspectives of other cultures from around the globe who also need to be more equally represented in the world body. That way, it would have a more holistic and wholesome view which would enhance its moral authority and command the respect and obedience of all other stakeholders in the health domain all over the world.

## References

Bearcroft, W. G. C. (1954). Zika virus infection experimentally induced in a human volunteer. *Transaction of the Royal Society of Tropical Medicine and Hygiene., 50*(5), 442–447.

Cheri, G., & Kyle, M. (2009). Comparative advantages of push and pull incentives for technology development: Lessons for neglected disease technology development. *Global Forum Update on Research for Health, 6*, 147–151.

Emanuel, E., et al. (Eds.). (2003). *Ethical and regulatory aspects of clinical research: Readings and commentary*. Baltimore/London: The Johns Hopkins University Press.

Ezeome, E. R., & Simon, C. (2010). Ethical problems in conducting research in acute epidemics: The Pfizer meningitis study in Nigeriaas an illustration. *Developing World Bioethics, 10*(1), 1–10.

Farar, J. (2015). *The Ebola vaccine we dared to dream of is here*. Available online: Accessed 14 March 2017.

Henao-Restrepo, et al. (2015). Efficacy and effectiveness of an rVSV-vectored vaccine expressing Ebola surface glycoprotein: Interim results from the Guinea ring vaccination cluster-randomised trial. *The Lancet, 386*(999), 857–866.

MacNamara, F. N. (1954). Zika virus: A report on three cases of human infection during an epidemic of jaundice in Nigeria. *Transaction of the Royal of Society Tropical Medicine and Hygiene, 48*, 139–145.

WHO. (2016). *Zika virus outbreak global response: Interim report*. Available online: Accessed 6 March 2017.

# Chapter 11
# Disease Outbreaks in Africa and the Response of African Governments

**Oyewale Tomori**

## 11.1 Historical Perspectives

One of the earliest records of disease outbreak in Africa dates back to the period 165–180 AD, when an unknown disease with symptoms similar to smallpox occurred in northern Africa (UMMC 1999). This was followed by plague disease which ravaged human populations from 746 to 747 AD. According to Alchon (2003), the plague is caused by a bacterium, *Yersinia pestis*. Humans can get the plague following a bite by a rodent flea that is a carrier of the bacterium. Alternatively they could be infected by handling an animal that is infected with it. Plague continued to ravage human populations up to the early nineteenth century, when the discovery and use of modern antibiotics brought the disease under control. However, human plague infections still occur significantly in parts of Africa and Asia (CDC 2017). The end of the nineteenth century and the beginning of the twentieth century saw the appearance of the influenza disease. Particularly severe were the global influenza pandemics of 1889–1890 and 1918–1920, during which one million and 75 million people, respectively, died. (Great Britain Local Government Board 1893; Patterson and Pyle 1991). Less severe influenza pandemics occurred between 1957 and 1958 (Asian flu, with two million deaths), and between 1957 and 1958 (Hong Kong flu, with 1million deaths) (Paul 2008).

O. Tomori (✉)
Nigerian Academy of Science, University of Lagos, Lagos, Nigeria



G. B. Tangwa et al. (eds.), *Socio-cultural Dimensions of Emerging Infectious Diseases in Africa*, https://doi.org/10.1007/978-3-030-17474-3_11

### 11.1.1 Cholera

Cholera that has been responsible for significant high morbidity and mortality throughout human history (Hays 2005). Millions of people died during the first cholera pandemic from 1816 to 1826, and seventh cholera pandemics which occurred in 1975. Cholera remains a disease of public health concern especially in Africa and Asia, with an on-going massive cholera epidemic in Yemen since 2016 (WHO 2017a).

### 11.1.2 Yellow Fever

Yellow Fever (YF) is a mosquito-borne virus disease, with an incubation period of 3–7 days, and an initial malaria-like acute onset. The disease runs a mild to fatal course, with either remission in 4–5 days or, death within 7–10 days (WHO 2016a). The severe disease is characterised by hepato-renal and neurotropic manifestations with or without haemorrhage. Mortality can be as high as 20–50% in hepato-renal disease. It is believed that YF originated in Africa since 3000 BC (CDC 2017). Through the slave trade (1526–1687), the disease was introduced into the Americas (Haddow 2012). Maya manuscripts dating back to 1648 contain the description of a disease with symptoms similar to yellow fever. Severe YF epidemics were reported to have occurred in two waves in the Americas. The first wave, from 1668 to 1699, swept through New York, Boston and Charleston. The second wave which ran from 1793 to 1878 occurred in Philadelphia, Savannah, New Orleans, Norfolk, Texas. Louisiana and Mississippi. The disease was introduced to Europe between 1700 and 1730; first in Spain and subsequently in the French and English sea ports. The first documented report of YF in Africa was in 1768 in St. Louis, Senegal. Outbreaks of the disease were subsequently reported across West Africa from Fernando Po to the Gambia between 1842 and 1878. In 1930, two YF vaccines were discovered and used in mass vaccination exercises between 1934 and 1953 to control outbreaks In West Africa (Tomori 2004; WHO 2016a). It was not until 1948 that the World Health Organization (WHO) commenced the official reporting of YF outbreaks (Fig. 11.1a, Tomori 2015b). However following attainment of independence by many of the West African countries, mass YF campaigns were stopped and the disease re-emerged with reports of major outbreaks between 1960 and 1990 in West Africa and as far east as Ethiopia (Vainio and Cutts 1998; Garske et al. 2014). Further spread of the disease was reported with outbreaks in Central and East Africa between 1990 and 2003 (Fig. 11.1b; Tomori 2015b). Following the introduction by the WHO, of an YF control strategy in West Africa, YF outbreaks escalated in Central and East Africa with reduced incidence in West Africa (WHO 2010). The YF control strategy used a three prong approach – a preventive mass campaign, introduction of YF vaccine into the routine immunization programme and an improved surveillance system for rapid YF outbreak detection. Consequently, the period 2008–2014, coincided with a definite shift of YF outbreaks to Central and

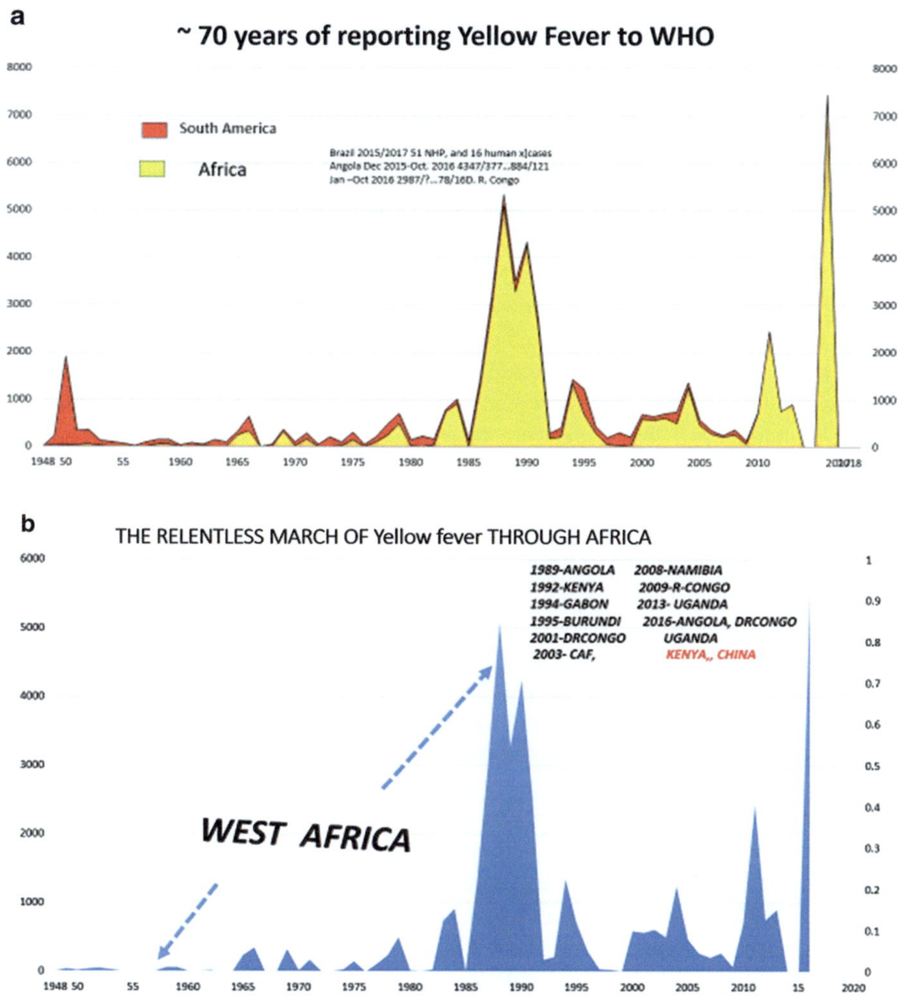


**Fig. 11.1** (**a**) Seventy years of reporting yellow fever outbreaks to the World Health Organization. (**b**) Shift of yellow fever Oubreaks from west to east and central Africa. (Tomori 2015b)

East Africa. In 2016, a severe urban YF outbreak which began in Luanda, Angola, later spread to the Democratic Republic of Congo, with infection and self-limiting exportation to China, Kenya and Mauritania (WHO 2017b).

### *11.1.3 Lassa Fever*

Lassa fever is endemic in many countries in West Africa including: The Republic Benin, Ghana, Guinea, Liberia, Mali, Sierra Leone, and Nigeria (CDC 2015). Lassa fever is an acute viral haemorrhagic illness and the causative agent, the Lassa virus, is transmitted to humans through contact with food or other household items that have been contaminated with the urine or faeces of a rodent that is infected with the virus. There is also the possibility Person-to-person and laboratory transmission especially in hospitals that do not have adequate infection prevention and control measures The incubation period of the disease ranges from 7 to 21 day. Case-fatality rate for Lassa fever is 1% (Richmond and Baglole 2003), whilst observed case-fatality rate among patients hospitalized with severe Lassa fever is approximately 15%.

Between 1969, when the disease was first discovered in Nigeria, and 2000, Lassa fever disease in Nigeria was limited to a few states in northern Nigeria occurring usually during the dry season. However, from 2001, the disease was reported in 10–21 of the 36 states in Nigeria and occurring throughout the year. For example, in 2016, there were over 1000 cases and 120 deaths reported from 28 states. In 2017 up to week 46, 19 States have reported 985 suspected cases and 126 deaths (NCDC 2017a), whereas in 1989, there were cases and deaths in 2 states, 29 cases and 12 deaths associated with nosocomial infections in a hospital Fisher-Hoch et al. (1995).

### *11.1.4 Ebola Virus Disease (EVD)*

Ebola virus disease (EVD), previously known as Ebola haemorrhagic fever, is a severe, often fatal illness in humans (CDC 2017b). The average case fatality rate for EVD is around 50% with case fatality rates often varying from 25% to 90% (WHO 2018). The Ebola virus is transmitted to humans via wild animals and spreads in the human population through human-to-human transmission. Early supportive care with rehydration and treatment of symptoms has the potential to improve survival. Till date, there is no licensed proven treatment for EVD but there exist a range of blood, immunological and drug therapies that are currently are under development. The first EVD outbreaks occurred in 1976 in remote villages in the Democratic Republic of Congo and Sudan and 602 cases and 431 deaths were recorded (Table 11.1) (CDC 2017c). Between 1976 and 2012, there were 22 EVD outbreaks in Africa, with 17,851 cases and 1159 deaths reported in 22 countries (DR Congo (5), Uganda (5) Congo (4), Gabon (4), Sudan (2), RSA (1) and CIV (1). The most severe and devastating epidemic of EVD occurred in West Africa (from 2014 to 2015. A total of 28,639 cases and 11,322 deaths were recorded in the 6 affected countries (CDC 2017c) – Guinea (3811 cases and 2543 deaths), Sierra Leone (14,214 cases and 3956 deaths), Liberia (10,675 cases and 4809 deaths), Nigeria (20 cases and 8 deaths), Mali (8 cases and 6 deaths) and Senegal (1 case and 0 death). Seven additional cases with one death, were exported to the USA (4 cases and 1 death) and one case each with no death in Spain, UK and Italy. An EVD outbreak in 2014, independent of the West African outbreaks, occurred in the DRC with 66 cases and 49 deaths. Eight cases and 4 deaths were recorded in the eighth EVD outbreak in DRC which occurred between May and July 2017 (CDC 2017c). The ninth EVD outbreak in the Democratic Republic of the Congo, started in April 2018 in the Bikoro Health Zone. Since the onset (on 4 April 2018), of the recent

**Table 11.1** Ebola virus disease 1976–2017[a, b]

| Year | Country | Ebola virus species | Cases | Deaths | Case fatality |
|---|---|---|---|---|---|
| April-May 2018 | Democratic Republic of the Congo | Zaire | 54 | 25 | 46.3 |
| May – July 2017 | Democratic Republic of the Congo | Zaire | 8 | 4 | 50% |
| 2015 | Italy | Zaire | 1 | 0 | 0% |
| 2014 | DRC | Zaire | 66 | 49 | 74% |
| 2014 | Spain | Zaire | 1 | 0 | 0% |
| 2014 | UK | Zaire | 1 | 0 | 0% |
| 2014 | USA | Zaire | 4 | 1 | 25% |
| 2014 | Senegal | Zaire | 1 | 0 | 0% |
| 2014 | Mali | Zaire | 8 | 6 | 75% |
| 2014 | Nigeria | Zaire | 20 | 8 | 40% |
| 2014–2016 | Sierra Leone | Zaire | 14124[a] | 3956[a] | 28% |
| 2014–2016 | Liberia | Zaire | 10675[a] | 4809[a] | 45% |
| 2014–2016 | Guinea | Zaire | 3811[a] | 2543[a] | 67% |
| 2012 | Democratic Republic of Congo | Bundibugyo | 57 | 29 | 51% |
| 2012 | Uganda | Sudan | 7 | 4 | 57% |
| 2012 | Uganda | Sudan | 24 | 17 | 71% |
| 2011 | Uganda | Sudan | 1 | 1 | 100% |
| 2008 | Democratic Republic of Congo | Zaire | 32 | 14 | 44% |
| 2007 | Uganda | Bundibugyo | 149 | 37 | 25% |
| 2007 | Democratic Republic of Congo | Zaire | 264 | 187 | 71% |
| 2005 | Congo | Zaire | 12 | 10 | 83% |
| 2004 | Sudan | Sudan | 17 | 7 | 41% |
| 2003 (Nov–Dec) | Congo | Zaire | 35 | 29 | 83% |
| 2003 (Jan–Apr) | Congo | Zaire | 143 | 128 | 90% |
| 2001–2002 | Congo | Zaire | 59 | 44 | 75% |
| 2001–2002 | Gabon | Zaire | 65 | 53 | 82% |
| 2000 | Uganda | Sudan | 425 | 224 | 53% |
| 1996 | South Africa (ex-Gabon) | Zaire | 1 | 1 | 100% |
| 1996 (Jul–Dec) | Gabon | Zaire | 60 | 45 | 75% |
| 1996 (Jan–Apr) | Gabon | Zaire | 31 | 21 | 68% |
| 1995 | Democratic Republic of Congo | Zaire | 315 | 254 | 81% |
| 1994 | Côte d'Ivoire | Taï Forest | 1 | 0 | 0% |
| 1994 | Gabon | Zaire | 52 | 31 | 60% |

(continued)

**Table 11.1** (continued)

| Year | Country | Ebola virus species | Cases | Deaths | Case fatality |
|---|---|---|---|---|---|
| 1979 | Sudan | Sudan | 34 | 22 | 65% |
| 1977 | Democratic Republic of Congo | Zaire | 1 | 1 | 100% |
| 1976 | Sudan | Sudan | 284 | 151 | 53% |
| 1976 | Democratic Republic of Congo | Zaire | 318 | 280 | 88% |

There is an ongoing epidemic of Ebola, the tenth outbreak in DR Congo since 1976. The outbreak was declared on 1 August 2018 in North Kivu. As of 14 April 2019, a total of 1264 EVD cases, including 1198 confirmed and 66 probable cases, were reported. A total of 814 deaths were reported (overall case fatality ratio 64%), including 748 deaths among confirmed cases
Numbers as of May 272,018
[a]CDC (2017c)
[b]WHO (2019)

outbreak, 50 confirmed or probable EVD cases and 25 deaths (giving a case fatality rate 50.0%) have been reported. (WHO 2018).

Effective control of an EVD outbreak would require a holistic approach involving but not limited to interventions such as: case management; infection prevention and control practices; surveillance and contact tracing; a good laboratory service; safe burial practices; and social mobilisation. Also, history shows that the role of community engagement in the management of EVD outbreaks cannot be overemphasised. These measures, however, often come up against countervailing socio-cultural beliefs, rituals and practices, such as those connected with death, burial, afterlife and welfare of the community (WHO 2018).

A recent WHO-led clinical trial aimed at testing a potential vaccine against EVD saw the participation reported that the candidate vaccine was highly protective against the Ebola virus (WHO 2017c). This vaccine is yet to receive regulatory approval. However, there is a commitment to conduct emergency ring vaccinations in the unfortunate event of an EVD outbreak in selected African countries including: the Democratic Republic of Congo; Sierra Leone; Liberia; Gabon; Guinea Bissau; the Republic of Guinea; Ivory Coast; Mali; Niger; Nigeria; Senegal; South Sudan; and Uganda. These emergency ring vaccinations will be carried out under the umbrella of the Expanded Access/Compassionate use. A ring EVD vaccination exercise was launched in affected Health Zones of the 2018 EVD outbreak in the DRC (WHO 2018). The exercise targeted health professionals, persons who have been in contact with confirmed EVD cases, as well as contacts of these contacts (Ibid).

### *11.1.5 Cerebrospinal Meningitis*

Cerebrospinal meningitis is a bacterial disease caused by several microorganisms; among which is, *Neisseria Meningitides* (Nm), the most common cause of bacterial meningitis. The disease is highly contagious and often occurs as seasonal epidemics

**Table 11.2** Cerebrospinal meningitis in Africa 1949–2017

| Year | Countries or Country | Cases | Deaths |
|---|---|---|---|
| 1949 | Nigeria | 49,081 | 7757 |
| 1950 | Nigeria | 56,185 | 7060 |
| 1995–2004 | 19 countries | 700,000 | 60,000 |
| 1996 | 20 countries | 250,000 | 25,000 |
| | Nigeria | 109,500 | 11,717 |
| 2012 | Nigeria | 1206 | 74 |
| 2013 | Nigeria | 871 | 47 |
| 2014 | 19 countries | 14,317 | 1304 |
| | Nigeria | 1176 | 81 |
| 2015 | 19 countries | 21,649 | 1577 |
| | Nigeria | 2711 | 131 |
| 2016 | 20 countries | 18,178 | 1576 |
| | Nigeria | 822 | 33 |
| 2017 | Nigeria | 14,005 | 1114 |

with the greatest burden being in in the meningitis belt of sub-Saharan Africa (WHO 2017d). In the meningitis belt, the highest morbidity due to cerebral meningitis is often recorded during the dry season, as the climatic and living conditions (e.g. crowding) as well as population movements tend to favour increased disease transmission. Between 1995 and 2004, outbreaks in the meningitis belt (Table 11.2) have resulted in close to 700,000 cases and 60,000 deaths (WHO 2005, 2014, 2015, 2016b, 2017d; Horn 1951; Mohammed et al. 2000; NCDC 2013, 2014, 2015, 2016a, b, 2017b). The largest recorded outbreak, in 1996, caused 250,000 cases and almost 25,000 deaths, with Nigeria alone reporting 109, 500 cases and 11,717 deaths (Mohammed et al. 2000). With the introduction, in 2010, of the Men-A conjugate vaccine (MenAfrivac) for mass preventive immunization campaigns in the meningitis belt, the occurrence of the disease has declined significantly (SAGE 2014). However, the risk of other types of Nm persists, with a recent outbreak in Nigeria, recording 14,005 cases and 1114 deaths (NCDC 2017b).

### *11.1.6 Other Disease Outbreaks*

Apart from the above listed diseases, Africa is home to other outbreaks of diseases, such as cholera, plague, Dengue haemorrhagic fever and Typhoid. The WHO African Region (AFRO) publishes a weekly bulletin on disease outbreaks and other emergencies in African countries. The edition of the bulletin for week 50 (10–15 December 2017) reports 2 new events (Fig. 11.2), 47 ongoing events, 41 disease outbreaks and 8 humanitarian crises (WHO-AFRO 2017a, b). On the cholera outbreaks in Zambia and Tanzania, the WHO AFRO weekly bulletin reports that "*…the incidence of cholera in Zambia is rapidly increasing, particularly in Lusaka District where transmission is intense. In Tanzania, the cholera outbreak is spreading to new*

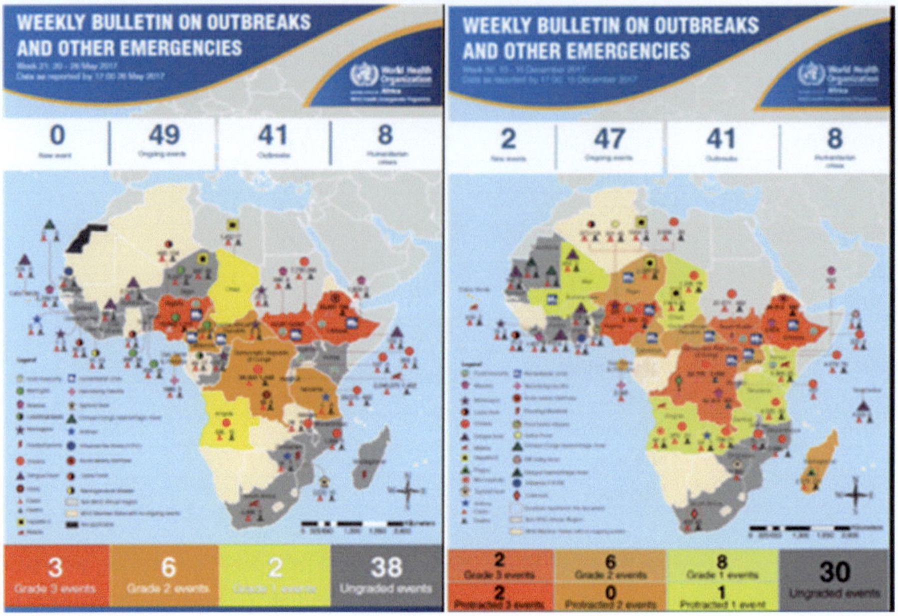


**Fig. 11.2** Outbreak and emergency situation in Africa. Left- Week 21 (20–26 May 2017) and Right -Week 50 (10–15 December 2017). (WHO-AFRO 2017a)

*areas, including Dar es Salam and Ruvuma Region. Cholera case fatality rates have remained very high in both countries, as well as in the Democratic Republic of the Congo, ranging from 3–5% (exceeding the 1% mark set by WHO)"* (ibid). The bulletin declares that national authorities are failing in their duties and recommends that *"the ongoing cholera outbreaks in Zambia and Tanzania require specific attention from the national authorities and partners"* (ibid). Meanwhile, response efforts to the cholera outbreak in the Democratic Republic of the Congo need to be scaled up and maintained. On the continuing deterioration of the *"humanitarian crisis in the Democratic Republic of the Congo, the bulletin joins UNICEF in warning that "more than 400 000 severely malnourished children could die within months unless emergency interventions are undertaken"* (ibid).

In Nigeria, the WHO is monitoring outbreaks of Lassa Fever, Yellow Fever, Cholera, Monkey pox, as part of the humanitarian crises caused by the *"protracted conflict which has resulted in widespread population displacement, restricted access to basic social services, including healthcare and protection needs, and a deepening humanitarian crisis"* (WHO-AFRO 2017a, b). Furthermore, in 2017, UNICEF estimates that about 400,000 children in north-east Nigeria are at risk of severe acute malnutrition and without treatment, it is estimated that one in five of those children are likely to die (Vittozzi 2017). The UNICEF report concluded that *the malnutrition situation in northeast Nigeria remains critical. The number of cases of children suffering from Severe Acute Malnutrition is extremely high, with the crisis in Borno state most acute. In 2016, working with partners, UNICEF treated 160,000 children suffering from Severe Acute Malnutrition in Borno, Yobe and Adamawa states. Although UNICEF has made significant progress in reaching children and their families with healthcare, treatment for malnutrition, safe water, sanitation and hygiene services, education and child protection, a persistent lack of funding continues to hamper the response effort* (Vittozzi 2017).

The state of affairs presented in the WHO AFRO bulletin for week 50 of 2017 is not an isolated event. It is a description of the day to day, common and regular endemic state of disease outbreaks and humanitarian disasters occurring all over Africa. How did Africa get to this miserable, deplorable, poor and wretched state of health? How come there is this pervading powerlessness and inability to control even the commonest diseases? It is an indictment of national authorities in Africa, who in perpetual fits of misplaced priorities, divert national resources to executing projects which fail to provide those basic essentials and facilities needed to provide better health and better protection for their citizens from the scourge of preventable and controllable disease outbreaks. Year in, year out, African countries lurch and stumble in dazed stupor as Ebola decimates sections of our populations, leaving survivors to the pain, agony and eventual annihilation by any of cholera, Lassa fever, malaria and numerous other diseases that have become contributors to the underdevelopment of African states. We must appreciate that the long history of poor governance in many independent Africa countries is the root cause of the deplorable state of humanitarian disasters arising from disease outbreaks.

## 11.2 Has Africa Always Been Unable to Take Care of Her Health and Incapable of Mounting effective Response for Combating Disease Outbreaks?

If Africa was ever able, it must have been only during the period when many African countries were under colonial subjugation/rule. For close to 50 years or more, many African countries have ostensibly operated as independent nations, free from colonial rule. Yet with every disease outbreak, African countries surrender their independence to donors and partners, as they seek assistance and aid to control even common disease outbreaks. Since 1976, when EVD was first discovered in Africa, and before the West African outbreak, there have been 24 other outbreaks, with a total of 2900 cases and 1583 deaths (CDC 2017a). Despite the number of EVD outbreaks in Africa, the West African outbreak, in terms of morbidity and mortality, was ten times worse that all of the EVD outbreaks reported in Africa since 1976. When the West African EVD humanitarian disaster was declared over by the WHO, there were 28,712 cases and 11,372 deaths (CDC 2017c). Several reasons were given for Africa's inability to learn from the lessons of the past and her inability to prevent repeats of histories of devastating disease outbreaks. According to Tomori (2015a, b), some of the reasons include:

- Unreliable disease surveillance system in most countries resulting in failure of early detection of outbreaks;
- Official national and community denial of the occurrence of most epidemics;
- Fragile and weak heath systems in most African countries leading to limited capacity to manage and contain epidemics;
- Cultural practices that favour the spread of the disease;
- Easy and uncontrolled mass movement of people between rural areas and urban centres, and across national and international borders;
- An unashamed dependency on foreign assistance.

### *11.2.1 Capacity Building for National Ownership*

Africa has experienced no less than 24 episodes of EVD outbreaks, since the first outbreak was reported in 1976 (CDC 2017b). One would imagine that by now, African countries would have learned the lessons and develop their capacity and competence to deal with EVD or other disease outbreaks. However, and unsurprisingly, Africa has, for the past 41 years relied heavily on international aid and assistance to solve a majority of its health crisis (Tomori 2015a, b). Unfortunately, these long years of reliance on international aid to support the continent's response to disease outbreaks has not yielded the desired result on building human and infrastructural capacity in Africa to effectively respond to disease outbreaks. This is aptly illustrated in a diary entry (published) of a WHO expert who has been at the forefront of several outbreaks of EVD and other viral haemorrhagic fever in Africa. He writes *"We received the first emails on the Guinea event on Friday 14 March. During the weekend, I was travelling in the DRC for a training course on how to take blood samples in Ebola. It was a 3-day training course"* (Formenty 2015). It is almost heart-breaking to read that in 2014, African health care professionals need to travel out of their countries to receive training on *'how to take blood samples in Ebola'*. Although the DRC often provides technical assistance to other African countries during outbreaks of EVD Muyembe-Tamfum et al. (2012), by and large, Africa has relied on foreign assistance and aid to solve her disease outbreak problems, and failed to create an enabling and a conducive local environment for her human resource capacity to function effectively (Tomori 2015a, b).

Arguably, foreign aid, by its nature and character, be it for economic purposes or health research, always tend to benefit the donor country more than the recipient country. A Director of a UK funded research centre in Africa, wrote this piece in an annual report of the center: *"Perhaps the most important achievement of the Unit during the past five years has been the training of a group of dedicated scientists and clinicians who have gone on to establish their own highly successful groups elsewhere in the tropics and in the UK and who continue to maintain the high reputation of the UK in tropical medicine"* (Greenwood 1995). Unfortunately, this is not an isolated case in Africa. A cursory review of the activities of externally funded health research centres in Africa reveals that researchers of the donor countries tend to benefit more from research collaborations than their African counterparts (Adubifa 2004). Although the dynamics may be slowly changing, in many of the international conferences that I have attended and for which issues concerning diseases of African origin, and diseases endemic in Africa are being discussed, most, if not all, of the participating researchers and presenters are non-Africans. Equally, outbreak of emerging and re-emerging infectious diseases have become opportunities for researchers in high income and research intense countries to fine-tune their skills thereby enabling them to be at the forefront of solving Africa's health problems, and by extension, doing for Africa what African researchers should be doing for Africa (Tomori 2015a, b). When African researchers are engaged in these collaboration, they are assigned the role sample collectors and eventually end up as impotent contributors to the control of disease outbreaks in their own countries and globally (Tomori 2015a, b).

For Africa to be prepared to manage and contain future outbreaks of EVD, the current heavy reliance and nature of external aid and assistance for health research collaboration must change (ibid). Africa must reorganize her priorities, and invest in health research and research capacity strengthening. Also, African governments must create an environment that allows its researchers to function with some degree of relevance and independence. On the other hand, high income countries should consider relinquishing their dominance and control of global disease surveillance and establish research collaborations that are based on mutual appreciation and respect for all partners (Tomori 2014). If African countries and high income countries where to do the suggested, the chances of Africa adequately responding to outbreaks will be maximised (Tomori 2015a, b).

## 11.3 African Governments and People's Health

While governments and scientific communities in the high income countries often devote considerable resources to addressing emerging infectious diseases, the reverse is the case in the resource-constrained countries of Africa, despite the fact that the region is especially prone to outbreaks of the diseases. In 2001, African Heads of State signed the Abuja Declaration and where member states pledged to increase their health budgets to at least 15% of the their annual national budget OAU (2001). Ten years after the Abuja Declaration, the African Union reported that only six AU member states had met set benchmark (Olajide 2010). Following an assessment by the WHO, 15 years after the Commitment was made, it was concluded that *"Most African governments have increased the proportion of total public expenditure allocated to health in the early 2000s. The average level of per capita public spending on health rose from about US$70 in the early 2000s to more than US$160 in 2014. Domestic resources for health in Africa accounted for about 76 [per cent] in 2014, and external aid has increased from 13 [per cent] to 24 [per cent] of total health expenditure over the same period"* (WHO 2016c). However, the report also estimated that of every US$100 of State fund, only US$16 is allocated to health, of which less than US$4 goes to the right health services. It also observed that funding of the health sector is inconsistent and unpredictable *(ibid).*

Many African governments still ascribe their lack of adequate funding for public health activates to the rampant poverty in their countries. But a look at the recent operations of many African countries will suggest that the real culprits are corruption and prolonged misplaced priorities. *The AIDS and Rights Alliance for Southern Africa*, a regional network of non-governmental organizations, runs a campaign that draws attention to the spending choices of African governments (AIDS and Rights Alliance for Southern Africa 2014). The alliance reports that some African governments, would rather devote exorbitant sums of national spending to frivolous expenditures rather than allocate it to health, education, and other basic services. Some examples include $500,000 expenditure on a luxury car for the king of Swaziland; A 48 million dollar spending for a private presidential jet for Uganda; $27 million dollars for a bronze statue in Senegal (Walker 2010); and the proposed new city gate to Abuja, which is estimated would cost the government of Nigeria, the huge sum of 395 million dollars (Agbo 2013). None of these nations has met its 2001 commitment in the Abuja declaration.

In most African countries, implementation of disease surveillance systems for the early detection of emerging pathogens remains defective (Tomori 2014). A recent assessment of disease surveillance and response in Kaduna State, Nigeria, showed that approximately 38% of the state's health facilities in Kaduna had no standard case definition for priority diseases, 71% lacked access to a computer and printer, and 81% did not analyse the data collected in their health facilities (Abubakar et al. 2013). Poor surveillance and data management can increase the time between the beginning of an outbreak and the first reported case, thereby limiting response. African governments have the capacity to provide such basic services, yet corruption and misplaced priorities makes it almost impossible for them to provide such services. For example, the African Union estimates that corruption costs African economies about $150 billion each year. Undoubtedly, a minute fraction of that amount could provide many African countries with efficient disease surveillance systems (Tomori 2014). African countries will have to wake up from their slumber and dependency.

## 11.4 Way Forward

A short while before and immediately after the WHO declared that the EVD outbreak in West Africa had been contained, many agencies, governments, and institutions all from outside Africa had already put together resources to assess lessons learnt from the EVD outbreaks and to map out strategies in the unfortunate event of another epidemics (Bell et al. 2016). However, the reports from Africa where mainly related to misuse of EVD funds (Paye-Layleh 2015; Sahid 2015). This was at a time when international agencies and donor governments were being blamed for reacting too slowly and not providing enough donations to combat the EVD disaster (Nierle and Jochum 2014; Grépin 2015). The questions that come to mind are: Is Africa prepared for the next EVD epidemic? What lessons have African countries learnt from the 2014 to 2015 EVD outbreak? Will Africa still be helpless and totally dependent on international agencies for assistance to control the future epidemic, which will surely come? Will scientists and governments from high income countries continue to control the processes of global disease surveillance system without meaningfully engaging African countries? Of course, the answers of a right thinking pessimist would be "no" to the first two questions and "yes" to the last two. For the contrary to occur, Africa must accept that her self-imposed poverty status is not due to a lack of resources, but rather to their misuse, and that it can be reversed (Tomori 2015a, b). This requires purposeful leadership and rightly guided followership. African leaders must regard health as a human right and the citizens must demand this right from their governments. Without good governance, there will never be a purposeful and citizen oriented leadership. With poor governance, funds allocated for health, education and other development activities are likely to be wasted, yielding poor outcomes. In addition, aid funds are more likely to be sucked into the vortex of corruption along with local and national resources (Paye-Layleh 2015; Sahid JS 2015). Civil society, and other stakeholders, must be frontline advocates for the establishment and institutionalization of good governance. During the first annual African governance forum, Kofi Anan, former UN Secretary General, said: *'there is no single issue of greater importance to the economic and political future of Africa than good governance, and it must command the full and lasting attention of Africans"* (ECA 1997). The comment was made 20 years ago, and it is even more relevant today for the development and health of the people of Africa.

### *11.4.1 Purposeful Leadership*

African Governments must provide a conducive and enabling environment with adequate resources for African researchers working together under the One Health concept to focus on local processes of pathogen emergence. Pathogens emerge under widely varying environmental, demographic, and socioeconomic circumstances (Tomori 2014). A pathogen's ability to emerge or re-emerge depends on several factors including but not limited to genetic changes or adaptation in the pathogen; environmental conditions; land use patterns;, international trade patterns, the neglect of public health services, and bioterrorism (Daszak et al. 2012). These factors and conditions interact differently in different parts of the world and therefore, the first step toward preventing and controlling outbreaks of emerging and re-emerging diseases will be to gain a thorough understanding of local processes of pathogen emergence. Once such an understanding is gained then governments, institutions, and researchers and healthcare professionals in Africa would have to commit themselves to clearly defined and proactive roles in the fight against emerging and re-emerging infectious diseases.

### 11.4.2 African Health Researchers

The African researcher or scientist would have to evaluate the needs of the countries where they operate and direct their research activities towards issues that are relevant to their and can positively impact on the daily life of populations in their countries of operation (Tomori 2015a, b). African researchers must take on the extra roles of guide, teacher, mentor, and beacon to their society. Therein lies the true relevance of the African researcher. International aid will not build the capacity for such desired relevance; it would have to be funded and groomed with home-based resources and through governments with the right priorities (ibid).

### 11.4.3 National Governments

It is also essential for all African countries to take "ownership" of their national disease surveillance systems as well as prevention and control of epidemics. This will allow for effective country-specific response measures (Tomori 2014). This will entail making a genuine political commitment providing adequate resources both financial and human. Taking a proactive role in combating disease will also require that African governments: implement appropriate emergency response plans; coordinate collaborative interactions between human and veterinary health surveillance systems; build and sustain the capacity of local health personnel to respond to disease outbreaks; ensure private sector involvement and establish a multidisciplinary approach to disease control (Tomori 2014).

### 11.4.4 Global Health Collaborations

Making the world safer from emerging and re-emerging infectious diseases requires global collaboration (Tomori 2014). It will entail a global collaborative efforts to develop and implement policies, for pathogen control and spread. It will require the sharing of real-time surveillance information that could support the detection of zoonotic diseases in animal populations before they appear in human populations. Also the contributions of Science-based nongovernmental organizations should be harnessed. This is because some of these organisations have a wide geographic reach and could help provide comprehensive surveillance and response capabilities (Tomori 2014). The fight against emerging and re-emerging disease is a complex and difficult one and would require genuine commitment from the different global health actors.

## 11.5 Conclusion

African countries individually and collectively through the AU, the WHO African Region, and other international and regional groups, have by resolutions and agreements, focused actions and adopted measures for the promotion and protection of the health of Africans. The enthusiasm of African leaders (including Ministers of Health) for adopting resolutions and making declarations on good governance was far less than for health and health matters. Over the past 10 years, African leaders have, on the average, adopted four resolutions/declarations per year on health and less than one on good governance (African Union 2017; WHO Afro 2017b). The surfeit of health resolutions, demonstrating more political "whiff" than will and commitment has led to Africa's health indices remaining much below accepted and acceptable standards. The clear lesson is that the health of African citizens will continue to suffer in the absence of good governance.

On a final positive note, two survivors of the EVD outbreak in Sierra Leone Ebola have sued the Sierra Leone government over mismanaged funds (Reuters 2017). This is a step in the right direction and a demonstration of positive use of citizen power. Our governments must be held accountable for their negligence and failure especially on issues adversely affecting the health of the people. On reflection, it appears that some of our leaders, through poor governance, may have produced more severe and longer lasting devastation than have been caused by past disease epidemics in Africa.

## References

Abubakar, A. A., Sambo, M. N., Idris, S. H., Sabitu, K., & Nguku, P. (2013). Assessment of integrated disease surveillance and response strategy implementation in selected Local Government Areas of Kaduna state. *Annals of Nigerian Medicine, 7*(1), 14–19.

Adubifa, A. O. (2004). *An assessment of science and technology capacity building in sub-Saharan Africa* (Special Paper Series 19). Nairobi: African Technology Policy Studies Network (ATPS).

African Union. (2017). *OAU/AU treaties, conventions, protocols & charters*. https://au.int/en/treaties. Accessed 19 Sept 2017.

Agbo, C. (2013). *Nigeria: New Abuja city gate to gulp N64 billion*. http://allafrica.com/stories/201310150454.html. Accessed 21 Dec 2017.

AIDS and Rights Alliance for Southern Africa. (2014). *The right to health*. Available at: www.arasa.info/index.php/info/fact-sheets. Accessed 26 Jan 2019.

Alchon, S. A. (2003). *A pest in the land: New world epidemics in a global perspective* (p. 21). University of New Mexico Press. ISBN:0-8263-2871-7.

Bell, B. P., Damon, I. K., Jernigan, D. B., Kenyon, T. A., Nichol, S. T., O'Connor, J. P., & Tapperoet, J. W. (2016). Overview, control strategies, and lessons learned in the CDC response to the 2014–2016 Ebola epidemic. *MMWR Supplement, 65*(3), 4–11.

CDC. (2015). *Lassa fever.* https://www.cdc.gov/vhf/lassa. Accessed 19 Dec 2017.

CDC. (2017). *Plague*. https://www.cdc.gov/plague/. Accessed 19 Dec 2017.

CDC. (2017a). *Yellow fever timeline of activities*. https://www.cdc.gov/travel-training/local/HistoryEpidemiologyandVaccination/HistoryTimelineTranscript.pdf. Accessed 21 Dec 2017.

CDC. (2017b). *Ebola virus disease*. https://www.cdc.gov/vhf/ebola. Accessed 21 Dec 2017.

CDC. (2017c). *Outbreaks chronology- Ebola virus disease*. https://www.cdc.gov/vhf/ebola/outbreaks/history/chronology.html#modalIdString_outbreaks. Accessed 21 Dec 2017.

Daszak, P., Zambrana-Torrelio, C., Bogich, T. L., Fernandez, M., Epstein, J. H., Murray, K. A., & Hamilton, H. (2012). Interdisciplinary approaches to understanding disease emergence: The past, present, and future drivers of Nipah virus emergence. *PNAS, 110*(Suppl 1), 3681–3688.

Economic Commission for Africa. (1997). *ECA First African Governance Forum*. http://www.africa.upenn.edu/Urgent_Action/apic_72097.html. Accessed 19 Sept 2017.

Fisher-Hoch, S. P., Tomori, O., Nasidi, A., Perez-Oronoz, G. I., Fakile, Y., Hutwagner, L., & McCormick, J. B. (1995). Review of cases of nosocomial Lassa fever in Nigeria: The high price of poor medical practice. *British Medical Journal, 311*(7009), 857–859.

Formenty, P. (2015). *Ebola diaries: First signals–March 2014*. http://www.who.int/features/2015/ebola-diaries-formenty/en/. Accessed 19 Dec 2017.

Garske, T., Van Kerkhove, M. D., Yactayo, S., Ronveaux, O., Lewis, R. F., Staples, J. E., Perea, W., Ferguson, N. M., & Committee, Y. F. E. (2014). Yellow Fever in Africa: Estimating the Burden of Disease and Impact of Mass Vaccination from Outbreak and Serological Data. *PLoS Medicine, 11*(5), e1001638.

Great Britain Local Government Board. (1893). Further report and papers on epidemic influenza, 1889–92: With an introduction by the medical officer of the Local Government Board. H. M Stationery Office.

Greenwood, B. M. (1995). From the Director: Gambia Medical Research Council Unit; Annual Report for 1995.

Grépin, K. A. (2015). International donations to the Ebola virus outbreak: Too little, too late? *BMJ, 350*, h376.

Haddow, A. J. (2012). The Natural History of Yellow Fever in Africa. *Proceedings of the Royal Society of Edinburgh Section B: Biology, 70*(03), 191–227.

Hays J. N. (2005). *Epidemics and pandemics: Their impacts on human history* (pp. 513). Santa Barbara: ABC-CLIO.

Horn, D. W. (1951). The epidemic of cerebrospinal fever in the northern provinces of Nigeria, 1949–1950. *Journal Royal Sanitary Institute, 71*(5), 573–589.

Mohammed, I., Nasidi, A., Alkali, A. S., Garbati, M. A., Ajayi-Obe, E. K., Audu, K. A., Abdulmumini, U., & Suleiman Abdullahi, S. (2000). A severe epidemic of meningococcal meningitis in Nigeria May 2000. *Transactions of the Royal Society of Tropical Medicine and Hygiene, 94*(3), 265–270.

Muyembe-Tamfum, J. J., Mulangu, S., Masumu, J., Kayembe, J. M., Kemp, A., & Paweska, J. T. (2012). Ebola virus outbreaks in Africa: Past and present. *The Onderstepoort Journal of Veterinary Research, 79*, 6–13.

Nierle, T., & Jochum, B. (2014). *Ebola: The failures of the international outbreak response*. http://www.msf.org/article/ebola-failures-internationaloutbreak-response. Accessed 21 Dec 2017.

Nigeria Centre for Disease Control. (2013). Federal Ministry of Health–Weekly Epidemiological Report: 2:52.

Nigeria Centre for Disease Control. (2014). Federal Ministry of Health–Weekly Epidemiological Report: 4 (1).

Nigeria Centre for Disease Control. (2015). Federal Ministry of Health – Weekly Epidemiological Report. 4: 52.

Nigeria Centre for Disease Control. (2016a) Federal Ministry of Health – Weekly Epidemiological Report: 6:5.

Nigeria Centre for Disease Control. (2016b). Federal Ministry of Health Weekly Epidemiology Report: 6:49.

Nigeria Centre for Disease Control. (2017a). Federal Ministry of Health Lassa fever outbreak weekly Situation Report No. 46–December 1, 2017.

Nigeria Centre for Disease Control. (2017b). Federal Ministry of Health – Nigeria Meningitis Outbreak, situation as of week ending 28 April 2017.

OAU. (2001). *Abuja declaration on HIV/AIDS, tuberculosis and other related infectious diseases-OAU/SPS/ABUJA/3*. http://www.un.org/ga/aids/pdf/abuja_declaration.pdf. Accessed 19 Dec 2017.

Olajide, A. (2010). *Ten year review: Abuja Declaration on health financing in Africa*. http://www.who.int/pmnch/media/membernews/2011/20110329_abujadeclaration.pdf. Accessed 18 Dec2017.

Patterson, K. D., & Pyle, G. F. (1991). The geography and mortality of the 1918 influenza pandemic. *Bulletin of the History of Medicine, 65*(1), 4–21.

Paul W. E. (2008). *Fundamental immunology* (pp. 1603). Philadelphia: Lippincott Williams & Wilkins.

Paye-Layleh, J. (2015). *Liberia audit report questions $673,000 in Ebola spending*. http://www.nytimes.com/aponline/2015/04/15/world/africa/ap-af-ebola-westafrica.html?_r=0. Accessed 21 Dec 2017.

Reuters. (2017). *Ebola victims sue Sierra Leone government over mismanaged funds*. https://www.reuters.com/article/us-health-ebola-leone/ebola-victims-sue-sierra-leone-government-over-mismanaged-funds-idUSKBN1E92NE. Accessed 21 Dec 2017.

Richmond, J. K., & Baglole, D. J. (2003). Lassa fever: Epidemiology, clinical features and social consequences. *The BMJ, 327*(7426), 1271–1275.

SAGE. (2014). *Roll out of the meningococcal A conjugate vaccine through mass vaccination campaigns in countries of the African meningitis belt current status, vaccine coverage, epidemiological and economic impact*. http://www.who.int/immunization/sage/meetings/2014/october/2.DJINGAREY_Session6_SAGE_Oct2014_FINAL_21Oct2014.pdf. Accessed 12 Dec 2017.

Sahid, J. S. (2015). *Sierra Leone's missing Ebola millions*. http://www.irinnews.org/analysis/2015/03/30. Accessed 20 Dec 2017.

Tomori, O. (2004). Yellow fever: The recurring plague. *Critical Reviews in Clinical Laboratory Sciences, 41*(4), 391–427.

Tomori, O. (2014). Winning the battle against emerging pathogens. A Nigerian Response. *Bulletin of the Atomic Scientists, 70*, 14–17.

Tomori, O. (2015a). Will Africa's future epidemic ride on forgotten lessons from the Ebola epidemic? *BMC Medicine, 13*, 116. https://doi.org/10.1186/s12916-015-0359-7.

Tomori, O. (2015b). *Epidemiology and risk of yellow fever in current context*. http://www.who.int/immunization/sage/meetings/2016/october/Session11-Part1-Epidemiology-and-risk-of-yellow-fever-in-current-context.pdf?ua=1. Accessed 25 Jan 2019.

University of Maryland Medical Center. (1999). *Plague of Athens: Another medical mystery solved at University of Maryland*. https://www.newswise.com//articles/plague-of-athens-medical-mystery-may-be-solved. Accessed 19 Dec 2017.

Vainio, J., & Cutts, F. (1998). *Yellow fever*. Geneva: World Health Organization (document WHO/EPI/GEN/98.11).

Vittozzi, K. (2017). *400,000 children in north-east Nigeria at risk of severe acute malnutrition*. https://www.unicef.org/infobycountry/nigeria_94178.html. Accessed 21 Dec 2017.

Walker, P. (2010). Senegalese president unveils £17m African Renaissance statue. *The Guardian*. www.theguardian.com/world/2010/apr/04/senegal-african-renaissancestatue. Accessed 21 Dec 2017.

WHO. (2005). *Enhanced surveillance of epidemic meningococcal meningitis in Africa: A three-year experience*. http://www.who.int/wer/2005/wer8037.pdf. Accessed 21 Dec 2017.

WHO. (2010). *Yellow fever initiative – providing an opportunity of a lifetime*. Geneva: World Health Organization. http://www.who.int/csr/disease/yellowfev/YFIbrochure.pdf. Accessed 19 Dec 2017.

WHO. (2014). *Meningococcal disease control in countries of the African meningitis belt*. http://www.who.int/wer/2015/wer9013.pdf?ua=1. Accessed 21 Dec 2017.

WHO. (2015). *Meningococcal disease control in countries of the African meningitis belt*. http://www.who.int/wer/2016/wer9116.pdf?ua=1. Accessed 21 Dec 2017.

WHO. (2016a). *Yellow fever*. http://www.who.int/csr/disease/yellowfev/en/. Accessed 21 Dec 2017.
WHO. (2016b). *Weekly epidemiological record*, 31 March 2017. 92(13): 145–164. http://apps.who.int/iris/bitstream/10665/254901/1/WER9213.pdf?ua=1. Accessed 21 Dec 2017.
WHO. (2016c). *Public financing for health in Africa: From Abuja to the SDGs*. https://apps.who.int/iris/bitstream/handle/10665/249527/WHO-HIS-HGF-Tech.Report-16.2-eng.pdf?sequence=1. Accessed 26 Jan 2019.
WHO. (2017a). *Cholera count reaches 500 000 in Yemen*. http://www.who.int/mediacentre/news/releases/2017/cholera-yemen-mark/en/. Accessed 21 Dec 2017.
WHO. (2017b) *The yellow fever outbreak in Angola and Democratic Republic of the Congo ends*. http://www.afro.who.int/en/media-centre/pressreleases/item/9377-the-yellow-fever-outbreak-in-angolaand-democratic-republic-of-the-congo-ends.html. Accessed 21 Dec2017.
WHO. (2017c). *Ebola ça suffit!- Phase III vaccine trial in Guinea*. http://www.who.int/medicines/ebola-treatment/q-a_ebola-ca-suffit/en. Accessed 21 Dec 2017.
WHO. (2017d). *Meningococcal meningitis*. http://www.who.int/mediacentre/factsheets/fs141/en/. Accessed 21 Dec 2017.
WHO. (2018). *Ebola virus disease: Democratic Republic of Congo external situation report 7*. https://apps.who.int/iris/bitstream/handle/10665/272728/SITREP-EVD-DRC-20180601-eng.pdf?sequence=1&isAllowed=y. Accessed 01 June 2018.
WHO-AFRO. (2017a). *Weekly bulletin on outbreaks and other emergencies week 50*. http://apps.who.int/iris/bitstream/10665/259709/1/OEW50-1015122017.pdf. Accessed 21 Dec 2017.
WHO-AFRO. (2017b). *Regional committee sessions*. http://www.afro.who.int/about-us/governance. Accessed 19 Sept 2017.
WHO. (2019). Ebola situation reports: Democratic Republic of the Congo. https://apps.who.int/iris/bitstream/handle/10665/311972/SITREP_EVD_DRC-20190416-eng.pdf?utm_source=Newsweaver&utm_medium=email&utm_term=click+here+to+download+the+complete+situation+report&utm_content=Tag%3AAFRO%2FWHE%2FHIM+Outbreaks+Weekly&utm_campaign=WHO+AFRO+-+Situation+Report+-+Ebola+Virus+Disease+Outbreak+in+DRC+-+Sitrep+37+%282019%29

# Chapter 12
# Africans in the Diaspora-The Hidden Force: Economics, Investment, Skilled Workforce and Public Health

**J. Radeino Ambe, Marion Koso-Thomas, Samuel G. Adewusi, and Muhammed O. Afolabi**

## 12.1 Introduction

Diaspora is an ancient Greek term for "dispersion or scattering." The term was also used in the late nineteenth century in narratives of the Jewish dispersal from Israel. Diaspora is defined as, the "movement, migration and or scattering of a people from their established or ancestral homeland (Merriam-Webster n.d.). Many scholars tend to agree that the *scattering* or *dispersal* of people from Africa was responsible for populating the globe. The advent of ancient and modern warfare, coupled with ecological and man-made disasters have contributed to dispersal, emigration, immigration and the continuing change of demographics in the world. The African Union (AU) defines the African Diaspora as:

> People of African origin living outside the continent, irrespective of their citizenship and nationality and who are willing to contribute to the development of the continent and the building of the African Union. (African Union n.d.).

J. R. Ambe (✉)
Department of Public Health, School of Nursing and Health Sciences, Capella University, Minneapolis, MN, USA

The Global Emerging Pathogens Treatment Initiative, Lagos, Nigeria
e-mail: jambe@capellauniversity.edu

M. Koso-Thomas
Global Health Researcher, Silver Spring, MD, United States

S. G. Adewusi
Lawyers Office of Samuel G. Adewusi, Silver Spring, MD, USA

Board of Trustees Nigerians in Diaspora Organization, Americas (NIDO Americas), Washington, DC, USA

M. O. Afolabi
Department of Clinical Research, London School of Hygiene & Tropical Medicine, London, UK



G. B. Tangwa et al. (eds.), *Socio-cultural Dimensions of Emerging Infectious Diseases in Africa*, https://doi.org/10.1007/978-3-030-17474-3_12

The African Diaspora is sometimes referred to as the “sixth region” of Africa. The estimated population of Africans in the Diaspora are: Latin America, 112.65 million; The Caribbean, 13.56 million; Europe, 3.51 million; and North America 39.16 million (World Bank 2012). As defined, most people do not choose to leave their homeland out of a sense of adventure, rather, they do so for life- preserving and or life-enhancing necessities. For example, Irish immigrants escaped the potato famine from Ireland, and became part of the Irish Diaspora in America. This occurred again as recently as 1973, when Ireland joined the European Union and lost many young skilled workers who migrated in search of work (Ages 2011). Similarly, convicts from London, to include those from the middle class, were sent to Australia in the 1800’s. After the convict period, it is unlikely that many voluntarily immigrated to Australia from the slums of London (Jupp 2004). Furthermore, the debates surrounding the definition of the word *diaspora* stems from the fact that this experience is rooted in the experience and consciousness of people who emigrated to new lands. According to Sandra Kim, it is a more *phenomenological* way of defining the word that gives a better understanding to the term, as this term really encompasses an *experience* lived by Diasporans (Kim 2007).

Diasporans typically engage their homelands through humanitarian relief, financial capital, investment capital and intellectual capital. Contrary to the Brain Drain theory, now with advances of smart phones and the internet, *Brain Gain* or *Brain Circulation* are the new terms used, as Africans in diaspora provide intellectual capital which return time and time again to assist whether temporarily, permanently and/or through virtual assistance via social media and cyberspace, enriching home countries (Chikezie 2015). Most diasporans will, out of a sense of what is right, obligation and altruism, reach out to help their homeland. Some will invariably forget the homeland and totally assimilate into the new destination culture and society after a period of acculturation. Acculturation has evolved and is now seen as a multidimensional concept which espouses both cultures; that of the home country as well as that of the host country (Ndika 2013). The choice made by the each individual diasporan depends on the circumstances that led to emigration, and whether or not the homeland contributed to the *scattering* of said diasporans.

## 12.2 Obligation: The Role of Diasporans to the Ancestral Homeland

It can be argued that diasporans owe no obligation to the ancestral homeland, especially, after the trauma of leaving. If the homeland is viewed as contributorily negligent or culpable in the actions or omissions that led to the dispersal. Based upon anecdotal and factual evidence, we can simply use the Jewish example as a model of the types of obligation that Diaspora owe to the homeland. Notwithstanding, the ambiguities related to the sense of obligations, many diasporans participate and contribute; much like the Jewish Diaspora, who set a shining example and defined the diaspora obligations to the ancestral homeland in the twentieth century. The list of obligations is not endless, encompassing financial remittances, the transfer of knowledge and technology, direct foreign investments, donations of medical equipment, non-perishable produce, clothing and kind, and the defending of interests of the homeland in adopted countries. Based on the altruistic nature of each diasporan, she/he chooses the level of obligations, if any at all, and whether to commit resources and time to assist the ancestral homeland. For Africans, there is an outpouring of support through professional and regional associations to the motherland.

**The Internet and Social Media** The internet has changed the way people communicate and the speed at which the interaction occurs. Although reference to Social Media is interspersed throughout the chapter, it is befitting to have a section in which some attention is given to the internet as it plays a crucial role in diasporan engagement and second generation diasporans who are showing interest in the countries of origin of their parents and grandparents. In the case of the African Diaspora, second generation diasporans are rallying support through social media as human rights advocates and facilitators for change; bringing new ideas and technological know-how. The internet avails diasporans the ability to connect over thousands of miles enabling like-minded diasporans the opportunity to work together to support countries of origin. PayPal and other internet based platforms to send and receive money have made it convenient and cheaper, across continents without exorbitant bank fees. Fund raising platforms such as GoFundMe enables the raising of funds for people all over the world. Social media and groups such as, *StopEbolaNow* and Ebola Social Media Coalition played a tremendous role in the dissemination of information and rallying of support during the Ebola outbreak. It is important to explicitly consider the leverage of the internet as a communication channel in the event of disasters. Not only does communication take place before an outbreak or disaster but also during and after, by using social media sites such as Facebook to help with the dissemination of information. Emergency plans and networks can be shared faster via the internet (Merchant et al. 2011).

### *12.2.1 The Hidden Forces: Economics, Investments and a Skilled Workforce*

In the year 2013, diasporan remittances to their home countries was in excess of 413 billion dollars (USD) (Ratha 2014). The importance of the diaspora investments cannot be over-emphasized. In the United States, data shows that the Chinese and Indian diaspora lead the pack in active direct foreign investments in their respective ancestral homelands. Both the Chinese and Indian diaspora are followed closely by the Jewish diaspora, and to some extent by the Nigerian diaspora. In the area of remittances to sub-Saharan Africa (sSA), the Nigerian diaspora will remit over $22 billion in 2017, according to World Bank estimates (World Bank 2017). Several trends point to the growing involvement of diasporans in the development of West

Africa. First, the financial volume of remittances sent to countries of origin continues to grow. Such growth is especially intense when families encounter emergency situations, such as in Sierra Leone, where there was an increase of funds sent to the country between 2013 and 2014 during the Ebola Virus Disease outbreak. These funds and resources had an impact which spread beyond the migrant family nucleus outwardly into communities. This can be seen in the example of homes built from these resources which produce a ripple effect to an increase of trade and other industries in the region (African Development Bank 2015).

Due to improved economic activities in certain countries with high incomes and part of the Organisation for Economic Co-operation and Development (OECD); there were higher remittances in 2017. It is estimated that in 2017, formal remittance to sub-Saharan Africa is projected to increase to about $38 billion from $34 billion in 2016. This shows an increase of 10% (World Bank Group 2017). Africans in the diaspora are investing in and expanding entreprenueral activity in their homelands through the passageway of migration. Both direct investment and entrepreneurial investment contribute to the building of economies in which policies need to be developed to harness the benefits (Ojo et al 2013).

There have been many factual stories of individual diasporans investing successfully in Africa. But in most cases, those investments are not large enough to fill the void of significant unemployment. Currently, except for Ghana, most sSA countries do not have coherent or targeted policies to attract Diaspora investments.

**Diaspora Bonds** These bonds are a debt instrument which can be issued by a private organization or a country to raise funds for specific purposes from its diaspora. Israel and India have large diaspora communities and both countries have harvested funds to fill gaps in the country's available resources using this flexible instrument. Since 1951, Israel has issued diaspora bonds for a menu of different needs, every year. India has used this method three times for raise funding, when they have had some difficulty in getting through to international capital markets. The combined amount raised by both countries is 44 billion dollars. These bonds offer effective risk management which make them attractive to Diasporans coupled with the sense of obligation or bias towards their home countries (Ketkar and Ratha 2011).

### *12.2.2 Consequences of the Exodus of Highly Skilled Emigration (Brain Drain) From Already Fragile Systems*

High skill emigration or brain drain that disperse or migrate from developing countries have serious financial consequences. In the modern age, knowledge and skills are capital. When highly skilled professionals emigrate from developing countries, the immigrants take away valuable capital that are not easily replaceable. To make matters worse, developing countries expend large sums of money to educate and train professionals who in turn leave for one reason or another. The dispersed professionals leave a vacuum of lost tax revenues and spending that are necessary to build strong economies.

Certain African countries have Diaspora affairs and commissions which give attention to bilateral relations and the development of policies for the Diasporans which invite them to participate through trade, tourism, image building, humanitarian work, as examples. Many of the governments have recognized *brain drain* and understand that it is difficult to stop people from leaving. They have come to a consensus that the countries their nationals are emigrating to and the countries of origin need to have a way to capitalize and benefit from the Diasporans. It has been shown that there are documented instances of migration contributing to provide a better outcome for the African country through the additional financial income, resulting economic development and the transfer of technology which reduces unemployment and poverty when correct policies are in place (Ethiopian Ministry of External Affairs 2013).

## 12.3 Diasporans and Altruism

In the area of humanitarian work, the diaspora from sub-Saharan Africa have worked individually and/or in groups through hundreds of associations; humanitarian, faith-based, tribal, alumni, home town associations and professional organizations – to strengthen and support each other in their new countries and to mobilize resources for the country they left behind. Many diaspora organizations could be further strengthened to serve as valuable intermediaries between traditional development actors, the homeland government, and the broader diaspora, playing a significant development role. Annually, these non-profit as well as professional organizations organize medical missions, training seminars and medical mobile clinics to their countries of origin.

The Afro-European Medical and Research Network (AEMRN) is an example of efforts by Diaspora to enhance skilled labour and invest in brain gain. AEMRN is a platform for professionals in the fields of education, medicine, engineering, nursing, and other faith-based disciplines can interact with the network at various levels. These professionals engage in projects in the spheres of health and food security in resource limited countries. AEMRN members identify, reach out, encourage and empower people to take part in continuous professional development programmes so that the stimulus of their learnt trade can be rekindled, improved and once again enable them to contribute to the development of their community and the world at large (AEMRN n.d.).

An example of a large diaspora group are Ethiopians who have been migrating for many years. According to Chacko and Gebre, in the 1970's and 1980's, well-educated Ethiopians initially emigrated to Australia, Europe and North America. This was then followed by a labour migration of Ethiopians with a lower socio-economic status to Middle Eastern countries (Chacko and Gebre 2013). In 2013, the Ethiopian government estimated approximately two million Ethiopian Diaspora were in other countries in Africa, Australia, Europe, Middle East and North America. The Ethiopian government acknowledges that the Diasporans in Europe and North America have more opportunities for better education and a higher income. They remit money to their families in Ethiopia and invest in different segments of the economy, support Ethiopia with knowledge and lobby for their homeland (Ethiopian Ministry of External Affairs 2013).

### *12.3.1 Public Health and Fragile Health Systems*

Given the fragile healthcare systems across sub-Saharan Africa and the dearth of health care professions in certain regions, many Diasporans have formed groups that lobby for and support programs on the continent of Africa. Most African governments have offices for Diaspora and many are actively engaged in activities across the globe. These are activities and the office of the diaspora is usually housed within the Ministry of External Affairs. Often Public Health activities are coordinated through the Ministries of Health and the Ministries of External Affairs.

### *12.3.2 Tapping the Diaspora During Difficult Times: The Ebola Outbreak*

When there are ecological disasters, the diaspora are galvanized into action to assist and help the ancestral homeland. When the Ebola outbreak took the countryside of Guinea by surprise, in December 2013, the world was extremely slow to respond despite best efforts from Médecins Sans Frontières (MSF) to draw the world's attention to the crisis and cry for mobilization. Through all of this, upon reflection, it is crucial to note the role that Africans in diaspora played during the outbreak that impacted the ultimate responses in the affected countries of Sierra Leone, Liberia and Guinea-Conakry. An emerging awareness of how Diasporans participate in the development of their countries of origin is increasing, especially in humanitarian, education and the public health spheres.

**Impact and Involvement of Diaspora Engagement** Although there are no definitive figures, many diaspora medical professionals from sSA, undoubtedly volunteered their services and skills during the Ebola outbreak in West Africa. According to the envoy from Sierra Leone, to the United Kingdom, health care professionals in the Diaspora travelled home during the outbreak to assist in the fight the epidemic. Many individuals walked, cycled, baked and sold cookies and cupcakes, with the goal of raising funds to help with the management of the Ebola outbreak. Others donated large sums of money, purchased supplies and equipment, sent clothing and shoes and other personal items through religious organizations and non-profits to the affected countries. For example, on September 30th, 2014, in New Jersey, United States of America, a 75-mile bike ride to raise $3300 took place to support Médecins Sans Frontières in their fight against EVD. Others formed non-profit organizations, like the five young individuals of Sierra Leonean descent; who formed EndEbolaNow.com which is a website that was instrumental in raising awareness through education and in raising funds for the fight against EVD. They teamed with Emergency USA and formed the hashtag #ShakeEbolaOff which was a dance campaign (Walton 2014). The Kono District Development Association in the United Kingdom put together personal protective equipment (PPE), chlorine powder and hand sanitizers and shipped the supplies to the Kono District, Sierra Leone. Supplies were distributed to 14 chiefdoms and communications on how to prevent the spread of the disease were successfully carried out.

**Liberia** There is an estimated 72,000 Liberians living in the United States. In July 2014, the Liberian Ambassador to the United States of America, responded to countless calls from Liberians in the United States asking for ways to assist their brothers and sisters on the ground. The Ambassador, Jeremiah Sulunteh asked Diasporans to donate to the Global Ministries who were about to ship a container of medical supplies during the month of August. He asked Liberians and well-wishers to assist with donating items for affected communities. He also stated that the embassy in Washington D.C. would set up a dedicated bank account for activities directed at supporting the management of EVD (Butty 2014a, b).

Liberians in diaspora galvanized through associations and actively used social media platforms to raise awareness and funds for the EVD outbreak in Liberia. Following the evacuation of non-essential personnel and family members from Liberia, by the State Department, the Liberian Vice President, Joseph Bokai, pleaded with Diasporans to call family members in Liberia and advise them to heed to calls put forth by the Liberian government. He appealed to Diasporans to educate their relatives about EVD especially as many Liberians were in a state of denial (Butty 2014a, b).

**Guinea (Conakry)** The EVD outbreak of 2014–2016, was the first of its kind in West Africa. The Guinean Community Association in the United States, actively participated in coordinating efforts to curtail the EVD outbreak by organizing, coordinating and supporting public health and community engagement activities in Guinea. The association was key in lobbying for assistance, from the United States, for a response to the affected region. Guinean Diasporans donated clothing, shoes, water and other items and pooled their resources to ship the merchandise home. Many used huge drums instead of cardboard boxes to ship the merchandise so that the drums could then be used to store clean, chlorinated water.

## 12.4 Narratives from the Field

**Sierra Leone (A Personal Narrative)** The following contribution is a personal narrative by Dr. Marion Koso-Thomas, a Diasporan in the United States. This narrative serves as an example of the impact and involvement of diaspora engagement during the Ebola Virus Disease outbreak of 2013–2016.

In August 2014, the Sierra Leone Ambassador to the United States invited Dr. Koso-Thomas to a town hall meeting in Washington, D.C where he proposed the formation of a Task Force to coordinate efforts of Sierra Leoneans in the metropolitan area. With the plethora of health experts in the region who were making inquiries of how they could contribute to curbing the epidemic, it was clear to him that there was an untapped potential. A physical therapist along with several physicians and nurses were invited to constitute the US-Sierra Leone Healthcare Coalition Taskforce. The group met with a U.S. based organization with collaborative work in Sierra Leone, and the State Department and attended briefings on the Hill to serve as a voice for advocacy. Though the Task Force was unable to directly deploy individuals with the relevant expertise, the intent was to provide the Ministry of Health and the government of Sierra Leone with support. The Task Force was able to compile a list of health care workers in the DMV, Delaware and Philadelphia metropolitan areas which quickly grew to over 100 names. The professionals listed had a range of the technical competencies, social, cultural, and language competencies that gave them the added advantage of being able to rapidly deploy, without the need for interpreters/translators and could also be an incredible resource for training their local counterparts. Unfortunately, the Task Force was unable to aid in the formal collective deployment of these volunteers; a challenge in the Ebola epidemic response which played a role in critical delays.

In February 2015, Dr. Koso-Thomas, a physician and public health professional whose native country is Sierra Leone, was invited by the Centers for Disease Control (CDC) to be deployed as an Infection Prevention Control (IPC) Specialist and Epidemiologist serving on the Ebola Emergency Response Team. As part of the team, she served on the District Ebola Response Command and Control Center (DERC) in Kambia which was one of the last resistant sites where the epidemic stubbornly persisted. Due to her expertise, she led IPC training for Category 1 and Category 2 staff of the Kambia District General Hospital and Epi investigation of EVD case (in collaboration with the World Health Organization).

## 12.5 Africans in Diaspora Within Africa

Many Africans working outside their home countries, yet within Africa, also contributed significantly to bring the outbreak of Ebola to a conclusive end. Following successful control of Ebola in Nigeria, there was a clarion call that the Government of Nigeria should share with other countries how they successfully achieved the control of the outbreak within a relatively short period with countries. The Ministry of Health of Lagos State, led by Honourable Commissioner, Dr. Jide Idris, invited volunteer health workers to share their expertise in neighbouring Sierra Leone, Guinea-Conakry and Liberia. This led to the deployment of several epidemiologists, nurses, paediatricians, laboratory scientists and community workers to Ebola-affected countries where they worked assiduously with the organisations and governments of the respective countries to bring the outbreak under control well before the time projected that it would end.

### 12.5.1 Post Ebola Outbreak: Another Personal Narrative

Dr. Muhammed Afolabi was working in one of the leading research institutions in The Gambia, West Africa, during the outbreak. Although, there was no outbreak of Ebola in The Gambia, the fear that it would enter the country kept everyone on their toes. Dr. Afolabi was looking for opportunities to contribute his quota to alleviating the unquantifiable human suffering wrought by the outbreak. The opportunity soon came when the head of his research organisation invited him to his office one afternoon to inform him that the organisation had been selected to be part of a consortium with the responsibilities of testing the safety and efficacy of an Ebola vaccine within 6 months. That sounded like an unbelievable feat, as it normally takes a minimum period of 10 ten years to test and roll-out a vaccine for any disease. However, due to the deadly nature of Ebola without a known cure or vaccine, the World Health Organization insisted on fast-tracking the development and testing of the vaccine to address the huge challenges posed by the virus.

Dr. Afolabi was chosen to coordinate the vaccine testing and evaluation for his organisation. Despite involvement in many other pressing research issues, he tackled the onerous task headlong working round the clock with other colleagues to develop and finalise the clinical trial protocol, study documents as well as ethical and regulatory approval from local, national and international committees. Sensitization efforts in the selected trial communities took place to ensure buy-in and meaningful engagement of the potential study participants and their families. Everything appeared set for the take-off of the Ebola vaccine testing, when the President of the country refused blatantly to give a nod for the trial to proceed. He did not see any reason why the organisation should be using his citizens as guinea-pigs to test Ebola vaccine especially when he thought he had a cure for it. Many advocacy efforts made to assuage his feelings proved abortive.

Towards the Fall of 2016, Dr. Afolabi joined a leading academic institution which was testing another Ebola vaccine among adults, adolescents and children in the northern district of Sierra Leone. This afforded him the opportunity to translate the knowledge and skills gained in his previous work place to ensure the research staff were properly trained, and good quality data collected. His greatest hope is that this current effort would lead to the licensure of an Ebola vaccine which can be deployed to stem the tide of Ebola whenever it rears its ugly head again, anywhere in the world.

In conclusion, Africans in diaspora play a critical role despite their physical absence from the continent and/or on the continent but away from their home countries. Many diasporans straddle the continent they live in and their home countries, travelling back to visit with family during important times and during the holiday seasons. They are comprised of people from all walks of life; from blue collar workers to white collar professionals in the fields of entrepreneurship, inventors, science, medicine and healthcare. No matter the diaspora's job in the new or host country, most Diasporans have the same goal of sending funds, books, electronics and clothing home to family and providing support for extended family, clans and hometowns. Financial remittances are a major infusion of foreign currency for some African countries. Diasporan investments and foreign exchange funding is critical to the development of economies in Africa due to the sheer magnitude of the influx in currency with a high increase during certain festive seasons. Although there are no conclusive figures, it appears that most diasporans have the interest of their countries of origin and that this is partly motivated by emotional attachments and familial obligations. This interest often manifests in their desire to contribute their knowledge, technical savviness, financial remittances and lobbying activities. Disaporans also lead and feature prominently in development projects in their home countries.

## References

African Development Bank Group. (2015). *Remittances from West Africa's Diaspora: Financial and social transfers for regional development*. https://www.afdb.org/en/blogs/measuring-the-pulse-of-economic-transformation-in-west-africa/post/remittances-from-west-africas-diaspora-financial-and-socialtransfers-for-regional-development-14614/. Accessed June 2019.

African Union. (n.d.). *The diaspora division*. https://au.int/en/diaspora-division

Afro-European Research and Medical Research Network. (n.d.). http://www.aemrnetwork.ch/index.php/en/

Ages, A. (2011). *The diaspora dimension*. Netherlands: Springer Netherlands.

Butty, J. (2014a). *Liberia diaspora mobilizing for Ebola relief*. Washington, DC: Federal Information & News Dispatch, Inc.

Butty, J. (2014b). *VP urges diaspora Liberians to help educate relatives about Ebola*. Lanham: Federal Information & News Dispatch.

Chacko, E., & Gebre, P. H. (2013). Leveraging the diaspora for development: Lessons from Ethiopia. *GeoJournal, 78*(3), 495–505. https://doi.org/10.1007/s10708-012-9447-9.

Chikezie, C. (2015, June). *The Ebola crisis and Sierra Leone, humanitarian practice network*. Retrieved from http://odihpn.org/magazine/the-ebola-crisis-and-the-sierra-leone-diaspora/

Ethiopian Ministry of External Affairs. (2013). *Diaspora Policy*. Retrieved from http://www.ethiopianembassy.org/PDF/diaspora%20policy.pdf

Jupp, J., & ProQuest Ebooks. (2004). *The English in Australia*. Cambridge/New York: Cambridge University Press.

Ketkar, S. L., & Ratha, D. (2011). VIEWPOINT: Diaspora bonds for funding education. *Migration Letters, 8*(2), 153–172. Retrieved from http://library.capella.edu/login?url=https://search-proquest-com.library.capella.edu/docview/1268704155?accountid=27965.

Kim, S. (2007). Redefining diaspora through a phenomenology of postmemory. *Diaspora: A Journal of Transnational Studies, 16*(3), 337–352. https://doi.org/10.1353/dsp.2007.0015.

Merchant, R. M., Elmer, S., & Lurie, N. (2011). Integrating social media into emergency-preparedness efforts. *The New England Journal of Medicine, 365*(4), 289–291. https://doi.org/10.1056/NEJMp1103591.

Merriam-Webster. (n.d.). https://www.merriam-webster.com/dictionary/diaspora

Migration and Remittances: Fact book 2011 World Bank. (2014). *African diaspora*. https://siteresources.worldbank.org/INTDIASPORA/Resources/AFR_Diaspora_FAQ.pdf

Ndika, N. (2013). Acculturation. *SAGE Open, 3*(4). https://doi.org/10.1177/2158244013515687.

Ojo, S., Nwankwo, S., & Gbadamosi, A. (2013). African diaspora entrepreneurs: Navigating entrepreneurial spaces in 'Home' and 'Host' countries. *The International Journal of Entrepreneurship and Innovation, 14*(4), 289–299. https://doi.org/10.5367/ijei.2013.0126.

Online Etymololgy Dictionary. (n.d.). Retrieved from https://www.etymonline.com/

The World Bank. (2012). African diaspora program. News & broadcasts. Retrieved from http://web.worldbank.org/archive/website01363/WEB/0__CO-81.HTM

Walton, A. (2014). Grassroots social media campaign aims to raise $1 million in the Ebola fight. *Forbes*. Retrieved from https://www.forbes.com/sites/alicegwalton/2014/10/21/social-media-campaigns-to-stop-ebola-gain-strength-celebrity-support/#1a86eab1fe1e.

World Bank Group. (2017, October). Migration and development brief 28 migration and remittances: Recent developments and outlook special topic: Return migration October 2017. https://www.afdb.org/en/blogs/measuring-the-pulse-of-economic-transformation-in-west-africa/post/remittances-from-west-africas-diaspora-financial-and-social-transfers-for-regional-development-14614/

# Chapter 13
# Insufficiency of Pathogen Focused Approaches Towards Managing Deadly Epidemics in Africa: Harmonising the Roles of Governments, Health Systems and Populations

**Samuel J. Ujewe and Alice Mungwa**

## 13.1 Introduction

In this chapter, we explore the insufficiency of the pathogen focused approaches often adopted by African governments in fighting deadly infectious disease epidemics. By "pathogen focused approach" we refer to strategies for preventing or managing medical emergencies, like the Ebola epidemic, which give undue emphasis to the epidemiological components. These often pay little to no attention to other varied aspects, like social, cultural and ethical dimensions of affected populations. We use the case of the West African Ebola epidemic to show that we can learn from how the virus thrives on close social networks in communities in managing future outbreaks. We also explore the grounds for a harmonised approach that leans on socio-cultural factors to inform health intervention policies and delivery in Africa. While we point to the need to incorporate socio-cultural approaches, a full description of the relevant framework is beyond the scope of this chapter. We emphasise the need to take seriously the social and cultural dimensions of local African contexts in relation to infectious diseases to attain robust interventions strategies.

To determine the insufficiency, the chapter shows the downsides of pathogen focused approaches, as exemplified in the response to the West African Ebola Epidemic. Reference will also be made to how different results were obtained in the 2018 Ebola epidemic in the DR Congo, where some attention was given to socio-cultural dynamics. Together, these point to the need for a harmonised approach in managing, controlling or preventing deadly infectious disease epidemics in Africa.

S. J. Ujewe (✉)
Canadian Institute for Genomics and Society, Toronto, ON, Canada

Global Emerging Pathogens Treatment Consortium, Lagos, Nigeria

A. Mungwa
Cameroon Bioethics Initiative (CAMBIN), Yaounde, Cameroon



G. B. Tangwa et al. (eds.), *Socio-cultural Dimensions of Emerging Infectious Diseases in Africa*, https://doi.org/10.1007/978-3-030-17474-3_13

Moon et al. (2015) offer ten essential reform strategies to be adopted globally before the next epidemic. While their proposed approaches are plausible, they mostly provide a vision to a global response, which African countries can draw from. This chapter, while drawing from the ten reforms, explores an approach that hinges on socio-cultural dimensions of pathogenic diseases on the African continent.

## 13.2 Deadly Pathogenic Diseases in Africa

The emergence of deadly pathogens has in recent years become synonymous with the name, Africa. While the challenges of HIV/AIDS linger, epidemics like Ebola, Yellow Fever and Cholera find fertile grounds to re-emerge, diminishing populations' health and well-being. The Ebola epidemic in West Africa recorded 28,646 cases and 11,323 deaths with Liberia, Sierra Leone and Guinea bearing the heaviest burden (WHO 2016). While claiming many lives, the crisis also had a psycho-social effect on affected persons, and severely diminished the socio-economic capacities of families, communities, and whole countries (UNICEF 2016; Van Bortel et al. 2016). Most notably, the virus thrives on close interaction within and between communities and across national borders (WHO 2015). Ebola thrives on available intra and inter communal networks to sustain its transmission chain, making the epidemic difficult to manage. This gained a vital consideration in managing the 2018 Ebola outbreak in DR Congo.

In the wake of the West African Ebola epidemic, much of the containment, control and prevention strategies were pathogen-oriented. The drive was to annihilate the transmission chain of Ebola, leading to great emphasis on the search for new drugs and vaccines to counter the disease. Yet, findings shows that the outbreak was not a factor of the Ebola virus alone, but also of weak structures and poor healthcare systems in the affected countries (Moon et al. 2015). Liberia and Sierra Leone, the two most affected countries, are still recovering from long and devastating civil wars, which destroyed basic health infrastructure, as well as the social and economic fabrics. The weak structures and systems meant that they were not prepared to cope with the sudden outbreak (Benton and Dionne 2015; Ravi and Gauldin 2014). The containment strategies deployed included technical approaches, like surveillance and quarantine, as well as intensive search for vaccines (The College of Physicians of Philadelphia 2014; Chan 2014; WHO Ebola Response Team 2014; Towers et al. 2014).

However, not much was invested in restoring the weak health systems, and addressing the social, cultural and economic factors fuelling the epidemic. The undue emphasis on technical strategies to stop the virus indicates that the governments of affected countries were inadvertently pushed towards investing in logistics and drug development, as the potential solutions to the problem. The downside to this approach has been the neglect of other crucial aspects of healthcare, like cultural practices, social determinants, ethical outlooks and socio-economic conditions of affected populations. Technical strategies drawn from modelled frameworks rooted in orthodox medicine, as employed during the Ebola epidemic in West Africa, are not suitable for all contexts across the globe. Peculiarities of African sociocultural contexts mean that addressing medical emergencies would require approaches informed by local knowledge and understanding of sociocultural subtleties. A robust response should consider not only technical strategies, but also take seriously the place of contexts in mapping intervention plans in medical emergencies. Beyond the pursuit of new medicines and vaccines, viable responses must proactively engage with local contexts. This will involve acknowledging and understanding varying sociocultural dimensions, and how they sustain disease outbreaks or determine the success of technical strategies being implemented. It will include strengthening health systems, regulating or encouraging certain kinds of social interactions and cultural practices, as well as enhancing socio-economic and environmental conditions.

## 13.3 African Governments, Health Systems, and the Pathogen Focused Approach

Recurrent outbreaks of deadly diseases diminish affected populations, and the primary responsibility to address them rests with Governments. African governments' responses may have evolved over time, but have been generally viewed to be severely inadequate. Some reasons for the lack of success by governments are shown by the inadequate coping mechanisms that they often adopt: from monitoring and reporting to the prevention and control of epidemics (Piot 2014; Dionne 2014). Specifically, most African governments tend to focus on the pathogenic aspect of deadly infectious disease epidemics (Khan 2015; Coltart et al. 2017), paying little to no attention to the social, cultural, ethical and economic dimensions. Yet, these aspects are crucial in preventing the occurrence of these diseases on epidemic scales, and restoring and sustaining the population's health.

The pathogen focused approach is a plausible strategy for containing or preventing epidemics, and was instrumental in ending the West African Ebola crisis. However, it is not sufficient for the well-being of affected populations. A sufficiency of well-being theory would argue that simply providing infrastructural facilities and drugs in affected areas would not be enough to address or prevent deadly epidemics:

> Sufficiency for any dimension of well-being will be relative to the level of social organisation and technological and scientific development in which that dimension must be realised. Because the ultimate focus of justice... is on what persons 'can do or be,' there simply is no way that such judgements can be made apart from some understanding of the background conditions. (Powers and Faden 2008, 60)

In public health, this would imply that the health and well-being of a population facing a deadly disease may not rest simply on building more health centres and procuring the relevant or available drugs. Rather, a sufficient approach would crucially understand the background social, cultural, anthropological and economic conditions influencing the spread of the disease. This should inform how the scientific and technological advancements are introduced into affected communities. For instance, despite the Yellow Fever vaccine being available for decades, there still are recurrent outbreaks of the disease in parts of Africa (Shearer et al. 2017). Why? Part of the problem is that the varying background conditions aiding the persistence of this disease have not been adequately understood and addressed. For instance, there may be ample stock of vaccines in global reservoirs, but these would require political will from governments to secure and distribute to at risk communities. There also has to be established population's trust in the health system to ensure uptake of locally available vaccines. Waiting to roll out mass supply of a vaccine during an outbreak, as with the 2016 Angola and DR Congo Yellow Fever cases (McNeil Jr 2017), is not sufficient for the well-being the relevant populations. A proactive engagement with populations, through sustained communication and regular vaccination exercise, will protect at-risk-communities and build trust in the health system. This would lead to earlier reporting in the case of an outbreak and enable quick containment.

Ebola is only one among many known and unknown diseases with epidemic capabilities. The newly developed Ebola vaccine may save lives, as has been demonstrated in the 2018 outbreak in DR Congo (World Health Organisation 2018). African health systems must be prepared to employ measures that go beyond building health infrastructure, procuring drugs and surveillance to avoid future outbreaks. They must: define the nature of the impact of considered strategies; explore various social and cultural dimensions that may fuel outbreaks or make available drugs or vaccines ineffective; and determine what surveillance means for the affected populations. The holistic approach would better help to prevent or manage future outbreaks of both known and unknown deadly pathogens.

### *13.3.1 Insufficiency of Governments and Health Systems' Responses*

Africa is a major hub for infectious diseases in the world, reporting 54 public health events in mid-2015, for instance, of which 47 resulted from infectious diseases (Fall and HSE Cluster 2015). The recent Ebola outbreaks bear significant political, social, economic, cultural, humanitarian and security challenges on the affected countries, their neighbours and the international community. As with most large scale medical emergencies, the responses of relevant governments were commendable to some, but condemnable to others. Lessons learnt from the West African Ebola epidemic would prove to be crucial for coordinating response to the 2018 outbreak in DR Congo (World Health Organisation 2018). One great challenge is that containing the outbreaks on both occasions would not be possible without sustained international intervention. This is shown by the absence of viable National Health Systems (NHS) in most the affected countries (WHO 2014b; Green 2018). Regarding the West African Ebola outbreak, the WHO notes that most countries had neither the capabilities nor the systems to respond quickly and effectively, allowing the outbreak to spread (WHO 2014b). The West African Ebola outbreak was unique in several dimensions, which permitted the spread before medical countermeasures could be applied. Hence, it may be too quick to blame the inadequacy of health systems as the major culprit. Also, the more recent outbreak in the DR Congo was better managed despite the country having equally bad health system (Green 2018).

The point is that complex disease outbreaks like Ebola must be equally matched by harmonised approaches to minimise their impact. Beyond the numbers of deaths and physical effects of the recent Ebola epidemics, there are psycho-social and socio-economic impacts on the affected populations. For instance, over 3300 children were orphaned by the West African Ebola epidemic (UNICEF 2014). Furthermore, Ebola is a traumatic illness both in terms of symptom severity and mortality rates. Those affected are predisposed to psychological effects from the trauma of the infection, fear of death and experience of witnessing others dying. And even after fighting off the disease, survivors also experience feelings of shame or guilt and stigmatization or blame from their communities (Van Bortel et al. 2016). The full impact of the disease can only be effectively addressed if done from a holistic approach.

### 13.3.2 Inadequacy of International Aid

According to a World Bank report, the loss of breadwinners in many families meant that living conditions were worsened for many. The socio-economic conditions were made worse as the affected countries faced isolation following closures of borders with other countries. This came with trade and travel restrictions on affected countries. In the three most affected countries, 10,000 schools were closed, putting more than two million children out of school. In Liberia, 46 per cent of the workforce lost their jobs within months of the outbreak. The outbreak affected every economic sector in Guinea, Liberia and Sierra Leone, undermining investment and trade, and engendering large scale job losses (Bank 2014).

Despite these challenges, much of the Ebola response approaches focused on the epidemiological dimension of the disease, and technical strategies towards containing it. At the onset of the West African Ebola epidemic, the WHO and the governments of Guinea, Liberia and Sierra Leone drafted the "Ebola Virus Disease Outbreak Response Plan for West Africa" (WHO 2014a). It proposed eight strategic actions plans for the WHO, including:

- providing leadership in coordinating international partners
- establishing a sub-regional operations coordination centre
- mobilising and deploying needed WHO staff, experts and consultants
- regularly disseminating updated information, and
- Continuously providing support to strengthen core capacities.

It also proposed ten national response plans for the governments of the affected countries, some of which include:

- mobilising government agencies and community, religious and political leaders to work towards improving awareness, psycho-social support, and understanding of the disease
- deploy additional qualified national staff
- commit additional financial resources
- strengthen surveillance, case finding, reporting and contact tracing, and
- Improve information and communication to communities on related matters, and to improve community participation.

The 18 strategic response plans outlined largely sway towards tackling the epidemiological aspects of the outbreak, and outline technical approaches as solutions. There is ample literature regarding the adverse social and economic effects of the outbreak (Novelli et al. 2018; Maconachie and Hilson 2015; Ippolito et al. 2015; UNDG 2015; Ordaz-Németh et al. 2017; Himelein and Kastelic 2015; Kastelic and Kastelic 2015; Himelein et al. 2015). These tend to corroborate the strategies employed in containing the epidemic. Yet, the literature on the socio-cultural implications and impact of the epidemic is sparse (Carrión Martín et al. 2016; Pellecchia et al. 2015; Whembolua et al. 2015). The sparse literature reflects the limited engagement with non-epidemiological factors to Ebola control. There is not much initiative around improving the living conditions of affected populations; economic recovery plans for families and communities; post-epidemic support for survivors and victims of Ebola; the ethical outlook of affected communities; and/or cultural adjustments in coping with Ebola and future epidemics. Yet, it has been shown that the Ebola epidemic has lasting effects on affected communities beyond the public health emergency period. These include social and psychological scars left on affected individuals; economic breakdowns among affected families, communities and countries; ethical/moral conflict in affected regions; as well as cultural shocks experienced by communities (Van Bortel et al. 2016; UNICEF 2014; Hamilton 2014; Thomas et al. 2015; BBC 2014).

### *13.3.3 Failed Strategies*

It is understandable that a more immediately effective strategy was needed to contain the Ebola crisis in West Africa. The point is that relevant pathogen/epidemiological approaches should be consolidated by those addressing underpinning social, economic and cultural conditions that trigger emergence or influence the spread of the diseases. Engaging a sociocultural approach in the process would enhance understanding, appreciation and uptake of other crucial technical strategies in affected communities. This will not only ensure a more effective management of an existing outbreak, but also prevent future occurrences of the same or similar disease outbreaks.

To provide an example, cholera has a long-standing vaccine, and has been eliminated from many countries across the globe (Khatib et al. 2012; Andre et al. 2008). Yet, the WHO continues to report several cholera outbreaks in Sub-Saharan Africa and a few other countries, even in 2018 (WHO 2018). In the face of medical emergencies, like Ebola, African governments and health systems tend to prioritise: logistics for tracing and quarantine, increasing response capacity with additional health workers, and research for a potential vaccine. The glaring social, cultural, ethical and economic dimensions of epidemics are not similarly prioritised. This is occasioned by heightened reliance on international support lead by high income countries in the West who operate using the aforementioned approaches. The shortcoming is that these approaching are mostly developed out-of-context and often forcibly adapted in African countries, and without due recourse to the wide sociocultural and socio-economic variances between African settings and Western settings.

Overwhelmed by the burden of deadly infectious diseases, African governments unquestionably adopt these strategies, as proposed by dominant international health agencies or affluent donor countries. Often these strategies are oriented towards proven scientific measures for eliminating or suppressing the pathogen. For instance, the West African Ebola epidemic saw a highly motivated campaign for a candidate vaccine to be use in affected countries. And despite public resistance to phase I trials in parts of West Africa, the candidate vaccines were tried and rolled out for use (Kpodo 2015; Sayburn 2014). The militaristic approach used in pushing forward the course for Ebola vaccines in West Africa was preceded by scientific evidence about the efficacy of the vaccine. These same vaccines were used in the 2018 Ebola outbreak in DR Congo (Kelland 2018). While vaccines are crucial for infectious disease control, their effectiveness as a strategy largely relies on several other factors, including social, cultural and economic conditions of affected regions or communities. Lessons may be learnt from the persistence of Cholera outbreaks in many African countries despite the availability of vaccines and other treatments.

The vaccine initiative towards ending Ebola in West Africa was globally applauded and commended by governments of the affected countries. In Ghana, where the public resistance against Ebola vaccine trials was most severe, the government reluctantly withdrew from partaking in the process (Kummervold et al. 2017). The resistance in Ghana was spurred by a lack of or inadequate engagement with the relevant communities in the process. In short, the sociocultural dimension of the vaccine trial was not taken seriously. A substantive community engagement in the proposed trial communities may have seen better appreciation or acceptance of the vaccine in Ghana. While the vaccine approach may be important for eliminating or reducing the potency of diseases like Ebola, it is only one step in the process. A discord between scientific measures, like vaccine development, and the affected populations' sociocultural outlook can make potentially effective strategies sterile. A harmonised approach is required to successfully end the reign of deadly pathogens in Africa.

A pathogen focused approach like the use of vaccines is, by itself, not sufficient. Consolidating scientific approaches with relevant social, ethical and cultural dynamics offers a more viable pathway out of deadly infectious disease epidemics in Africa. Taking this step would require harmonising the roles African governments and health systems with social, ethical, cultural and economic dynamics in the affected regions or communities. This would mean that while African governments and health systems attempt to understanding the scientific nature of these diseases, the strategies they adopt must be informed by the affected populations' socio-cultural outlook and socio-economic conditions that influence potential epidemics.

In what follows, we describe the structure of African communitarian societies, their understanding of disease, and how these may influence infectious disease outbreaks.

## 13.4 Structure of African Societies

Defining the term "African" often poses a challenge, given that Africa is geographically vast with diverse cultural heritage. Despite this diversity, the different ethnicities are united by commonalities that give them a remarkable family resemblance analogous to the family resemblance of groupings that are in some way remarkably different from one another but all justifiably bracketed under the term "Western" (Tangwa 2017). For instance, one can point to the glaring emphasis on vital participation, sharing and dependency as crucial aspects of many African ethnicities.

Despite the effects of modernisation, a strong sense of kinship still exists among African populations. This calls for a vital participation in matters that affect others within one's network of relationships:

> Kinship is reckoned through blood ties and betrothal – engagement and marriage – and controls social relationships between people in a given community: "the kinship system is like a vast network stretching laterally in every direction, to embrace everybody in a given local group… (Mbiti 1990, 102)

According to Ujewe (2016), kinship situates the African person within a web of a wider social network. He notes, for instance, that it is common practice in Nigeria for a person to refer to his wife's parents or relatives as family; also, one's siblings would refer to his/her spouse's family as family, to whom they have certain obligations. The event of one marriage reshapes an entire web of social relationships within and between African communities. Every individual is involved in constantly making and reshaping the nature of these relationships, and a person's life evolves with every change in the communal structure. While not everyone in a given society may be related through kinship, the existing network of relationships has wider societal implications, embracing the whole of humanity (Ujewe 2016). The embeddedness of persons within the networks of social relationships also defines the nature of commitments owed to others, and the kinds of loyalty obliged.

Consequently, individual persons are in a sense morally obligated to participate in matters that affect others within their network of social relationships. As a norm, family members are obligated to share in the burdens of other members, simply in virtue of being of the same family. Note that the African idea of family extends beyond one's parents and siblings and includes other relatives. The obligation is carried through the wider family to whole communities, depending on the nature of existing demands or needs (Ujewe 2012). Thus, the values of sharing and dependency are engrained as moral imperatives in African societies:

> The natural relationality of the individual immediately involves one in some social and moral roles in the form of obligations, commitments, and duties (or responsibilities) to other members of his or her community which the individual must fulfil. Social or community life itself, a robust feature of the African communitarian society, mandates a morality that clearly is weighted on duty to others and to the community; it constitutes the foundation for moral responsibilities and obligations. (Gyekye 2011)

The obligations to participate and share in matters affecting others is consolidated by a (inter)dependency ideal that exist in the social structure. It is considered morally reprehensible, for instance, for one to live an economically superfluous life, while his family (siblings or other relatives) live in abject poverty. The community expects that the morally upright person would be one that balances his or her well-being against those of others within their network of relationships (Ujewe 2016). The communitarian ideal of interdependency is facilitated or regulated by the African ethic of responsibility:

> The success that must accrue to a shared or cooperative living depends very much on each member of the community demonstrating a high degree of moral responsiveness and sensitivity to the needs and well-being of other members. This should manifest in each member's pursuit of his responsibilities. (Gyekye 1997, 67)

The emphasis here is that one always has in mind a motivation to seek the good of the whole community or society to which they belong. In so doing they also seek their own good as well as build a firm basis for their own lasting social benefits, making the welfare of the whole community the highest good to seek (Gyekye 1996). The social obligations engendered by the ideals of vital participation and interdependency also have a crucial role in the African understanding of health and illness. This also informs how African populations approach issues of public health emergencies.

## 13.5 Understanding of Health and Illness

African understanding of health and illness spans beyond the physiological constitutions emphasised in orthodox medicine. Health and illness are viewed from a dual perspective, where natural and existential conditions are recognised as causally linked. Harmony with oneself, community and the metaphysical world is a key determinant of good health (Ujewe 2016):

> The African conception of health is all-embracing... health is not just about the proper functioning of bodily organs. Good health... consists of mental, physical, and emotional

> stability for oneself, family members, and community. This integrated view of health is based on the African unitary view of reality. (Omonzejele 2008, 120).

> ...health does not simply mean the absence of disease; it incorporates balance and harmony between the individual and his or her social surroundings, including harmony with the self. Disease results from the breakdown in relatedness, including disharmony between the individual and the rest of the universe. (Mkhize 2008, 39) .

This understanding of and approach to health and illness persists, as shown by the established practices and high subscription to traditional medicine in countries like Nigeria and South Africa. Specifically, people tend to seek traditional remedies where Western medicine is unable to provide satisfactory explanations or treatments for certain ailments (Manda 2008; Omonzejele 2008). The persistence of the holistic view of health means that it also shapes populations' attitudes towards seeking healthcare; it determines the effectiveness of policies and intervention plans.

The existence of the "African" understanding health and illness, coupled with the mode of socialisation, means the approach to and understanding of public health issues would be similarly inclined. Consider the case of the Ebola outbreak in West Africa. The international standard approach involved identifying and quarantining suspected or actual cases, and further developing a vaccine. Yet, many of the narratives from Ebola survivors show that many persons got the disease in the process of fulfilling their communal and social obligations. These included caring for ill family members or orphaned children who were unknowingly infected. One other prominent point of contact was burial ceremonies, the attendance of which is basic social obligation among kins in African societies. Effectively managing the epidemic would go beyond simply banning traditional burials, for instance. Communal obligations must be understood in light of the population's understanding health and illness. This will inform a comprehensive and more effective approach in managing current and future outbreaks.

For the populations caught in the middle of the outbreak, simply identifying and quarantining suspected cases, and developing new drugs and vaccines is not sufficient. To them, "health is a much more complex concept, and healing from affliction or misfortune is more than a technique for eliminating a scourge or contagion" (Tangwa 2017, 104). The understanding of health and illness is shaped by their social, ethical and cultural realities that play significant roles in fuelling the chain of transmission for diseases like Ebola.

Thus, approaches to curb infectious diseases like Ebola should be shaped not only by physiological factors, but also by the socio-cultural experiences of the affected populations. One can argue, for instance, that the HIV/AIDS pathogen is not specifically what makes the disease dreadful in Africa today. Rather the disease's associated social, ethical, economic and cultural consequences trigger deadlier contingent consequences. The point is not to deny the deadly nature of the disease itself, but rather to show the existential dimensions of HIV/AIDS that may be causing more damage than the physiological considerations that dominate scientific research. Associating HIV/AIDS to sexual immorality (Familusi 2011; Twesigye et al. 2005), for instance, fuels stigma, compounding the pain and suffering of affected persons. While antiretroviral therapy (ART) has been developed to suppress HIV, one major challenge remains that of broad uptake by affected populations. A demographic survey shows that the uptake of HIV testing in sub-Saharan Africa remains low, despite the disease's high prevalence on the continent (Staveteig et al. 2013). Even among the educated and wealthy classes, who generally have better access to healthcare, uptake is not encouraging (Staveteig et al. 2013; Cremin et al. 2012). Also, Alcorn (2015) shows that large numbers of people who turn up for testing, when diagnosed with HIV, either never make it to the clinic to be assessed for antiretroviral therapy eligibility, or do not return when told that they are not yet eligible. This shows that the low uptake of HIV testing or ARTs is not primarily a result of limited facilities or drug availability, but also of a complex of several other determinants. Among these the socio-cultural determinants play a significant role.

To successfully tackle deadly infectious disease in Africa, it is important to take seriously the role of cultural communities and the socio-ethical dimensions shaping them. A viable approach would seek to integrate current pathogen focused approaches, such as quarantine for Ebola, testing and ART for HIV, and vaccine development for both diseases, with socio-culturally informed approaches that "speak the languages" of the relevant African contexts. While African governments and health systems work towards expanding treatment facilities and logistics, they must also harmonise these projects with the populations understanding of health, as informed by their social, ethical and cultural environments.

## 13.6 Embracing a Harmonised Approach

Considering the foregoing, we propose that a harmonised approach be adopted in addressing the scourge of deadly infectious diseases in Africa. This will offer more effective outcomes by consolidating strategies already being used. The approach will seek to address the multidimensional underpinning of disease outbreaks. It will go beyond tackling the pathogen by using purely scientific or technical strategies to giving equivalent attention to other background social, cultural, socio-ethical and economic issues that provide favourable conditions for the emergence or spread of such pathogens.

A harmonised approach recognises that the pathogen focused method has significant benefits in the management of deadly infectious diseases. We have seen how the discovery of vaccines and the invention of advanced medical technologies have played strategic roles in eliminating diseases around the world. Some diseases that were endemic in many parts of the world decades ago are now on the brink of elimination, since the relevant vaccines were discovered. As of July 2018, only 12 new case of the wild polio virus were recorded worldwide for the year (GPEI 2018). It is worth noting that the drive towards polio eradication suffered severe setbacks in Nigeria due to the existence of other factors. These range from socio-cultural and religious factors to salient socio-economic conditions surrounding the worst affected regions of the country (Yahya 2007; Jegede 2007). Hence, significant medical advancements and production of life-saving drugs are not sufficient. It is important to take other background conditions seriously. This is what a harmonised approach specifically aims to address.

The harmonised will approach recognises the crucial place of drugs and advances in medicine in managing, eradicating or eliminating deadly infectious diseases in Africa. Yet, it will also emphasise the socio-cultural dimension's essential place in the effectiveness of life-saving vaccines, drugs and technical strategic. A harmonised framework informed by sociocultural medical countermeasure during medical emergencies like Ebola must include and aim to address the following:

- Engaging with the family structure in the local contexts, understanding its dynamics and using this knowledge to inform technical procedures
- Acknowledge the place of communal networks and how these can play crucial roles in both escalating the epidemic and enhancing the effectiveness of technical intervention strategies
- Representations of the local understanding of the disease and perceptions related to the varied symptoms, and understanding how these are crucial to the success of any intervention strategy deployed
- Understand the appropriate communication patterns in affected communities, and use this knowledge to inform guidelines for disseminating information about the disease and it risks to local populations
- Account for the local understanding of health risks associated with the disease and how this may induce public fear, engender stereotypes in affected communities, and influence non-compliance to available interventions

We have seen, for instance, that the effectiveness of polio vaccines was hampered by the non-inclusion of socio-cultural and religious dimensions in the affected regions. Similarly, the rejection of the Ebola vaccine trial in Ghana stresses the need to crucially engage the socio-cultural outlooks of the relevant communities for a successful intervention. In fighting deadly infectious diseases, understanding and adequately considering varied socio-cultural backgrounds of affected populations are crucial for any meaningful success.

A broad description of the harmonised approach and the relevant guidelines are beyond the scope of this chapter. They will form the subject of future research, and constitute the outcome of a different publication.

## 13.7 Conclusion

We have argued in this chapter that while significant resources are being invested by governments and the international community in combating deadly infectious disease in Africa, the approaches employed are largely pathogen focused, and are insufficient. We have shown that the inefficiency of African health systems and poor infrastructural facilities play a role in sustaining disease outbreaks, making it difficult for governments to contain them. In a bid to effectively address the problem, the focus should not be limited to fixing the healthcare systems and infrastructure. Rather, significant attention should also be given to other background conditions, like social, cultural, economic and ethical dynamics that fuel the incubation of the diseases or spread of epidemics. To provide a holistic solution to Africa's frequent recurrence of infectious disease outbreaks, we propose a harmonised approach, as opposed to the dominant pathogen focused approaches deployed. If adequately developed and deployed, the new approach will provide a holistic solution towards eliminating these diseases from Sub-Saharan Africa.

## References

Alcorn, K. (2015, July 21). *Innovative approaches to linkage to care boost clinic visits, HIV treatment uptake in African study*. https://www.aidsmap.com/Innovative-approaches-to-linkage-to-care-boost-clinic-visits-HIV-treatment-uptake-in-African-study/page/2986249

Andre, F. E., Booy, R., Bock, H. L., Clemens, J., Datta, S. K., John, T. J., Lee, B. W., Lolekha, S., Peltola, H., & Ruff, T. A. (2008). Vaccination greatly reduces disease, disability, death and inequity worldwide. *Bulletin of the World Health Organization, 86*, 140–146.

Bank, The World. (2014). *The economic impact of the 2014 Ebola epidemic : Short and medium term estimates for West Africa*. 91219. The World Bank. http://documents.worldbank.org/curated/en/524521468141287875/The-economic-impact-of-the-2014-Ebola-epidemic-short-and-medium-term-estimates-for-West-Africa

BBC. (2014, September 19). Ebola health team killed in Guinea. *BBC News*. sec. Africa. http://www.bbc.com/news/world-africa-29256443

Benton, A., & Dionne, K. Y. (2015). International political economy and the 2014 west African Ebola outbreak. *African Studies Review, 58*(1), 223–236.

Carrión Martín, A. I., Derrough, T., Honomou, P., Kolie, N., Diallo, B., Koné, M., Rodier, G., Kpoghomou, C., & Jansà, J. M. (2016). Social and cultural factors behind community resistance during an Ebola outbreak in a village of the Guinean Forest region, February 2015: A field experience. *International Health, 8*(3), 227–229. https://doi.org/10.1093/inthealth/ihw018.

Chan, M. (2014). Ebola virus disease in West Africa—No early end to the outbreak. *New England Journal of Medicine, 371*(13), 1183–1185.

Coltart, C. E. M., Lindsey, B., Ghinai, I., Johnson, A. M., & Heymann, D. L. (2017). The Ebola outbreak, 2013–2016: Old lessons for new epidemics. *Philosophical Transactions of the Royal Society B: Biological Sciences, 372*(1721), 20160297. https://doi.org/10.1098/rstb.2016.0297.

Cremin, I., Cauchemez, S., Garnett, G. P., & Gregson, S. (2012). Patterns of uptake of HIV testing in Sub-Saharan Africa in the pre-treatment era. *Tropical Medicine & International Health, 17*(8), e26–e37.

Dionne, K. Y. (2014, July 15). Why west African governments are struggling in response to Ebola. *Washington Post*. https://www.washingtonpost.com/news/monkey-cage/wp/2014/07/15/why-west-african-governments-are-struggling-in-response-to-ebola/

Fall, Ibrahima-Soce, and HSE Cluster. (2015). WHO Africa: Outbreak Bulletin. Vol. 5 Issue 2. World Health Organization (WHO).

Familusi, O. O. (2011). Human sexuality in African thought and the HIV/AIDS scourge. *LUMINA, 22*(2), 1–1.

GPEI. (2018). *This week: Polio this week as of 10 July 2018*. http://polioeradication.org/polio-today/polio-now/this-week/

Green, A. (2018). Ebola outbreak in the DR Congo: Lessons learned. *The Lancet, 391*(10135), 2096. https://doi.org/10.1016/S0140-6736(18)31171-1.

Gyekye, K. (1996). *African cultural values: An introduction*. Philadelphia: Sankofa Publishing Company.

Gyekye, K. (1997). *Tradition and modernity: Philosophical reflections on the African experience*. Oxford: Oxford University Press.

Gyekye, K. (2011, Fall). African ethics. In E. N. Zalta (Ed.), *The Stanford encyclopedia of philosophy*. Stanford: Metaphysics Research Lab, Stanford University. https://plato.stanford.edu/archives/fall2011/entries/african-ethics/

Hamilton, R. (2014, August 21). The economic impact of Ebola. *BBC News*, sec. Business. http://www.bbc.com/news/business-28865434

Himelein, K., & Kastelic, J. G. (2015). *The socio-economic impacts of Ebola in Liberia*. Washington, DC: The World Bank Group.

Himelein, K., Testaverde, M., Turay, A., & Turay, S. (2015). *The socio-economic impacts of Ebola in Sierra Leone*. Washington, DC: World Bank.

Ippolito, G., Puro, V., & Piselli, P. (2015). Ebola in West Africa: Who pays for what in the outbreak. *The New Microbiologica, 38*(1), 1.

Jegede, A. S. (2007). What led to the Nigerian boycott of the polio vaccination campaign? *PLoS Medicine, 4*(3), e73.

Kastelic, K. H., & Kastelic, J. G. (2015). *The socio-economic impacts of Ebola in Liberia: Results from a high frequency cell phone survey round five*. Washington, DC: The World Bank Group.

Kelland, K. (2018, May 21). First Ebola vaccines given as WHO seeks to beat Congo outbreak. *Reuters*. https://www.reuters.com/article/us-health-ebola-vaccinations-congo/first-ebola-vaccines-given-as-who-seeks-to-beat-congo-outbreak-idUSKCN1IM18Q

Khan, A. (2015, July 27). Dealing with African epidemics needs more than just a health response. *The Conversation*. http://theconversation.com/dealing-with-african-epidemics-needs-more-than-just-a-health-response-44481

Khatib, A. M., Ali, M., von Seidlein, L., Kim, D. R., Hashim, R., Reyburn, R., Ley, B., Thriemer, K., Enwere, G., & Hutubessy, R. (2012). Effectiveness of an oral cholera vaccine in Zanzibar: Findings from a mass vaccination campaign and observational cohort study. *The Lancet Infectious Diseases, 12*(11), 837–844.

Kpodo, K. (2015, June 10). Ghana halts Ebola vaccine trial due to community protests. *Reuters*. https://www.reuters.com/article/us-health-ebola-ghana/ghana-halts-ebola-vaccine-trial-due-to-community-protests-idUSKBN0OQ2SG20150610

Kummervold, P. E., Schulz, W. S., Smout, E., Fernandez-Luque, L., & Larson, H. J. (2017). Controversial Ebola vaccine trials in Ghana: A thematic analysis of critiques and rebuttals in digital news. *BMC Public Health, 17*(August), 642. https://doi.org/10.1186/s12889-017-4618-8.

Maconachie, R., & Hilson, G. (2015). Ebola and alluvial diamond mining in West Africa: Initial reflections and priority areas for research. *The Extractive Industries and Society, 2*(3), 397–400.

Manda, L. D. (2008). Africa's healing wisdom : Spiritual and ethical values of traditional African healthcare practices'. In R. Nicolson (Ed.), *Persons in community: African ethics in a global culture*. Scottsville: University of Kwazulu-Natal Press.

Mbiti, J. S. (1990). *African religions & philosophy*. Oxford: Heinemann.

McNeil, Jr. D. G. (2017, December 22). Yellow fever epidemic in Africa shows gaps in vaccine pipeline. *The New York Times*. sec. Health. https://www.nytimes.com/2016/12/05/health/yellow-fever-africa-vaccine.html

Mkhize, N. (2008). Ubuntu and harmony : An African approach to morality and ethics. In R. Nicolson (Ed.), *Persons in community: African ethics in a global culture*. Scottsville: University of Kwazulu-Natal Press.

Moon, S., Sridhar, D., Pate, M. A., Jha, A. K., Clinton, C., Delaunay, S., Edwin, V., Fallah, M., Fidler, D. P., & Garrett, L. (2015). Will Ebola change the game? Ten essential reforms before the next pandemic. The report of the Harvard-LSHTM independent panel on the global response to Ebola. *The Lancet, 386*(10009), 2204–2221.

Novelli, M., Burgess, L. G., Jones, A., & Ritchie, B. W. (2018). "No Ebola… still doomed"–the Ebola-induced tourism crisis. *Annals of Tourism Research, 70*, 76–87.

Omonzejele, P. F. (2008). African concepts of health, disease, and treatment: An ethical inquiry. *Explore: The Journal of Science and Healing, 4*(2), 120–126.

Ordaz-Németh, I., Arandjelovic, M., Boesch, L., Gatiso, T., Grimes, T., Kuehl, H. S., Lormie, M., Stephens, C., Tweh, C., & Junker, J. (2017). The socio-economic drivers of Bushmeat consumption during the west African Ebola crisis. *PLoS Neglected Tropical Diseases, 11*(3), e0005450.

Pellecchia, U., Crestani, R., Decroo, T., Van den Bergh, R., & Al-Kourdi, Y. (2015). Social consequences of Ebola containment measures in Liberia. *PLoS One, 10*(12), e0143036.

Piot, P. (2014). *Ebola's perfect storm*. Washington, DC: The World Bank Group.

Powers, M., & Faden, R. (2008). *Social justice: The moral foundations of public health and health policy*. New York: Oxford University Press.

Ravi, S. J., & Gauldin, E. M. (2014). Sociocultural dimensions of the Ebola virus disease outbreak in Liberia. *Biosecurity and Bioterrorism: Biodefense Strategy, Practice, and Science, 12*(6), 301–305.

Sayburn, A. (2014). WHO gives go ahead for experimental treatments to be used in Ebola outbreak. *BMJ, 349*(August), g5161. https://doi.org/10.1136/bmj.g5161.

Shearer, F. M., Moyes, C. L., Pigott, D. M., Brady, O. J., Marinho, F., Deshpande, A., Longbottom, J., et al. (2017). Global yellow fever vaccination coverage from 1970 to 2016: An adjusted retrospective analysis. *The Lancet Infectious Diseases, 17*(11), 1209–1217. https://doi.org/10.1016/S1473-3099(17)30419-X.

Staveteig, S., Wang, S., Head, S. K., Bradley, S. E. K., & Nybro, E. (2013). *Demographic patterns of HIV testing uptake in Sub-Saharan Africa*. Calverton: ICF International Calverton.

Tangwa, G. B. (2017). Giving voice to African thought in medical research ethics. *Theoretical Medicine and Bioethics, 38*(2), 101–110.

The College of Physicians of Philadelphia. (2014, November 19). *Ebola virus disease and Ebola vaccines | History of vaccines*. https://www.historyofvaccines.org/content/articles/ebola-virus-disease-and-ebola-vaccines

Thomas, M. R., Smith, G., Ferreira, F. H. G., Evans, D., Maliszewska, M., Cruz, M., Himelein, K., & Over, M. (2015). *The economic impact of Ebola on Sub-Saharan Africa: Updated estimates for 2015*. Washington, DC: The World Bank Group.

Towers, S., Patterson-Lomba, O., & Castillo-Chavez, C. (2014). Temporal variations in the effective reproduction number of the 2014 West Africa Ebola outbreak. *PLoS Currents, 6*. https://doi.org/10.1371/currents.outbreaks.9e4c4294ec8ce1adad283172b16bc908

Twesigye, E. K., Benedicts, A. S., & Benedicts, M. W. (2005). The ethics of HIV/AIDS and the rise of an apocalyptic mariologist movement for the restoration of the ten commandments: The challenge of HIV/AIDS to Christian theology. *Scriptura: International Journal of Bible, Religion and Theology in Southern Africa, 89*(1), 456–468.

Ujewe, S. J. (2012). *Ought-onomy and African health care: Beyond the universal claims of autonomy in bioethics*. Dunedin: University of Otago. otago.ourarchive.ac.nz

UJEWE, S. J. (2016). *Just health care in Nigeria–the foundations for an African ethical framework*. Preston: University of Central Lancashire. Clok.uclan.ac.uk

UNDG, United Nations Development Group. (2015). *Socio-economic impact of Ebola virus disease in west African countries: A call for national and regional containment, recovery and prevention*. Dakar: United Nations.

UNICEF. (2014, October 7). *Ebola orphans: West Africa's abandoned children*. UNICEF USA. https://www.unicefusa.org/stories/ebola-orphans-west-africas-abandoned-children/19831

UNICEF. (2016, July 12). *Impact of Ebola*. UNICEF. https://www.unicef.org/emergencies/ebola/75941_76129.html

Van Bortel, T., Basnayake, A., Wurie, F., Jambai, M., Koroma, A. S., Muana, A. T., Hann, K., Eaton, J., Martin, S., & Nellums, L. B. (2016). Psychosocial effects of an Ebola outbreak at individual, community and international levels. *Bulletin of the World Health Organization, 94*(3), 210.

Whembolua, G. S., Kambamba, D. K., Conserve, D., & Tshiswaka, D. I. (2015). *Socio-cultural factors associated with epidemics: The case of 2014 Ebola outbreak*. Washington, DC: The World Bank Group.

WHO. (2014a). *Ebola virus disease outbreak response plan in West Africa – a call for action*. Washington, DC: The World Bank Group.

WHO. (2014b, August 8). *WHO | Statement on the 1st meeting of the IHR emergency committee on the 2014 Ebola outbreak in West Africa*. WHO. http://www.who.int/mediacentre/news/statements/2014/ebola-20140808/en/

WHO. (2015, January). *WHO | Factors that contributed to undetected spread of the Ebola virus and impeded rapid containment*. WHO. http://www.who.int/entity/csr/disease/ebola/one-year-report/factors/en/index.html

WHO. (2016, March 30). *Ebola situation report – 30 March 2016 | Ebola*. http://apps.who.int/ebola/current-situation/ebola-situation-report-30-march-2016

WHO. (2018). *WHO | Cholera*. WHO. http://www.who.int/csr/don/archive/disease/cholera/en/

WHO Ebola Response Team. (2014). Ebola virus disease in West Africa—The first 9 months of the epidemic and forward projections. *New England Journal of Medicine, 371*(16), 1481–1495.

World Health Organisation. (2018, May 23). *Ebola virus disease – Democratic Republic of the Congo*. WHO. http://www.who.int/csr/don/23-may-2018-ebola-drc/en/

Yahya, M. (2007). Polio vaccines—"no thank you!" barriers to polio eradication in Northern Nigeria. *African Affairs, 106*(423), 185–204.

# Part IV
# Ethics and Policy in the Context of EIDs

# Chapter 14
# Context and Ethical Challenges During the Ebola Outbreak in West Africa

**J. Radeino Ambe and Francis K. Kombe**

## 14.1 Introduction

Public health ethics is seen from the view of communities and populations. The ethical considerations related to forced quarantine *i*mpinges on the rights of individuals to protect the wellbeing of the greater public, in an effort to curb an epidemic, a pandemic or to ensure that neither starts. In these situations, ethical conflicts are bound to occur because public health and the safety of the community often trumps individual rights. This chapter will examine the ethical questions pertaining to public health ethics that arose from the Ebola outbreak of 2014/2015. During the outbreak, it is said that the United States of America went through extraordinary lengths to give two tow of it citizens, experimental drugs, outfit a plane with an incubation pod and monitors; airlift them out of the "red zone" to a special, ward at Emory University hospital which houses the most sophisticated infectious disease unit in the United States. Many people were outraged that the individual rights of these two citizens appeared to be more important than that of the public. The fear of Ebola Virus Disease spreading in the country turned to hate mail hurled at doctors at Emory. (Usborne 2014). The practice of forced quarantine will be a focus of the discussions as the risks of emerging and re-emerging infectious diseases increase with modern travel that transports people, to different continents within a few hours via airplanes, ships and trains that cross borders at exceedingly increasing speeds. With this "speed travel" comes the speed of rapid transport of

J. R. Ambe (✉)
Department of Public Health, School of Nursing and Health Sciences, Capella University, Minneapolis, MN, USA

The Global Emerging Pathogens Treatment Initiative, Lagos, Nigeria
e-mail: jambe@capellauniversity.edu

F. K. Kombe
African Research Integrity Network (ARIN), Kilifi, Kenya



G. B. Tangwa et al. (eds.), *Socio-cultural Dimensions of Emerging Infectious Diseases in Africa*, https://doi.org/10.1007/978-3-030-17474-3_14

communicable, infectious diseases, bio-hazards and toxic, biological agents; across borders. In the United States of America, rules and regulations that govern the use of quarantine are in place to safeguard the public against the transmission of infectious diseases to the general public.

This chapter attempts to explain differences between medical and public ethics, using quarantine, as an example. It also explains the differences between quarantine and isolation. There are existing laws, regulations, as well as, ethical considerations that affect health practice and practitioners when a forced quarantine occurs. Examples from the countries around the world are used for discussion purposes in an effort to express a global experience and to outline historical perspective.

## 14.2 International Law

Historically, international law played a key role in global communicable disease by providing guidelines for the control of diseases as well as playing a major role in the surveillance of global communicable diseases. During the nineteenth century, in lieu of a world global health body which could harmonize the different laws within European nations, international law dominated the field. There were inconsistent regulations on quarantine until the exchange of information and the establishment of international health organizations (Aginam 2002). Communicable diseases shape global health since pandemics and epidemics know no borders. International law has been of importance since it reduces cross-border vulnerability to these diseases.

### *14.2.1 Quarantine and Isolation*

In 1377, the first known record of modern day quarantine was introduced in Dubrovnik, on Croatia. In 1424, the first *lazeretto* was opened in Venice because of the Plague. It was on the island of Santa Maria di Nazareth. In 1467, the system in Venice was adopted by Genoa (Tognotti 2013). The origin of the word "quarantine" is said to be from Venetian Italian and a variant of the term "*quaranta giorni*" which was used as a designated period of 40 days that ships were isolated before crew and passengers could come ashore during the Plague and Black Death (CDC n.d.). Quarantine is government enforced and can apply to humans, animals and can be used at borders or within countries. Clearly, this is the historical perspective of quarantine from a global north perspective. Isolation is when a sick person is kept separate from others. This differs from quarantine where people who have been exposed but are not ill, are separated from the general public.

#### 14.2.1.1 Patrick Sawyer: Ebola Virus Disease in Lagos[1,2]

On July 20th 2017, a Liberian national, by the name of Patrick Sawyer, flew to Lagos, the former administrative and current commercial capital of Nigeria from Monrovia with a brief stopover in Lomé in Togo. Although there are no accurate statistics on the population of Lagos, in 2016, the National Population Commission of Nigeria, stated that the population of Lagos was over 21 million. Lagos became the largest city on the continent of Africa, surpassing Cairo back in 2012 (World Population Review n.d.). Patrick Sawyer arrived in Lagos with the intention to proceed to Calabar, Nigeria, for a government conference. Some reports state that he was seeking the healing ministry of one of the Nigerian pastors, in Calabar, because he knew he was sick and possibly had Ebola Virus Disease (EVD). Mr. Sawyer's actions were reported to have been deliberate; as he reportedly evaded health warnings and the health protocols for the spread of infectious disease and lied to the staff at the hospital about not having contact with anyone who had EVD. Patrick Sawyer had nursed his sick sister who was confirmed to have EVD. She later succumbed to the disease. According to Patrick Sawyer's wife, he evaded contact with people at the Monrovia airport. In an interview with Mrs. Sawyer, she stated that her husband travelled to Nigeria because of the better health system. He knew he was ill and wanted to be treated (Mai-Duc 2014). Patrick Sawyer was the index case, (the first known case) of EVD in Nigeria. Professionally, Patrick Sawyer was a lawyer and the National Public Health Officer for Arcelor-Mittal, headquartered in Luxembourg. Patrick Sawyer was a naturalized American citizen with his family residence in the state of Minnesota, although he was consulting for the government of Liberia, at the time (Mai-Duc 2014). Information regarding Mr. Sawyer's education and social status is worthy of note, as it rules out the case of a person who may not know or understand the lethal and highly infectious nature of EVD. Against this backdrop, one can only assume that Patrick Sawyer, as the public health officer knew he was not supposed to travel and therefore should have quarantined himself to avoid exposing others to risk of contracting EVD.

Patrick Sawyer underscored the tension that might arise in balancing self-determination and autonomy of individuals and protecting the greater good of the society at large. Considering the social, health and psychological impact the Sawyer case had in Lagos and Nigeria at large, there is no doubt that the potential benefits for self-quarantine would certainly have outweighed by far, the individual rights of Mr. Sawyer. However, the debate on whether or not one should self-quarantine themselves is more complex than what many can imagine. For example, in the event that a person does not self-quarantine, important questions may arise about the

[1] https://www.premiumtimesng.com/investigationspecial-reports/166560-exclusive-how-liberian-govt-cleared-patrick-sawyer-to-travel-to-nigeria-while-under-observation-for-ebola.html

[2] https://www.premiumtimesng.com/news/166660-ebola-why-patrick-sawyer-travelled-to-nigeria-wife.html

ethical considerations for having that person under mandatory quarantine in an effort to protect the public from the spread of an outbreak? In the event that mandatory quarantine is considered, questions may equally arise regarding infringing and violating their individual rights? At face value, these questions and considerations may sound simple, yet too complex to resolve!

#### 14.2.1.2 West Point: Government of Liberia

On August 20, 2014, the Liberian government, led by President Ellen Johnson-Sirleaf, imposed a 21 day quarantine in an effort to contain the EVD outbreak, on a sprawling area known as West Point. The Liberian government were at a loss as to how to contain the outbreak and the decision to cordon off this community, a week after the government had declared the outbreak a public health emergency, did not go well with the international community. West Point, a lower socio-economic slum of about 800,000 people, came under strict military enforced quarantine after a holding center for suspected Ebola disease victims was ransacked. Seventeen suspected EVD patients escaped; mattresses and infected materials were stolen. The government of Liberia felt the need for barbed wire and wooden checkpoints to go up around West Point. In a Time magazine interview, President Johnson-Sir leaf cited the attack on the holding center as the reason for the quarantine. She further went on to say that the attack "put the entire community at risk, hence the government had to protect them from themselves." (MacDougal 2014). President Johnson-Sirleaf was making reference to the residents of West Point.

West Point residents struggle to eke out a living by trade and barter such as, selling their catch of fish for the day, to people in wealthier neighborhoods. Contrary to international advice, President Johnson Sirleaf, imposed mandatory quarantine enforced by the military. The Liberian government got caught up in the fear and the turmoil of the Ebola epidemic which led to violent clashes. There were many scuffles with the police and West Point residents threw bottles and stones at the authorities, attempting to escape the makeshift checkpoints. Liberian security forces opened fire on the rioting crowd and killed a 15-year-old, Shakie Kamara,[3] wounding two other teenagers in the resulting melee. There was no autopsy performed on Shakie Kamara and the Ministry of Defence forces took possession of his body (MacDougall 2014). The quarantine imposed area was cordoned off for a total of 10 days (Butty 2014). On Friday, August 30th, the quarantine was lifted amongst much jubilation.

[3] https://www.nytimes.com/2014/08/30/world/africa/quarantine-for-ebola-lifted-in-liberia-slum.html

#### 14.2.1.3 Thomas Eric Duncan: Texas Health Presbyterian Hospital[4,5]

Thomas Eric Duncan, a 42 year-old man from Liberia, although feeling ill, flew to Texas in the United States. He went to Texas Presbyterian Hospital. After arriving at the hospital and complaining about symptoms, he was given antibiotics and some other medications and released from the hospital. He had no medical insurance. Thomas Duncan vomited on the sidewalk outside his apartment and was again taken to the same hospital. Upon arrival this time, he was admitted. Tests were run and they came back positive for Ebola Virus Disease.

Thomas Duncan's family and the staff of Texas Presbyterian Hospital faced a 21 day quarantine because they had been exposed to Thomas Eric Duncan who came from Liberia with EVD. There was a series of events that led to the fear that not only was Thomas Duncan discriminated against, but also the African community, many of whom had to be quarantined.

Reports suggest that Thomas Duncan was treated unfairly and unfortunately died on October 8, 2014 however, there is no empirical evidence to prove it. According to the Washington Post newspaper, some Ebola patients were rushed to advanced medical facilities contrary to what happened with Thomas Duncan. Duncan's family stated that he did not receive the expected standard of care owing to his lack of medical insurance, his race and poor background. The family stated that they requested for everything that they thought would save his life and a family member asked if he could donate blood, but this request was not heeded by the hospital staff. The hospital made an out of court settlement with the family on the strength that Duncan should have been admitted the first time he was taken to the hospital. (Moyer 2014). Had Duncan been hospitalized and quarantined appropriately, by staff who were wearing PPE, others would not have been exposed to EVD or infected with EVD and the questions would not have arisen.

The Director of the National Institute of Allergy and Infectious Disease which is part of the National Institutes of Health (NIH), stated that the hospital made a mistake by not admitting Duncan during his first visit. However, he stressed that he did not think that Duncan was treated differently compared to others (referring to allegations of Duncan being black, poor and uninsured (Moyer 2014). In this case, the ethics pertaining to economic support and the delivery of care would need to be questioned (Kominski 2014). According to the director, some of the staff who had cared for Thomas Duncan became infected because some of their skin on their necks and face was exposed. They also did not wear shoe covers which made them vulnerable to the deadly infection of Ebola virus disease (Jaffe 2014). Two nurses, Nina Pham and Amber Vinson, both exposed to Thomas Eric Duncan, tested positive for EVD. The two nurses were just two out of one hundred workers who had contact with Thomas Eric Duncan at Texas Presbyterian Hospital.

---

[4] https://www.thedenverchannel.com/news/u-s-world/dallas-texas-ebola-patient-thomas-duncan-dies-at-texas-health-presbyterian-hospital

[5] https://www.washingtonpost.com/news/post-nation/wp/2014/10/08/texas-ebola-patient-has-died-from-ebola/?utm_term=.609115f8a0ce

#### 14.2.1.4 Carnival Cruise Ship[6]

On October 17, 2014, a Carnival cruise ship with 4000 passengers headed back to the United States after not allowed to dock in Cozumel, Mexico. This happened because a laboratory technician who handled Thomas Eric Duncan's biological samples was on board the ship. Although the laboratory technician showed no symptoms, she was to self-monitor. After 3 days of the cruise, the lab technician and her husband self-quarantined. On arrival at Belize, the United States requested permission for her to board a flight back to the United States, however the Belizean government denied that permission. Other passengers were allowed to disembark. The laboratory technician and her spouse self-quarantined from Thursday until the ship docked in Texas the following Sunday. Nevertheless, the nation of Mexico isolated this ship by not allowing it to dock on their shores. Belize, refused passage for this passenger to board a flight back to the United States. In addition, some students who had been on the ship were kept out of school. This is an example of how people can be stigmatized as a result of suspected contact with EVD (Bever 2014).

Ethical conflicts were inevitable especially in the United States of America. The reason for this is the history and environment of the United States which allows for the expression of individual rights. Quarantine puts healthy people who are not yet exhibiting symptoms of a communicable disease into a very confined and restricted environment. Most people who enter quarantine usually never become sick (Wynia, 2007).

#### 14.2.1.5 Nurse Kaci Hickox[7]: Civil Rights Violations, Liberty, Due Process and Systematic Change.

In the Autumn of 2014, states to include Maine, New York and New Jersey took onstricter standards for returning health care workers than was required by the United States federal government. On October 22, 2014, Governor Christie announced enhanced Ebola preparedness plans for the state of New Jersey. Two days later, Governors Christie (New Jersey) and Cuomo (New York) passed mandatory quarantine for health care workers returning from working with patients with EVD in West Africa. The former U.N Secretary General, Ban-Ki Moon cautioned against these restrictions because healthcare workers were critical to the efforts in curbing EVD. (Sherwood and Jenkins 2014).

Kaci Hickoxarrived at Newark Liberty International Airport, on October 24, 2014, from Sierra Leone where sheworked with Médecins sans frontiers (MSF) during the EVD outbreak. She passed through the new screening for all travellers from West Africa, as she transited to a connecting flight enroute to Maine. Her temperature was taken with a temporal scanner which showed elevated temperature readings

---

[6] https://www.independent.co.uk/news/world/americas/ebola-cruise-ship-in-utter-panic-as-mexico-and-belize-refuse-to-let-it-dock-9804428.html

[7] https://www.nbcnews.com/storyline/ebola-virus-outbreak/kaci-hickox-maine-nurse-quarantined-ebola-scare-sues-new-jersey-n449491

however when taken orally her temperature was normal. She had been questioned aggressively for several hours by several people upon arrival at the airport; taken with several police cars in tow, sirens and lights on, and held illegally,in a tent on hospital grounds, against her will (Sherwood and Jenkins 2014). Kaci Hickox was forced into mandatory quarantine in New Jersey and held against her wishes for three dayswithout legal counsel. Two tests for EVD were found to be conclusively negative.

When Kacy was released, she went back to Maine where she was toself-quarantine, as mandated by the state, for a total of 21 days. Kaci Hickoxwent for a bike ride with her boyfriend defying state voluntary quarantine guidelines. The American Civil Liberties Union and lawyers for Kaci Hickox, filed afederal civil rights law suit stating her civil rights had been violated. Shesoughtboth compensatory and punitive damages. In October, 2014, a judge in the state of Maine overturned the state's forced quarantine and reversed a court order however ordered that Kaci Hickox self-monitor, take her temperature daily and get travel approved by state officials. Governor LaPage (Maine) stated that the judge put Kaci Hickox rights above public safety. (Nicks 2014).

Systematic changes concerning quarantine in the state of New Jersey are intended to be a new guideline to be used for other states. These include the concern that forehead scanners can be inaccurate and an oral reading is preferable, right to communication, right to legal counsel prior to hearings, the right to privacy, as long these do not interfere with the needs of the public (Santora 2017).

### *14.2.2 Quarantine Strategy*

A good quarantine strategy would take into consideration all members of the public to include those under quarantine. It would ensure that when a quarantine is imposed,people have access to liberty and due process (Santora 2017), in addition to the basic necessities such as water and food. It would also be critical to ensure the people have access to health care that would curtail the spread of the communicable diseases to others within a population. The strengths of quarantine lie in the power of the state to impose it. However, the flip side of this is that it can be a weakness as it is important to have checks and balances such as a committee made up of multiple heads of institutions saddled with the responsibility of engaging those affected at various levels, rather than one person or entity making unilateral decisions. This would keep the balance of fairness. The United States has a federal law and institutions such as the Center for Disease Control (CDC) which have been authorized to take action in the event of quarantine. Africa now has an organization as the African Union and the CDC partnered to form the new Africa CDC (Africa CDC 2017). The strategy for Africa and quarantine is that it has to embody the African culture and must include stakeholder engagement. Failure to do so will result in a failed quarantine that could cost the public dearly.

#### 14.2.2.1 Community Engagement

It is important to consider community engagement during an outbreak and most especially when quarantine is considered necessary, such as the case of West Point. Unfortunately, most national governments easily engage the military to reinforce quarantine, without considering sensitizing the affected communities on the value and importance of the exercise. Lack of community and stakeholder sensitization can create tensions between the government and the affected community, human rights activities and civil societies who may resist a potentially beneficial intervention. Community engagement should be considered to avoid unnecessary tension. The World Health Organization Country representative for Liberia had previously advised that community consent was necessary prior to the quarantine of West Point. However, this was not sought by the Liberian government, thereby contributing to the civil unrest.

#### 14.2.2.2 Other Ethical Considerations

Professionals working in field of healthcare have an immense responsibility to act professionally whether they work with individual patients or with populations or communities. Professional ethics is part and parcel of the duty of professionals in the domain who are responsible for those who have entrusted the professionals with their health. This is a complex field to navigate most especially because there is no current framework for ethics in public health (Wilson and Mabhala 2009; Kass 2001). There is a risk of the transfer of deadly infectious disease, as was seen with the Severe Acute Respiratory Syndrome (SARS) in 2013 and the 2014 EVD outbreak in West Africa. This risk, also carries with it the possibility of threats of bioterrorism, by nature (Tognotti 2013).

**Stigma and Shame** In Africa, another ethical consideration of quarantine is related to the associated stigma of those who are quarantined. For example, survivors of EVD in West Africa were initially ostracized and shunned by their own community members, and in some cases by their own families. Survivors often experienced psychosocial trauma such as feelings of guilt, isolation and shame, as well as stigmatization. Survivors were also frequently attacked, evicted and threatened by community members. Many were excluded from their communities and their properties burned and destroyed because the communities believed they still harboured the deadly virus and could infect others.

**Right to Life** Should citizens of more affluent countries be given priority by their countries and saved from the burden of disease by being airlifted out of a grave situation, whilst others are unable to get basic treatment and left to die? (Kass 2014). This individualistic view examines considerations that focus on autonomy while public health ethics supports the rights of the community. Essentially, everyone has a right to life. While the experience of life differs dramatically between different contexts, there is a general appreciation that optimal quality of life should comprize of a healthy life, free from disease, including any form of physical and psychological distress. Against this backdrop, every human being, regardless of their socioeconomic background, ought to have an optimal life experience. Health care provides a means towards restoring the divergent quality of life to its optimal standard. Unfortunately, this was never the case during the EVD outbreak. The outbreak saw numerous cases where individuals from specific nationals received preferential treatment over others. Thus, individuals from well-resourced countries, those who were affluent or who came from wealthy families were more likely to receive the best quality of health care compared to the poor black persons from resource-poor countries where the health systems were already dilapidated and severely constrained. In fact, it is fair to say that the outbreak exposed the pathetic disparities that exist between the well resourced and poor resourced countries and individuals more profound.

**Culture and Traditions** Survivors of EVD were stigmatized, in part because cultural beliefs such as the concept of having been bewitched, brought by those who were afflicted, affected survivors and their families(Van Bortel et al. 2016).It is clear that the African perception of a personhood or self, lies within how or where that persona can be found. Since there are no logs or manuscripts chronicling the journey of self, persona and humanness; disease and death, this can only be found in African philosophy and evidenced by the way the African people live and breathe, the essence of African "ness" and how they perceive themselves. Although traditional African societies have been eroded by the Western values, health had a high value and this value was what made other avenues in life possible (Tangwa 2000). Quarantine within the West African context also falls right in the middle of treading within the delicate balance of tradition and cultural, vis-a-vis public health. For example, the way Africans perceive the concept of health and illness, death and the dying and personhood, as a whole differ, significantly from the public health construct, which borrows heavily from the western epistemology. Despite its good intentions, quarantine is likely to create tensions with individual rights as well as general African culture and traditions.

## 14.3 Government Blunders

The Liberian government made several blunders, the first recorded one concerning quarantine was the case of Patrick Sawyer, outlined above. Sawyer was able to travel to Nigeria when he was supposed to have been on the no-fly list, under observation and in self-quarantine. This mistake which could have been corrected at several pointsprior to Sawyer's leaving Liberia and his arrival in Nigeria. This error, put the people of Lagos metropolis at high risk of EVD, causing the infection of 20 people out of whomeightdied.

In Monrovia, 17 patients escaped from a holding center for suspected EVD patients. After the escape, the Liberian government through the Ministry of Information, claimed the patients were rounded up and taken to the John Fitzgerald Kennedy Hospital; a claim which a doctor at the hospital denied. The quarantine of West Point was also a disaster with the use of force; batons, sticks and teargas as well as bullets, to control the rioting by the unarmed residents. This led to some human rights activist expressing dismay at the unjustified shooting of a teenager in an epidemic situation. This show of force was totally unwarranted (MacDougall 2014).

## 14.4 Conclusion

Public health ethics is geared towards communities and populations, unlike medical ethics which supports the rights of individuals (Kass, 2001). Ethical considerations related to public health can be seen through two main views. These views are from that of the healthcare worker and the associated professionality of that worker. Ethical considerations in regards to public health and the practice of quarantine primarily centers on the loss of freedom for the individual being quarantined. West Africa is a region that is susceptible to emerging infectious diseases. It is crucial that the region examines its surveillance system, restrictions concerning biological specimens, and has a true model to ensure that fairness and equity prevails. The quarantine of West Point under military guard is an example of how leaders make decisions against international advice, out of fear and disregard for people of lower economic classes who are helpless and do not have a voice. The decision to impose a mandatory, military enforced quarantine at a time of such fear; interrupted livelihoods of people who were already at a serious economic disadvantage some of whom are yet to recover. A lot has happened in the field of Public health since the Ebola outbreak of 1976, in the Central African nation of Zaire (now known as the Democratic Republic of the Congo), in a remote rainforest and a village known as Yambuku, when Peter Piot discovered the Ebola virus and provided epidemiological evidence of the path of the virus. (Boseley 2014). The examples shared in this chapter, show how an outbreak can spill over to neighbouring towns, villages and countries, like the situation with both Patrick Sawyer who flew to Lagos, Nigeria and Thomas Duncan who flew to Texas, United States.

Professionals, working in field of healthcare and public health have an immense responsibility to act professionally whether they work with and treat patients individually or if they are public health professionals dealing with populations of people in communities, regions or at a national level. Professional ethics is part and parcel of the duty of professionals in the domain who are responsible for those who have entrusted the professionals with their health. This is a complex field to navigate most especially because there is no current framework for ethics in public health. (Wilson and Mabhala 2009; Kass 2001). There is a very real risk of the transfer of deadly infectious disease, as was seen with the Severe Acute Respiratory Syndrome (SARS) in 2013 and the 2014 EVD outbreak in West Africa. This risk, also carries with it the possibility of threats that are bioterrorist by nature (Tognotti 2013).

## References


Africa Center for Disease Control. (2017). Retrieved from https://www.au.int/web/en/africacdc. Accessed 21 Dec 2017.

Aginam, O. (2002). International law and communicable diseases. *Bulletin of the World Health Organization, 80*(12), 946–951.

Bever, L. (2014). *After ebola scare, some cruise ship passengers kept out of Oklahoma school*. Washington: WP Company LLC d/b/a. The Washington Post.

Boseley, S. (2014). Stories of 2014: Peter Piot: The scientist who helped to raise the alarm over ebola. *The Guardian (London, England).*

Butty, J. (2014). *Liberia's ebola quarantine affecting livelihoods*. Lanham: Federal Information & News Dispatch, Inc.

Center for Disease Control (CDC). (n.d.). Retrieved from https://www.cdc.gov/quarantine/history-quarantine.html. Accessed 21 Dec 2017.

Jaffe, S. (2014). US federal health agencies questioned over ebola response. *The Lancet, 384*(9953), 1489–1490.

Kass, N. E. (2001). An ethics framework for public health. *American Journal of Public Health, 91*(11), 1776–1782. https://doi.org/10.2105/AJPH.91.11.1776.

Kass, N. (2014). Ebola, ethics, and public health: What's next? *Annals of Internal Medicine, 161*(10), 744–745.

Kominski, G. F. (2014). *Changing the U.S. healthcare system: Key issues in health services policy and management* (4th ed.). San Francisco: Jossey-Bass. ISBN: 9781118128916.

MacDougall, C. (2014). Liberian governments blunders pile up in the grip of Ebola. *Time Magazine*. http://time.com/3247089/liberia-west-point-quarantine-monrovia/. Accessed 21 Dec 2017.

Mai-Duc, C. (2014). Suspected U.S. Ebola victim in Nigeria had planned to visit Minnesota. *LA Times.*

Moyer, J. (2014). *Ebola victim Thomas Eric Duncan's family has settled with Dallas hospital*. Washington: WP Company LLC d/b/a. The Washington Post. http://search.proquest.com.library.capella.edu/docview/1624819213?accountid=27965. Accessed 21 Dec 2017.

Nicks, D. (2014). Time Magazine. Health. http://time.com/3550960/ebola-quarantine-maine-kaci-hickox/. Accessed 9 July 2018.

Santora, M. (2017). *New York Times*. https://www.nytimes.com/2017/07/27/nyregion/new-jersey-accepts-rights-for-people-in-quarantine-to-end-ebola-suit.html. Accessed 9 July 2018.

Sherwood, D., Jenkins, C. (2014). Nurse Kaci Hickox and the state of Maine settle quarantine lawsuit. *Scientific American*. https://www.scientificamerican.com/article/nurse-kaci-hickox-and-state-of-maine-settle-quarantine-lawsuit/. Accessed 9 July 2018.

Tangwa, G. B. (2000). The traditional African perception of a person: Some implications for bioethics. *The Hastings Center Report, 30*(5), 39–43.

Tognotti, E. (2013). Lessons from the history of quarantine, from plague to influenza A. *Emerging Infectious Diseases, 19*(2), 254–259.

Usborne, D. (2014). *Atlanta hospital receives hate mail for treating aid workers stricken by Ebola*. http://www.independent.co.uk/news/world/americas/atlanta-hospital-receives-hate-mail-for-treating-aid-workers-stricken-by-ebola-9645199.html. Accessed 21 Dec 2017.

Van Bortel, T., Basnayake, A., Wurie, F., Jambai, M., Koroma, A. S., Muana, A. T., & Nellums, L. B. (2016). Psychosocial effects of an Ebola outbreak at individual, community and international levels. *Bulletin of the World Health Organization, 94*(3), 210.

Wilson, F., & Mabhala, M. (2009). *Key concepts in public health*. London: Sage. ISBN: 9781412948807.

World Population Review. (n.d.). Lagos Population. Retrieved from http://worldpopulationreview.com/world-cities/lagos/

Wynia, M. K. (2007). Ethics and public health emergencies: Restrictions on liberty. *The American Journal of Bioethics, 7*(2), 1–5.

# Chapter 15
# Scientific Response to Deadly Novel Epidemics: The Role of Good Clinical Practice

**Francis K. Kombe, Jennyfer Ambe, Gibril Ndow, and Korlia Bonarwolo**

## 15.1 Introduction

It has been argued that participation in biomedical research is above and beyond the call of duty. As such, individuals and communities have an obligation to participate in biomedical research, as a public good (Schaefer et al. 2009). On the other hand, those who participate in research are exposed to different levels of harm. To ensure optimal protection to those involved in research, several universal guidelines, including the Nuremberg code, the Declaration of Helsinki, Belmonte report and the Council for International Organizations of Medical Sciences (CIOMS) were developed and ratified, following the infamous German Nazi experiments (Department of Health 2014; Macrae 2007). The International Conference on Harmonization (ICH) Good Clinical Practice (GCP) guideline was developed with a focus to protect the rights of human subjects participating in clinical trials and to ensure the scientific validity and credibility of the data collected in human clinical studies (Dixon 1999; Guerra 2011; International

F. K. Kombe (✉)
African Research Integrity Network (ARIN), Kilifi, Kenya

J. Ambe
Global Emerging Pathogens Treatment Initiative, Mainland Hospital, Lagos, Nigeria

Department of Public Health, School of Nursing and Health Sciences, Capella University, Minneapolis, MN, USA

G. Ndow
Medical Research Council Unit The Gambia at London School of Hygiene & Tropical Medicine, Banjul, The Gambia

Institute of Global Health Innovation, Division of Integrative Systems Medicine & Digestive Diseases, Faculty of Medicine, Imperial College London, London, UK

K. Bonarwolo
Global Emerging Pathogens Treatment Initiative, Mainland Hospital, Lagos, Nigeria



G. B. Tangwa et al. (eds.), *Socio-cultural Dimensions of Emerging Infectious Diseases in Africa*, https://doi.org/10.1007/978-3-030-17474-3_15

Conference on Harmonization of Technical Requirements for the Registration of Pharmaceuticals for Human Use 1996). Unfortunately, its development focused on clinical trials conducted in the United States, Europe, and Japan. As such, despite being an international guideline, its application in other regions of the world, has often failed to match the ground realities of conducting research in different context, such as Africa and other resource-poor settings, where resources are severely constrained and the socioeconomic status and level of education grossly limited. This situation may further be exacerbated in a disease outbreak, such as the Ebola outbreak in West Africa. This chapter seeks to discuss whether GCP could be used to adequately protect potential research participants during a dangerous disease outbreak.

## 15.2 The Story of Mama Kadzo

Mama Kadzo, the mother of 8 children, returns home late evening to find her youngest daughter Matsezi, aged four, lying in the tiny, wooden family bed with her body feeling unusually hot and shivering. It is not unusual for Mama Kadzo to return home from her casual day jobs and find one of her eight children complaining of a headache or chills. Her usual response is to run to the nearest retail shop in her neighbourhood for a maramoja tablet, a common brand of painkiller that she would crash and give to the child to take with some water. Then the following morning before leaving the house in search of another casual job, she would normally touch the cheek of the sick child with the back of her hand to see if they were still running a temperature. If they were, Mama Kadzo would give them another dose of maramoja before dashing out of the house in search of another casual job that would guarantee the family some ugali to be served with whatever edible leaves the neighbouring bush would provide in the evening.

On this particular evening, Mama Kadzo found Matsezi's body extremely hot! She gave her the usual dose of maramoja and supervised her feed with the rest of the children. Matsezi, unfortunately, vomited her meal almost immediately, prompting Mama Kadzo to monitor her closely all night, checking her temperature and observing her movements as she slept. This was especially important to ensure Matsezi's condition did not deteriorate while Mama Kadzo was fast asleep, owing to how tired she was that day given that she had been lucky to be allowed to work in a newly established construction site just a few kilometres from her home.

It was about 4.30 am when the call for the Fajr *prayer* from the *Ustadh* at the nearest mosque rented the air. As is her usual habit, Mama Kadzo touched Matsezi by the cheek before gasping at how hot she felt. All the same, she said a short prayer then left the house for a short call. She had planned to return briefly to do her house chores before leaving for her casual job that day.

"Maama eeh, Maama eeh, Maama eeh!" the voice of Mkasi; Mama Kadzo's 15 year-old daughter, filled the air as the twilight sky was just about to give way to the rising sun. Mama Kadzo interrupted her short call and ran back to the tiny,

Makuti thatched house to find out what had suddenly gone wrong. True to her suspicion, she found Matsezi convulsing with her eyes rolled back and looking scary. "Oh Jesus Christ, what is wrong with you Matsezi?", Mama Kadzo lamented in shock as if Matsezi was able to respond.

### *15.2.1 Mama Kadzo Arrives at the Local Hospital*

In the wake of Mama Kadzo's confusion, coupled with wailing children, alarmed the neighbours who rushed to see what had befallen Mama Kadzo's home. A neighbour suggested taking Matsezi to the local county referral hospital and offered her motorcycle to carry Mama Kadzo and Matsezi to the hospital. They arrived at exactly 8.30 am and were immediately helped into the doctor's room by the motorbike rider and other patients who were concerned about Matsezi's condition. During the two-hour ride to the hospital, Matsezi had vomited and convulsed several times. The doctor reviewed and recommended to have Matsezi admitted in the paediatric ward, further worrying Mama Kadzo whose only hospital experience was the half-hour admission that preceded the death of her husband. Mama Kadzo's husband had broken his spine after falling from a *mnazi* (traditional palm tree) while taping palm wine and was pronounced dead, a few hours after being admitted. Before this day, Mama Kadzo had always taken any unwell child to the traditional healer in her neighbourhood instead of the hospital. The whole hospital scene was therefore scary and intimidating for Mama Kadzo.

### *15.2.2 Invitation to Participate in a Drug Trial*

When they arrived at the hospital's paediatric ward, Mama Kadzo was approached by a nurse named Ningoma who directed them to an unoccupied bed and asked her to undress Matsezi. Sister Ningoma then took a few vital signs including body temperature, weight, oxygen levels, blood sugar, and a blood sample. She encouraged Mama Kadzo to stay calm as a doctor was going to be with her shortly and that all would be done to take care of her child. Given the circumstances, these words were very reassuring to Mama Kadzo. She finally sat patiently and waited for further direction from the next person. The ward was full, and she could not help looking at what other parents were going through as they cared for their children. Even as she wondered about what was going to happen to her sick child, her mind drifted and started thinking about her children and what would happen to them during the period she would be nursing Matsezi in the ward. Endless questions lingered on her mind as she nervously waited for the doctor, *"Who will take care of them?, who will bring food to them?, who will take the goats out of the house today?, tomorrow?, the next day....? who will ensure their safety?"*

In a neighbouring bed, a sick child was gasping for breath in a flurry of activity, as the child's mother and nurses helplessly struggled to keep her alive. It was a terribly frightening experience, for a little one to be struggling to live, yet death was at her door. Parents are supposed to die before their children, thought Mama Kadzo. More thoughts of sick children, most especially Matsezi and what would become of her flooded her mind. Mama Kadzo tried her best to think positively and remain optimistic but death was right before her eyes.

*"What is this sickness that is stealing our children?, why are people dying and you are not saving them?"* wailed the mother who just lost her little girl. "Please help us save our children, they should not die before us!"Mama Kadzo was brought back to reality by a *"Hello Mama Matsezi"*, greeting that came from a neatly dressed young man who introduced himself as Mr. Tinde. Mr. Tinde's voice, after the traumatic experience, was calming. She felt that her wait was over and there was finally some help. Mr. Tinde went on to say he was a fieldworker interested in talking to Mama Kadzo about the condition of Matsezi. Worried but reassured, a ray of hope pierced her heart as she sat upright to listen to Mr. Tinde's message. "Yes, doctor, what is wrong with my child? Will she be well? When do you think we can be discharged?" Mama Kadzo's inquisitive voice rented the room.

Mr. Tinde emphasized that all would be done to help baby Matsezi. He, however, informed her that from the initial investigations, Matsezi had been found to be suffering from a severe, highly fatal disease that had no known treatment. There was, however, an ongoing research at the county referral hospital trying to find if a new drug was an effective cure for the disease and he would like to invite Mama Kadzo to be part of a group of individuals who would volunteer as part of this trial. Mr. Tinde further explained that children enrolled in the study would be in two groups, one group receiving the new drug being investigated and the other group not receiving the new drug. Neither the researchers nor Mama Kadzo would know which arm of the research Matsezi would be randomly allocated. Participating in the research, he said, would help investigators and the country at large find a cure for this dangerous and deadly disease.

*"Do you agree to participate in this trial or do you have any questions or concerns that you would like me to address?"* posed Mr Tinde as he waited for Mama Kadzo's response.

*"Eeeeeh? No, it is okay. I don't have any questions. All I want is my child to get better so I can get out of this place as soon as I can. I am ready doctor… I am fine. It's OK, go ahead and give my daughter whatever drug that you can give her to assist her"*, said Mama Kadzo.At this point, a neatly typewritten form was presented to Mama Kadzo. Mr. Tinde read each section of the form, asked if Mama Kadzo had any further questions, and then asked her to sign the consent form that would effectively enrol Matsezi to participate in the clinical trial to find a cure for this new deadly infectious disease!

## 15.3 What Is the Role of Ethics and Good Clinical Practices in Guiding Scientific Response to Deadly Novel Epidemics?

Mama Kadzo's story reflects what thousands and thousands of people, especially in Africa, are likely to experience in the wake of an epidemic. To date, the world has experienced more than 200 epidemics, with the first documented epidemic having occurred over 700 years ago.[1] Despite such a long history, epidemics almost always strike when least expected, at times when levels of preparedness are lowest. Consequently, most epidemics cause merciless deaths and immeasurable suffering, sometimes wiping over 90 percent of the affected population. The worst epidemic ever to happen in the world killed around 100 million people, constituting over 60 percent of the population in Europe at the time. Because of the untimely and fatal nature of epidemics, they are usually compounded with a lot of fear, anxiety and reactionary decisions. In most cases health systems are taken by surprise and significantly overwhelmed, often resulting in delayed or inefficient responses and reactions aimed at "putting out fires". On the other hand, communities become vulnerable and over-dependent on the limited resources offered by the government. Where no effective response strategy is agreed upon in time, communities quickly lose trust and confidence in their governments and health care systems, resulting in discontent, name calling and blame games.

### *15.3.1 The Role of Clinical Research During an Epidemic*

The critical role which clinical research can play in finding immediate and long-term solutions for an epidemic cannot be overemphasized. Clinical research plays an important and inevitable role in identifying new interventions and establishing the safety and effectiveness of such interventions. Randomized controlled clinical trials have often been described as the gold standard to answer important scientific and health care questions (Odom et al. 2005; Victora et al. 2004). However, in order for the results from such studies to be trustworthy, reproducible and reliable, it is important that such studies both employ scientifically sound methodologies as well as adhere to international ethical standards and Good Clinical Practice (GCP), collectively known as Good Clinical Research Practice (Guerra 2011; ICH 2016; International Conference on Harmonization of Technical Requirements for the Registration of Pharmaceuticals for Human Use 1996).

According to the World Health Organization (WHO), Good Clinical Research Practice is a process that involves the use of internationally established ethical and scientific quality standards for the design, conduct, recording and reporting of clinical research involving the participation of human subjects (World Health

[1] https://en.wikipedia.org/wiki/List_of_epidemics

Organization 2005). Researchers who comply with GCP guidelines are more likely to respect the rights and well-being of research participants hence promote trust in research enterprise and ensure a high level of research integrity.

### *15.3.2 Why Is It Important to Adhere to GCP Guidelines When Conducting Research During an Epidemic?*

Epidemics are characterised by fear and anxiety. In Mama Kadzo's case, for example, witnessing the death of a child in the paediatrics ward followed by Matsezi's being diagnosed with the same fatal incurable illness was overwhelming. For many in her position, the extreme fear of losing their loved one makes them vulnerable. The additional concerns about the welfare of her other children at home and her previous hospital experience made her even more desperate. Mama Kadzo knew very well that the chances of surviving a serious illness were very slim in this rural health setting with poor facilities, inadequate resources and frequent stock-outs of essential medication.

In addition, those who are well equally fear for the unknown; as they may be afraid of getting infected with the killer bug due to the increased burden of caring for their relatives.

Depending on the severity of the disease, its mode of transmission and fatality, an epidemic can cause significant alarm in neighbouring communities, entire regions or even globally. Inevitably, serious epidemics with the potential of affecting large populations quickly become newsworthy. The ensuing media coverage, if controlled effectively, can be used to address prevailing concerns and educate the public about protective and rapid response measures. Unfortunately, information in the media (especially in social media) are often compounded with rumours and misconceptions about the epidemic, creating unnecessary fear and inciting mass panic both in the general public as well as among trained healthcare personnel.

It is in this type of situation that generates fear for potential exploitation of those who are eligible to participate in clinical trials. For example, potential research participants may not have the capacity to internalize and comprehend the information given to them during the consent process. This may be because they may be mentally unstable or they may be too desperate to do anything that offers them any little hope of living one extra day.

Mama Kadzo gave consent for Matsezi to participate in the clinical trial when she clearly; based on the comment she made, did not understand what exactly was going on and what Matsezi would go through, most probably as a result of the anxiety she herself was experiencing. Mama Kadzo's story is very similar to what many potential research participants are likely to go through when being involved in research during an epidemic. Situations may arise when the conditions under study are so severe that the index research participant is rendered incapable of giving a true informed consent. In such circumstances, proxy consent from the closest relative, including the spouse or legal guardian/representative may be sought. Either way, when individuals have to make decisions in an environment that is compounded with such extreme fear and anxiety, it is unlikely that such decisions would be rational. It, therefore, may be of little difference to obtain consent from a proxy. It is difficult to imagine that participation in that circumstance would be purely voluntary. Indeed, the concept of voluntariness is one of the most important ethical aspects related to the principle of autonomy or respect for persons in research (Grant and Sugarman 2004). According to Robert Nelson et al., voluntariness encompasses two necessary and jointly sufficient conditions, including intentional action and the absence of controlling influences (Nelson et al. 2011). In their arguments, Robert Nelson et al. described voluntariness in terms of the degree of control an individual has over his or her own behaviour. Other international guidelines, including the Nuremberg code also put emphasis on the ability for a research subject to maintain a free power of choice, without the intervention of any element of force, fraud, deceit, duress, over-reaching, or other ulterior form of constraint or coercion" (Nelson et al. 2011; Weindling 2004). In the situation described above, there is a high possibility that a participant or/and their legal representatives who give proxy consent might insist on participation because they are feeling helpless, hopeless and desperate, which is expected especially when there are no existing alternative options.

Having said that, it is also important to note that an epidemic may offer unique and sometimes the only opportunity for testing new products and therapies. This is due to their untimeliness and sometimes, an acute prevalence that may last for only a few days, weeks or months. Because of this, researchers involved in testing products and interventions during an epidemic intervention are prone to potential conflict of interest. For example, a researcher might be extremely desperate to get enough participants before the epidemic weans. It is this paradox of the-desperate-participant-and-the-desperate-researcher, that calls for the need to ensure clinical trials strictly follow international principles of GCP and that Research Ethics Committees (REC) are extremely keen when reviewing protocols for clinical trials to ensure research participants are adequately protected and researchers remain as objective as possible.

Thus, Good Clinical Practice guideline is the clinical trial researchers' "Bible" that prescribes the ethical and scientific "Fourteen Commandments" in the conduct of clinical research. By following the principles of GCP, researchers ensure that their actions are driven by rationality and not their emotions which are likely to be subjective and biased at such times. On the other hand, adhering to the principles of GCP ensures that research participants will be respected and protected, will not be exposed to undue risk, and that the integrity of the data collected will be assured. As stated in the WHO, GCP guidelines 2002, "adhering to the principles of GCP does not only serves the interests of the researchers but also protects the rights, safety and well-being of subjects and ensures that investigations are scientifically sound and advance public health goals" (World Health Organization 2005).

One of the most important features of GCP guidelines is that apart from being informative to researchers during research planning and protocol development, it clearly spells out the responsibilities of all stakeholders in a clinical trial planning and execution. These include the sponsors, clinical investigators, Independent Ethics Committees/Institutional Review Boards [IECs/IRBs], monitors and contract research organizations [CROs). In addition, the guidelines provide for what needs to be put in place prior, during and after the clinical trials. For example, the guidelines put a lot of emphasis on risk identification, ensuring appropriate study design, use of statistical methodology and selection of the study population during the development of the protocol. There is also a lot of emphasis on the development of Standard Operating Procedures, such as, informed consent, quality assurance, monitoring and recording of Severe Adverse Events (SAE) and ensuring there are enough tools to facilitate the conduct of a quality, clinical trial. Other areas that the guidelines put a lot of emphasis on include Safety management and reporting; Quality assurance of the trial performance and data; Enrolment of subjects into the study, including recruitment, eligibility, and informed consent; Reporting the trial; Management of the investigational products, including quality, handling and accounting; regulatory and ethical approval of the protocols, qualification and training of the clinical trial staff among others.

According to the WHO GCP guidelines 2002, all clinical trials must adhere to 14 principles of GCP. These principles include; (1) the need for research involving humans to be scientifically sound and conducted according to the basic ethical principles i.e. respect for persons, beneficence, and justice; (2) the need for research involving humans to be scientifically justified and described in a clear, detailed protocol; (3) the need to identify any foreseeable risks and discomforts and any anticipated benefits for individual research participants as well as the society prior to the initiation of the clinical trial; (4)the need for research involving humans to be initiated only if the anticipated benefits for individual research participants and society outweigh the risks; (5) the need for research involving humans to receive independent ethics committee/institutional review board (IEC/IRB) approval/favourable opinion prior to initiation; (6) the need for research involving humans to be conducted in compliance with the approved protocol; (7) the need to obtain informed consent from every research participant prior to research participation; (8) the need for research involving humans to be continued only if the benefit-risk profile remains favourable; (9) the need for research involving humans to be conducted by qualified and duly licensed medical personnel who should take responsibility of the medical care of research participants; (10) the need for research involving humans to be carried out by individuals who are qualified and licensed (where necessary) by education, training, and experience to perform their respective task; (11) the need to ensure all clinical trial information is recorded, handled, and stored in a way that allows its accurate reporting, interpretation, and verification; (12) the need to ensure confidentiality of records that could identify research participants is protected; (13) the need to ensure investigational products are manufactured, handled, and stored in accordance with applicable Good Manufacturing Practice (GMP) and used in accordance with the approved protocol and finally (14) the need to ensure systems with procedures that assure the quality of every aspect of the trial are implemented.

While the GCP guidelines provide a very systematic tool to protect participants and promote ethical conduct as well as the integrity and quality of data in clinical trials, it is easy to notice that the guidelines are premised on an ideal scenario where there is prior systematic development of the protocol, review and approval before implementation and close-up of the clinical trial. Unfortunately, epidemics leave little room for such systematic planning and implementation. As alluded to above, during an epidemic, the environment becomes messy, systems break down and everyone is thrown in a panicky and reactionary mood. And more often than not, this situation affects every stakeholder in the research enterprise. Moreover, such a situation can easily get out of hand and control if there weren't already systems in place to guide the process.

Thus, while GCP provides an extremely important tool through which clinical trials can be reviewed, approved, get quality assurance and monitored for scientific and ethical soundness, it is equally important to appreciate that the reality on the ground during an epidemic is very delicate to allow for such a systematic and smooth flow. There is, therefore, a need to compliment the good principles of GCP with locally applicable approaches that can strengthen the conduct of clinical trials under such a sensitive environment. In fact, it is fair to say that it is high time the current GCP guidelines were revised to take into account new and emerging trends in the research enterprise. For example, the current GCP guidelines are strikingly silent on approaches that have recently been described as a cornerstone to the successful implementation of clinical trials, especially in Africa. Approaches such as the use of different models of community consultation and engagement have been seen to add both intrinsic and instrument value in the conduct of clinical trials (Marsh et al. 2008; Weijer and Emanuel 2000; Folayan et al. 2015). In addition to adhering to all the principles prescribed in the guidelines, involving the community, explaining the research to people who are prone to infection and getting their buy-in to conduct the research would not only ensure that community concerns are addressed in the planning and implementation of the research, but would also ensure that trust in the study and the research team is build. Although this process should not replace the informed consent process, support or resistance for a clinical trial from the larger community may give a strong indication on whether or not it is acceptable to carry out such kind of a study in the community and can serve as a benchmark for obtaining informed consent from those who get infected during the epidemic.

The big question is, at what point should community consultation get conducted? To this end, we propose a three-tier approval process. In some African settings, for example, clinical trials are approved by the relevant regulatory authority after conditional approval from the Research Ethics Committees (RECs). In the same manner, RECs could be allowed to give conditional approval that would give permission to the clinical research team to conduct rapid community consultations and engagement and submit the report to the REC before full approval is granted. This way, community consultation and engagement would become an integral part of conducting clinical trials, which would go a long way, not only to address fears and concerns from the community in a more neutral environment (i.e. before one is infected and admitted to a hospital); but would greatly contribute in strengthening the informed consent process, that is marred by a lot of uncertainty, tensions and fears when conducted in a hospital setting, during an epidemic. Doing this would take into account the traditional views, culture and expectation of the community in the consenting process. This process could also provide a unique opportunity to sensitize the community about the disease in question, fill in important knowledge gaps, which is common during a novel epidemic. If we take the example of Mama Kadzo for example, the situation could have been different if she had prior knowledge about the epidemic and what to expect on admission. Deliberate efforts to share vital information about the disease could help in addressing potential fears and anxiety that affect effective communication and hinder true informed consenting process when recruiting research participants in an epidemic. In doing this, it is also important to appreciate the importance of multi-sectoral collaboration and partnership during an epidemic. Partners' efforts, for example, while sensitizing the community about the epidemic, the Ministry of Health (MOH) personnel may use the opportunity to share information about any planned clinical research studies, so long as they are well informed about such studies. In other words, the process of community consultation and engagements should be as inclusive as possible so that all key stakeholders are aware and well informed hence can be used to complement the efforts of the clinical research teams in building trust and getting the community informed about the clinical study in advance. It is particularly important to ensure that communities understand that there is no direct or immediate benefit to participant in clinical studies conducted during an epidemic.

## 15.4 Conclusion

Finally, it is important to realize that epidemics place a disproportionate burden on the poor of the poorest people and countries. According to Ruth Faden of Johns Hopkins University, this poses the greatest moral challenge, especially with regards to how to respect commitments to social justice in the face of the overwhelming and entrenched inequalities (Dickens and Cook 2003). It is therefore important to ensure that the poorest and vulnerable are dully protected and that those affected by an epidemic are involved in planning and developing principles and policies that uphold the rights and interests of disadvantaged groups and in deciding how such principles can be included in planning for strategic responses against the epidemic.

**Disclaimer** All names used in this chapter are fictitious and therefore do not belong to any particular individuals. They are however common Mijikenda names, hence some people may relate to them within the Mijikenda community context. Obtaining consent from such individual is therefore not applicable.

## References

Department of Health. (2014). The Belmont report. Ethical principles and guidelines for the protection of human subjects of research. *The Journal of the American College of Dentists, 81*(3), 4.

Dickens, B. M., & Cook, R. J. (2003). Challenges of ethical research in resource-poor settings. *International Journal of Gynecology & Obstetrics, 80*(1), 79–86.

Dixon, J. R. (1999). The international conference on harmonization good clinical practice guideline. *Quality Assurance, 6*(2), 65–74.

Folayan, M. O., Peterson, K., & Kombe, F. (2015). Ethics, emergencies and Ebola clinical trials: The role of governments and communities in offshored research. *The Pan African Medical Journal, 22*. https://doi.org/10.11694/pamj.supp.2015.22.1.6216.

Grant, R. W., & Sugarman, J. (2004). Ethics in human subjects research: Do incentives matter? *Journal of Medicine and Philosophy, 29*(6), 717–738.

Guerra, S. Á. (2011). Harmonization of quality standards for clinical trials. ISO-9001 standard and guide of good clinical practice. *Armonización de Estándares de Calidad Para Ensayos Clínicos. Norma ISO 9001-Guía de Buena Práctica Clínica.*

ICH. (2016). E6 (R2) Guideline for good clinical practice. *Guidance*. https://doi.org/10.1056/NEJMp1012246.

International Conference on Harmonization of Technical Requirements for the Registration of Pharmaceuticals for Human Use. (1996). ICH E6 guideline for good clinical practice. *ICH Harmonised Tripartite Guideline*. https://doi.org/10.1056/NEJMp1012246.

Macrae, D. J. (2007). The Council for International Organizations and Medical Sciences (CIOMS) guidelines on ethics of clinical trials. *Proceedings of the American Thoracic Society, 4*(2), 176–179.

Marsh, V., Kamuya, D., Rowa, Y., Gikonyo, C., & Molyneux, S. (2008). Beginning community engagement at a busy biomedical research programme: Experiences from the KEMRI CGMRC-Wellcome Trust research programme, Kilifi, Kenya. *Social Science & Medicine, 67*(5), 721–733.

Nelson, R. M., Beauchamp, T., Miller, V. A., Reynolds, W., Ittenbach, R. F., & Luce, M. F. (2011). The concept of voluntary consent. *The American Journal of Bioethics, 11*(8), 6–16.

Odom, S. L., Brantlinger, E., Gersten, R., Horner, R. H., Thompson, B., & Harris, K. R. (2005). Research in special education: Scientific methods and evidence-based practices. *Exceptional Children, 71*(2), 137–148.

Schaefer, G. O., Emanuel, E. J., & Wertheimer, A. (2009). The obligation to participate in biomedical research. *JAMA, 302*(1), 67–72.

Victora, C. G., Habicht, J.-P., & Bryce, J. (2004). Evidence-based public health: Moving beyond randomized trials. *American Journal of Public Health, 94*(3), 400–405.

Weijer, C., & Emanuel, E. J. (2000). Protecting communities in biomedical research. *Science, 289*(5482), 1142–1144.

World Health Organization. (2005). Handbook for good clinical research practice (GCP): Guidance for implementation.

# Chapter 16
# Scientific Response to Deadly Novel Epidemics: The Role of Health Research Ethics

**Francis K. Kombe, Jennyfer Ambe, and Gibril Ndow**

## 16.1 Introduction: Ethical Considerations During an Epidemic

Bioethics is an important inter-disciplinary and rapidly emerging field. The concept of biomedical ethics emanates from the process of doing right and good action in the biological and medical setting (Veatch 1999). In general, ethics has been defined as the moral principles governing or influencing conduct. *Ethics* is the science of criteria, norms, and values for human action and conduct (Beauchamp and Childress 2001). It is engaged in reflection and analysis of morals concerning whether an act is good or bad and how it influences our basic quest for meaning, our search for humanity, and our attempt to create a humane society (Engelhardt 2011). Its intention is to safeguard human dignity and to promote justice, equality, truth, and trust. On the other hand, *Medical ethics* is not only about the moral behaviour of clinicians, but about ethics and health care (Andorno 2009; Jacobson 2007). It can be described as a reflection on moral actions within the framework of health care. Its objective is to promote health, to care, to heal, to alleviate pain, and to prevent suffering (Jacobson 2007).

F. K. Kombe (✉)
African Research Integrity Network (ARIN), Kilifi, Kenya

J. Ambe
Global Emerging Pathogens Treatment Initiative, Mainland Hospital, Lagos, Nigeria

Department of Public Health, School of Nursing and Health Sciences, Capella University, Minneapolis, MN, USA

G. Ndow
Medical Research Council Unit The Gambia at London School of Hygiene & Tropical Medicine, Banjul, The Gambia

Institute of Global Health Innovation, Division of Integrative Systems Medicine & Digestive Diseases, Faculty of Medicine, Imperial College London, London, UK

 
G. B. Tangwa et al. (eds.), *Socio-cultural Dimensions of Emerging Infectious Diseases in Africa*, https://doi.org/10.1007/978-3-030-17474-3_16

Major international guidelines for the conduct of medical research identify three universal principles which should guide the conduct of research. These include the principles of autonomy, beneficence/maleficence and justice (Department of Health, Education, and Welfare and National Commission for the Protection of Human Subjects of Biomedical and Behavioral Research 2014). Historically, these principles were developed following a series of inhumane medical research with the goal of safeguarding the rights and dignity of research participants.

In 1947, the Nuremberg Code was created as a result of the unethical experiments carried out during World War II at Nazi war camps by German physicians. Consequently, these physicians were tried and charged at the Nuremberg Military Tribunal. Ten codes were developed during the trial that set forth the ethical principles that guide the conduct of research involving humans (Code 1949). The Universal Declaration of Human Rights (December 10th 1948) was also adopted and proclaimed by the United Nations after the atrocities of World War II and it further reiterated the human factor involved in medical experiments (Howard-Jones 1986; Macrae 2007).

The Declaration of Helsinki was developed in 1964 by the World Medical Association (WMA) which put a lot of focus on the protection of the rights of human subjects. Subsequently, WMA developed the Declaration of Helsinki that involves ethical principles aimed at guiding physicians and other participants in medical research involving human subjects (Declaration 2013; World Medical Association 2008). The Declaration of Helsinki emphasises the duty of the physician to promote and safeguard the health of the people. In 1979, The Belmont Report was developed by the National Commission for Protection of Human Subjects of Biomedical and Behavioural Research which identified the three main ethical principles which have come to be known as the universal ethical principles and include (Department of Health, Education, and Welfare and National Commission for the Protection of Human Subjects of Biomedical and Behavioral Research 2014):

1. **Respect for Persons**: This principle acknowledges the dignity and freedom of every person. It requires obtaining informed consent from research subjects (or their legally authorised representatives)
2. **Beneficence**: This principle requires that researchers maximise benefits and minimise harms (non-maleficence) associated with research. Research-related risks must be reasonable in light of the expected benefits.
3. **Justice**: This principle requires equitable selection and recruitment and fair treatment of research subjects.

Worthy of note is that, although the development of the principles was well intended, their application in different contexts has been the subject of debate for several decades. Understandably, these debates have been well-intentioned, given the diversity of communities and circumstances where these principles are applied, including where there are huge power imbalances between researchers and research participants as well as deficiencies in health systems, huge health burden, economic disparities which expose communities involved in research to unique and varied forms of vulnerability that require more rigorous protection than provided for by the mainstream ethical framework.

Indeed, most of the ethical issues related to research in public health emergency situations are the same as those already addressed in general ethics guidelines governing biomedical research. Problems are however likely to arise with regards to perceptions of risks, benefits and trust which must be taken into account in the ethics review process; a heightened need for attention to organizational values like accountability and transparency; and the fact that, there may not be sufficient time for standard ethics review processes which in many countries can sometimes take months (Morrison et al. 2009). It is essential that clinical trials conducted during an emergency observe all the necessary ethical review processes. Importantly, oversight and regulatory authorities must be particularly keen to ensure research participants are not put under unreasonable risks and are adequately respected and protected. If there is any step that should be exempted or avoided, such a decision should rest on the appropriate regulatory authority or Research Ethics Committee (REC) instead of the individual researcher/Principal Investigator. On the other hand, regulatory authorities and RECs should come up with ways that will ensure a fast but good quality review is conducted before approval is granted.

Finally, there is a critical need to ensure REC members are adequately trained and that nations and regions have adequate capacity to conduct thorough ethics review. Existing gaps may be complimented through the use of novel methods of ethics review such as online review platform (www.rhinno.net), outsourcing of reviewers from external experts who have the knowledge, experience and expertise to carry out the required review and able to appreciate the urgency of the review. Importantly, Researchers, public health agencies and other stakeholders should work together to develop short courses, degree programmes and other training modalities aimed at building skills and capacity of local researchers and regulatory authorities to ensure optimum protection of research participants. For Africa where epidemics have the greatest impact, it is important to ensure that funding agencies direct appropriate support towards capacity building to ensure a timely and robust review is conducted during an epidemic.

## 16.2 Challenges with Mainstream Bioethics Frameworks

There is no doubt that mainstream ethical frameworks rely heavily on a western epistemology. For example, although aimed at protecting individuals involved in research, the principle of autonomy puts a lot of emphasis on an individual's ability to make a free and informed choice; and places the individual as an independent and autonomous agent. As such, it assumes that once the individual has been given all the necessary information, is deemed to be of sound mind and competent capacity to comprehend the information given; and makes an independent choice free of any influencing factors, then that individual's decision is deemed final. In her book *Moral Prejudices: Essays on ethics*: Harvard University Press; Baier (1995) notes that this approach assumes equalization of power. Unfortunately, it fails to take into account situations where some individuals may lack full autonomy because of certain positions, roles prescribed to them by the community or certain conditions that may make them feel powerless and unable to exercise their full autonomy. In such circumstances, applying the principle of autonomy in its strict form may not augur well with the tradition and expectation of such a community or make the particular individual any better, in exercising their autonomy. Furthermore, if bioethics is concerned with the moral principles associated with doing what is right or good, then it is important to appreciate that what is good or right depends on the context and what the people believe is right or good in that context. For example, it is acceptable all over the world that respecting people is generally a good thing. However, the way one community shows respect may differ greatly with how another community shows respect. This is true for many actions and behaviour in life, which may be acceptable in one community but remain unacceptable or even an abomination in another community.

According to the internet encyclopedia of philosophy, the traditional but deficient view concerning ethical reasoning and decision making in applied ethics is that one simply "applies" a particular ethical theory such as utilitarianism or deontology in a given context in order to solve the moral problem in question (Bacon et al. 2008). This top-down approach of ethical reasoning and decision making adheres to the idea that ethics is quite similar to geometry, in that it presupposes a solid foundation from which principles and general rules can be inferred and then applied to concrete cases independent of the details of the particular case. The locus of certitude, that is, the place of the greatest certainty for principle ethics---approaches using one master principle---concerns its foundation; the reasonableness of the ethical decision is passed on from the foundation itself.

**What Needs to Be Done?**

The above examples demonstrate how difficult it is to have universal bioethical principles. This calls for the need to develop an indigenous African framework that will take into account some of the context-specific issues related to conducting research in Africa. A few attempts have been made to develop or advocate for the development of more culturally sensitive guidelines, including Yoruba, indigenous groups in New Zealand, Canada and Australia and the Aboriginal communities.

This chapter presents a framework for ethical conduct of research in indigenous African contexts. We believe that this framework will be used to guide all researchers and research ethics committee on the best practices in conducting research in Africa.

**Why Is It Necessary to Have an Africa Indigenous Framework for Bioethics?**

According to Onuoha (2007), a bioethics framework is supposed to be a system that informs all bioethical practices and choices. In addition, it should guide ethical evaluations of the actions, decisions and policies of individuals, groups and organisations and must provide the ground for the articulation of duties, obligations, and expectations of those involved in making bioethical decisions (Onuoha 2007). Despite the existence of what is claimed to be universal bioethical rules and principles, these principles do not resonate with the holistic view held by African cultures (Chukwuneke et al. 2014; Onuoha 2007). For example, the way Africans perceive the concept of health and illness, death and the dying and personhood as a whole differs significantly with the western construction of the same. As such, biomedical ethical principles developed in the west have been known to be highly individualistic, with a strong leaning towards the western culture but failed to incorporate the pluralistic and communal nature that defines the majority of the Africa culture and epistemology. During an epidemic or any calamity for that matter, most African communities tend to be more cohesive and come together to offer moral support and demonstrate their togetherness and brotherhood. Such behaviour, while offering moral support might promote the spread of highly infectious diseases. Without this understanding, any principles applied in this context that might be seen to negate the prevalent African spirit might be construed to lack respect for the cultural values of the community and be divisive. Understanding this behaviour can lead to developing effective ways through which the community can be well engaged, feel respected and be more responsive to any proposed intervention during an epidemic.

The need to develop an indigenous African bioethics guideline is also informed by the process from which the universal principles were developed. In addition to the principles being individualistic and western-culture oriented, the process followed to develop these principles talks nothing about how Africa as a region or continent was involved. For example, major international guidelines on ethical conduct of research link the genesis of biomedical ethical principles to the infamous atrocities conducted in the early 1900 and during the First World War, including the Tuskegee and the Nazi experiments. Accordingly, during the trial of the Germany Nazi physicians, some 10 codes were identified as key in the conduct of research involving humans. These codes were later modified and developed to what came to be known as the universal ethical principles. Importantly, throughout the process, the contribution of African philosophers and experts in developing these codes is completely missing. In fact, the codes were developed during an era when Africa was still perceived as the "dark" continent, with absolutely nothing to offer in the process. Thus, the process assumes Africa as merely a recipient rather than an active and equal partner in developing the guidelines. This presumes Africans as a whole are at a disadvantage and unable to participate in the process. It is no wonder therefore that the codes do not take into account the African culture, value and epistemology.

There is no doubt that the African continent makes a significant contribution to the medical research field. Recent decades have seen a massive increase in the number of studies and clinical trials being conducted in Africa. With the majority of these studies being transnational studies that are funded by the West but implemented in Africa, it makes sense that the claimed universal ethical principles, which guide the conduct of such a large volume of research in the region take into account the unique cultural and world view of the African continent. Unfortunately, there is a huge gap regarding the extent to which the current ethical guidelines take this into account. The discussion presented in this chapter provides insights on how this gap can be filled. There is no doubt that the international ethical guidelines have been extremely important in shaping the conduct of research in the world. In fact, the whole world can take pride in conducting more ethically sound research as a result of the existing ethical guidelines. However, given the dynamics of research, it is high time that an indigenous African bioethics framework was developed that can take into account important dimensions that influence bioethical practices in the African context, including but not limited to ethnicity, culture and language; all of which differ significantly from the West. Importantly, such a framework must be sensitive of and respect the pluralistic and communal nature of the Africa culture and be based on Africa's own ethnological, cultural, and philosophical underpinnings.

To do this effectively, it is important that such guidelines appreciate the diversity of African cultures. African bioethics guidelines should be premised on the understanding that Africa operates under a context of unique cultural, economic and researcher-participants power dynamic where the majority of transnational clinical studies take place.

## 16.3 Guideline/Framework for Conducting Research in Africa

Important principles to be considered when conducting research in Africa, especially during an emergency epidemic include;

### *16.3.1 Respect for the Community Hierarchies and Leadership*

The Mijikenda community, which is a collection of nine tribes; and one of the biggest tribal groupings in Kenya have a saying that goes "*sikiro karikira kitswa*", which literally means, an ear can never grow longer past the head. This saying is often used to send a strong message regarding family and community hierarchies that are not written anywhere yet every member of a family or a community is expected to adhere to. Many a time, this saying is used to warm people when they try to override the decision of older people in the family or community. In such cases, it doesn't matter how old you are; when someone above your age tells you something, their decision is final. This saying applies in most African communities. For example, most people in Africa believe that when an adult gives the final decision and a young person overrides that decision, something bad will happen to the young person, including that decision backfiring or a bad incidence happening against them. Thus, in this community, the final decision maker in any serious matter regarding the family or any member of the family is usually the most senior member of the family.

Although this example relates specifically to the Mijikenda community, most African societies have a very deep respect for familial or communal hierarchies. In most African settings, elders are believed to possess immense wisdom which allows them to critically consider all corners of the world before making their decision. In addition, because of their age, elderly family members have a lot of general life experiences-with a rich knowledge base which they are expected to utilize to facilitate decision making. This is why elderly men and women are often consulted to tackle complex issues in the community. It is also for this reason that young people are required to defer decision making to the elderly members of their families, even when the person is an adult and able to decide on their own.

This is an important principle to be observed when conducting research in Africa. Observing this norm will ensure families involved in research remain harmonious after research comes to an end. This is also a show of respect for the values withheld by families or communities involved in research. Although the universal ethical principles advocate for individual autonomy, it is important to apply this principle within the acceptable African norms and values. For example, when implementing research in a given community, it would be important for the researcher to first obtain permission from the highest traditional ruler of the region before approaching the individuals for individual consent. Additionally, where for example, the head of a household refuses to allow members of their household to participate in a given study, it should be the duty of the research team to find out why the old man refused and come up with ways through which the expectations of such people can be included in the research planning and their concerns addressed. Perhaps one may argue that this process is too tedious and practically complex to implement. Of course, this is likely to be the case when there is a lot of focus on getting studies implemented as oppose to putting emphasis on the actual process of implementing such projects. It is especially important to realize that studies that follow procedures that are acceptable in the community, such as the one described above, are more likely to be seen as respectful to the community hence better able to win the community trust and receive overwhelming support from community leaders and members. This may ultimately make recruitment of research participants easy, reduce mistrust and promote uptake of research outputs after the study. Similar approaches have recently been advocated for by proponents of community engagement and community-based research approaches.

It is also important to understand that a human being in the African context is not merely an individual who is autonomous, independent and mentally competent and able to make an independent decision. In fact, a human being is considered to be of sound and stable mental state; competent; and a reliable adult if such a person is able to articulate the societal hierarchies and defer issues such as critical decision making to the social entities bestowed with the moral and legitimate authority to make such decisions. For this reason, a person who ignores the existing channels of decision making is considered to be disrespectful and undermine the decision-making authorities. This construction of personhood is embedded in all aspects of life, including upbringing of children, ownership of property, ill and good health just to mention but a few. For example, although the key responsibility of child upbringing rests on the parents, when a child misbehaves, anyone in the community has a right to reprimand or punish the child without obtaining permission from the biological parents. This holistic and pluralistic construction of the person has important implications on decision making. People who have very close ties to a village, for example, might feel much respected and develop trust in the research team if they knew the village elder was already informed and gave permission for everyone to give consent. Understanding these contractions and perceptions can help researchers to appreciate the entire cobweb of interconnectivity among people in the community and provide space to discuss alternative decision-making mechanisms which the community deems most appropriate and acceptable, which is paramount especially in delicate and sensitive matters affecting the community.

We would, therefore, like to advocate for a more inclusive approach to community entry, consultation and informed consent seeking in which, hierarchies for community leadership and entry are identified and followed in order to enhance respect for the structures which the community reserved respect for, before seeking individual consent. In addition, where discordance arises between the prescribed community hierarchies and the target individuals, research teams should solve such differences amicably and only involve the target individuals when doing so is likely to promote harmony between the parties involved. This is a much wider and a more inclusive construction of the principle of respect, acceptable in many parts of the African continent.

### 16.3.2 Health and Illness

Most communities in Africa believe that health and illness are both associated with God's will. For example, across East and West Africa, a number of communities believe that one lives a healthy life because God/Allah has allowed them to be healthy and they become ill when God/Allah wishes them to be so. Accordingly, God/Allah operates in a spiritual manner, hence, although no one can see God, he is present everywhere. In certain parts of Africa, they believe God exists in the form of spirits that take different shapes, including fellow human beings, birds, plants, and other living things. These spirits operate in two main distinct categories, namely, evil spirits and angels/good spirits. Evil spirits are responsible for causing ill health while good spirits (sometimes called Angels) are responsible for good things, including health. Thus, when one gets sick or experiences a bad incidence in life, it means they have committed some bad acts that made God angry or someone prayed to God that they get sick or experience such a bad incidence. It is for this reason that some communities believe that no medicine-traditional or biomedical-has healing powers unless God grants such powers. In fact, most people believe that doctors and all traditional healers are merely a conduit through which God sends his healing to individuals who have ill health. It is therefore common for people to say "*mulungu nde andekuhoza*" meaning God is the one who will heal you, soon after a treatment has been administered to a sick person, even when they are not believers per se. This implies that regardless of how good your treatment is, actual healing comes from God.

The belief that good health and ill health all come from God also implies that people who cause ill health and those who treat, all must pray to God for such action to happen including witchcraft. It is all a matter of who has the strongest faith. Importantly, there is a strong connection between ill health and evil spirits or evil power. Thus, when one becomes sick, its either they have some evil spirits or some witchdoctor exerted some evil power in them. For this reason, most people believe an effective treatment should involve negotiating with the bad spirits to leave the sick person's body or extorting them by force through some medicine. Of course, underlying this whole process are either direct or indirect prayers to God.

This belief system on the origin of health and illness has a strong influence on the health-seeking behaviour of the indigenous community. It is for this reason, for example, the Mijikenda community from Kenya, in East Africa; rather take their children suffering from cerebral malaria to the traditional healer as opposed to the hospital. To them, cerebral malaria is caused by a bad spirit that gets into the child through a flying bird called *yuni*. When *yuni* flies over a child, the bad spirit enters the child and the child starts convulsing. During convulsions, if the child is given an injection, the injection aggravates the spirit and the spirit then kills the child. They are therefore better off taking the child to a traditional healer who will negotiate with and peacefully take the spirit out of the child before giving the child an oral concoction.

Although not exactly related, similar views related to the existence of bad and good spirits are also held by those following Christianity and Islamic values. Although Christians rarely consult traditional healers, almost all religions in many African settings believe in extorting evil spirits as part of the healing process. Interestingly, quite a number of communities believe in the healing powers of traditional medicine men.

The above epistemology may sound primitive but is important to understand and consider in developing ethical principles that respect indigenous African cultural values. In so doing, it is important that such principles take into account how such indigenous knowledge and values can be incorporated into any framework developed. For example, the knowledge possessed by traditional healers and what they practice in treating people during an epidemic should be considered and incorporated into any public health education and future interventions that may be developed towards the treatment of the prevailing condition/disease. Acknowledging the original source of this knowledge in a publication is a good way of showing respect to the indigenous community and sharing the benefits of the research output; while pursuing alternative methods of managing the disease. In addition, understanding the link between health and illness; good and evil spirits and the power of the will of God towards good and poor health may enhance how discussion and messages aimed at restoring an individual's psychological and full health could be formulated.

Indigenous African bioethics guidelines, therefore, should underscore the need for researchers to take time to understand from the community perspective how they conceptualize health and illness and consider these constructs into any interventions they develop. Importantly, as primitive as these concepts may sound, it is important that anyone conducting clinical research in the affected community acknowledges the existence of the indigenous knowledge and credit it in publication if they utilize such information in any way in the process of their research. It is also important to understand that, before the introduction of biomedicine in the community, the community had respect for life and followed an indigenous health system that took care of all their health needs. Rubbishing this system as primitive only serves to ridicule the community that has been part of these practices since time immemorial. Using a dialogic approach that allows both traditional and biomedical worldviews to prevail is likely to nature a more harmonious co-existence of both views. This way, an environment filled with mutual respect and understanding is likely to prevail. It may also be important to understand why so many indigenous people trust traditional medicine men. Trust is an important component of value ethics that must be natured between researchers and the community at all times, and more so during an epidemic. Understanding what constitutes trust and what attributes the community considers essential in nurturing trust is essential in ensuring researchers who work in the community use the same attributes to develop appropriate levels of trust with the community members.

### *16.3.3 Gender*

There is a notion that most African settings undermine the status of women. This is a notion that is often misinformed. Many African men are brought up in a belief system where men are expected to provide for and protect women. As such, there is a tendency for men to undertake the most challenging roles in the society and leave the light or less challenging roles to the women. Because of the need to protect women, women's roles have often been overshadowed by the men's prominence in undertaking their roles. Over time, most African women have been brought up in families where the role of women is defined as the 'nurturer'. On the other hand, most parts of Africa believe that a respectful woman is one who listens to and is less aggressive compared to their male counterparts. Part of this submissiveness involves the ability to consult with spouses and senior members of the family before making decisions, understandably because most families in the old days lived in extended families and making certain decisions that had serious implications on the family would be too heavy a responsibility for any one person to undertake, especially given that women often joined their matrimonial families. The requirement for women to consult their spouses and avoid making unilateral decisions is also related to the issue of familial hierarchies discussed above. Unfortunately, recent debates around this issue have been reduced it to a gender and women exploitation issue, a view that is often misguided and misinformed.

One issue that Africans have guarded selflessly is the importance of their family ties. Most African settings believe in the need to promote, protect and respect the family unit. Importantly, the woman is considered as a critical element of the family. Within the Giriama community, in Kenya for example, there is a saying that goes "*mudzi ujengwa ni muche*" meaning, a home is built by a woman. This implies that the woman is the key pillar of a family. Contrary to the popular western belief about African women as being submissive and oppressed, there is a very huge responsibility the society places on women, which entails ensuring the family is always well kneaded together and at peace. This responsibility is often unspoken but no doubt the most important role in a family. In fact, many people believe that a happy family and disciplined children usually reflect the behaviour and family management skills of the woman in the family. So important is the responsibility of a woman towards maintaining the family ties that the Giriama have a saying that implies that if a woman decides, she can break an entire family (not just her home) in a day. One important way that is believed to keep the family, especially amongst the rural communities in Kenya is the need to continuously consult among family members. Understandably, this promotes collective responsibility, mutual respect and harmony in families and avoids unnecessary disagreements and tensions. Unfortunately, the inability for women to make outright decisions in order to consult their spouses or significant family members has often been blown out of proportion and reduced to feminine talk.

As stated previously, mainstream bioethics guidelines were developed with the western cultural context in mind. As such, there is an assumption that every potential research participant would be an independent autonomous agent who would be able to make free and informed unilateral decision. Obviously, this does not apply in certain settings in Africa. There is, therefore, a need for researchers to create a dialogic space between spouses and family members and facilitate them to reach consensus regarding their participation.

Within extended families with married couples; many decisions concerning the wife are made in conjunction with the wife. However, advice and final words may be from the husband. On this basis, rather than regarding family consultations as a manifestation of the women oppression and indecisiveness, this should be encouraged, respected and natured as an important African family value. Where necessary, information about studies should be given to both spouses, where the researcher's role becomes to facilitate and allow the couple to make informed choices.

Excluding husbands from influencing the decision making of their wife, for example, only serves to create doubts, anxiety and unnecessary tensions during participation. These types of tensions should be avoided as much as possible by ensuring researchers proactively create space for consultation and collective decision making among significant family members and spouses, even if the target participant is an independent woman.

### *16.3.4 Power Differences*

Much of the discussion around power differences between researchers and research participants, especially during epidemics, relates to congested and constrained health systems which often lack adequate supplies to meet the health needs of the population. As such, people involved in research may find themselves in a situation where the research product constitutes the only health care accessible to them. Such situations make the already vulnerable populations; by virtue of being poor, even more vulnerable. In addition, researchers may be seen to belong to certain elite social classes. This may make research participants feel powerless and unable to refuse whatever is asked of them, not forgetting that participants may not even have the mental capacity to comprehend the information being given to them, due to the conditions they are going through at the time. This scenario was well presented in the case of Mama Kadzo in the previous chapter. But a less obvious aspect related to power differences relates to communication and complexities of communication tools used. It is an undisputed fact that all participants need to be given all the necessary information before making an informed decision. However, understanding such information requires having a great level of competence, and sometimes specific speciality in a given area of study. Although not always obvious, the use of technical language and medical jargon often renders research participants totally helpless as they struggle to understand the different concepts presented. This is a common mistake made by many clinical-research personnel!

While GCP guidelines and the principle of respect for persons emphasize the need for a truly-informed consent, little is said about how to achieve this principle. It is important to appreciate that most people in Africa may have low literacy level. As such, they are linguistically challenged in comprehending complex terminologies which are usually used in clinical research protocols. On the other hand, it is important to understand that low literacy level does not denote stupidity or foolishness. In exactly the same way that foreigners struggle to understand the local language, so do local people struggle to understand complex medical terminologies. It is therefore important to ensure indigenous language is used to communicate key concepts in the research. To facilitate this process, research teams must utilize available resources such as local idioms, terms and analogies to ensure the messages being communicated are understood and that potential participants are able to relate to these messages. For example, instead of using technical terms to explain research (a term that is often misunderstood) community members could be asked to explain how they discovered a local plant is useful in treating a certain illness. Their explanation could then be used to facilitate explanations about medical research. Through this process, the community would be better able to understand the research being conducted and be able to contribute toward it in a more meaningful way.

Another important aspect related to power imbalance is lack of resources on the part of the community involved in research. This may mean that, while the research team's priority may be to find a cure for a certain epidemic, the community may have a different priority altogether. It is important that researchers planning to conduct research in Africa do so in consultation with the community. In addition, such consultation should endeavour to empower the community and improve their general wellbeing through support from the research team. This may be achieved by ensuring the target community is involved in the planning and implementation of the research as well as in disseminating the research finding. Using employees drawn from the community involved in the research may ensure there is more trust in the research being conducted. On the other hand, employing such cadre of staff impact positively towards the living standards of the community involved. Carrying out community consultation should not be done as a public relations activity but as an integral part of the research project. This way, views and ideas gathered through the process of consultation can be used to directly inform the study team on the best ways to improve the conduct of the research. Additionally, projects identified by the process of consultation that had not been previously thought of as part of the research project may be added to cater for the community needs and expectations. This way, the community will be able to feel respected as equal partners in planning and executing the research as opposed to being treated as recipients of the research.

## 16.4 Conclusion

This chapter has argued for the need to have an inclusive and Afro-centric approach in the application of the universal ethical principles. In addition, the chapter has presented some limitations associated with the existing guidelines and proposed several ways through which the principles can be made more sensitive and responsive to the indigenous African culture and moral principles that promote the value system and aspirations of all Africans within and without the continent. In doing so, this chapter tried to use as many local examples as possible, including how the various principles can be applied on the ground. Although the proposed framework may not address all challenges; given the wide-ranging diversity within and without African national boundaries; this chapter provides insights on how researchers can conduct clinical research in Africa that takes into account the true African context where the research will be conducted. The authors stress that public participation in the crafting of such a framework and guidelines will be important in creating popular acceptance of the difficult choices that must be made during an epidemic.

## References

Andorno, R. (2009). Human dignity and human rights as a common ground for a global bioethics. *Journal of Medicine and Philosophy, 34*(3), 223–240.

Bacon, F., Calvin, J., Lipsius, J., Luther, M., Knowledge, M., & Montaigne, M. D. (2008). *Internet encyclopedia of philosophy*. Retrieved February, 24, 2008.

Baier, A. (1995). *Moral prejudices: Essays on ethics*. Cambridge, MA: Harvard University Press.

Beauchamp, T. L., & Childress, J. F. (2001). *Principles of biomedical ethics*. Oxford: Oxford University Press.

Chukwuneke, F. N., Umeora, O. U. J., Maduabuchi, J. U., & Egbunike, N. (2014). Global bioethics and culture in a pluralistic world: How does culture influence bioethics in Africa? *Annals of Medical and Health Sciences Research, 4*(5), 672–675.

Code, N. (1949). *The Nuremberg Code. Trials of war criminals before the Nuremberg military tribunals under control council law* (Vol. 10, pp. 181–182). Washington, DC: US Government Printing Office.

Declaration, H. (2013). World medical association declaration of Helsinki: Ethical principles for medical research involving human subjects. *JAMA, 310*(20), 2191–2194.
Department of Health, Education, and Welfare, & National Commission for the Protection of Human Subjects of Biomedical and Behavioral Research. (2014). The Belmont Report. Ethical principles and guidelines for the protection of human subjects of research. *The Journal of the American College of Dentists, 81*(3), 4.
Engelhardt, H. T. (2011, Sep). Core competencies for health care ethics consultants: In search of professional status in a post-modern world. HEC forum (Vol. 23, No. 3, p. 129). Springer Netherlands.
Howard-Jones, N. (1986). CIOMS ethical code for animal experimentation. *ICLAS Bulletin*.
Jacobson, N. (2007). Dignity and health: A review. *Social Science & Medicine, 64*(2), 292–302.
Macrae, D. J. (2007). The Council for International Organizations and Medical Sciences (CIOMS) guidelines on ethics of clinical trials. *Proceedings of the American Thoracic Society, 4*(2), 176–179.
Morrison, C. A., Horwitz, I. B., & Carrick, M. M. (2009). Ethical and legal issues in emergency research: Barriers to conducting prospective randomized trials in an emergency setting. *Journal of Surgical Research, 157*(1), 115–122.
Onuoha, C. (2007). "Bioethics across borders." An African perspective. *Uppsala Studies in Social Ethics, 34*, 210–211.
Veatch, R. M. (1999). The foundations of bioethics. *Bioethics, 13*(3–4), 206–217.
World Medical Association. (2008). Medical association declaration of Helsinki: Ethical principles for medical research involving human subject. Edinburgh: 52nd WMA General Assembly (online) URL, Tomado desde: http://www.wma.net/e/policy/17-c_e.html. El, 15(07), 04.

# Chapter 17
# Criminalisation and "Reckless" Ebola Transmission: Theorizing Ethical Obligations to Seek Care

**Morenike Oluwatoyin Folayan, Bridget Haire, Kristin Peterson, Aminu Yakubu, Jemee Tegli, and Brandon Brown**

## 17.1 Introduction

The Ebola Virus Disease (EVD) outbreak in Liberia, Sierra Leone and Guinea – referred to as the Mano River States – was a major international crisis. It was the 27th EVD outbreak, and the outbreak resulted in the death of five times as many people as every other known EVD outbreak combined (Folayan and Haire 2016; World Health Organisation 2016). In addition to the Mano River States, which were worst affected by the EVD epidemic, numerous countries outside of the region and the continent reported cases (Centres for Disease Control and Prevention 2015). The World Health Organization initiated a global response, which was its largest operation in its 70 year history (World Health Organisation 2015). By the 27th of March 2016, 28,610 cases had been reported and 11,308 persons had died from Ebola infection.

M. O. Folayan (✉)
Department of Child Dental Health and Institute of Public Health, Obafemi Awolowo University, Ile-Ife, Nigeria

B. Haire
School of Public Health and Community Medicine, UNSW, Kensington, Australia

K. Peterson
Department of Anthropology, University of California, Irvine, CA, USA

A. Yakubu
National Health Research Ethics Committee, Federal Ministry of Health, Federal Secretariat, Abuja, Nigeria

J. Tegli
UL-PIRE Africa Center, University of Liberia, Monrovia, Liberia

B. Brown
Department of Social Medicine and Population Health, UCR School of Medicine, Riverside, CA, USA



G. B. Tangwa et al. (eds.), *Socio-cultural Dimensions of Emerging Infectious Diseases in Africa*, https://doi.org/10.1007/978-3-030-17474-3_17

The centuries-old practices of isolation and quarantine were central to the EVD response in this outbreak (Chertow et al. 2014). However there were other practices that also contributed to the successful control of the 2014–2016 and other past outbreaks. These included providing protective clothing to health care workers, contact tracing and monitoring, public education and awareness-raising on EVD infection, as well as providing support to community members to conduct safe burial practices and home care for infected individuals (Heymann 2014).

Separation of infected and exposed individuals from the unexposed is a classic public health response. It is especially important in the absence of specific therapy or amenable healthcare facilities to house and nurse those infected. However, presenting to an isolation facility may not be an acceptable option for all those with EVD-related symptoms. During the recent epidemic, some individuals exposed to EVD actively sought to evade quarantine and treatment facilities; some also crossed borders either in denial of their potential infection or sought adequate healthcare elsewhere (World Health Organisation 2014a).

Outbreaks in Nigeria, Senegal, Mali, Spain and the United States had index cases originating from the Mano River States. The index cases in Nigeria, Senegal, and United States had all knowingly been in contact with persons infected with EVD. The index cases in Nigeria and the United States ostensibly provided false information at the port of entry into those countries (Felix 2014). These cases precipitated discussions about the criminalization of EVD transmission. The Government of Liberia threatened to prosecute the Liberian EVD patient hospitalized in the U.S. on the 25th of September, 2014 due to the fact that he knew he was exposed to the virus and yet he left the country (United Nations 2014).

In this paper, we will discuss the putative obligations of those who know they have been exposed to EVD, and the criminalization of EVD infection. Additionally, we highlight issues that may arise in resolving some of the ethical dilemmas associated with criminalisation of 'reckless transmission' of EVD infection. We will take into consideration the impact of the political-economic situation and the state of the health systems and structure in the EVD zone on the decision about seeking care for EVD infection. We will also analyse the socio-cultural context of the response to the epidemic and consider the social implications of criminalising EVD infection.

## 17.2 The Ebola Virus Disease in Context

The major concerns with EVD are its high case fatality and its high infectiousness. In the outbreak in Mano River States, EVD associated mortality was exacerbated by failures of health facilities to provide basic care (O'Hare 2015). As described by Boozary et al. (2014), health care systems in affected countries were insufficient to provide basic primary care, let alone respond to an emergency of the magnitude and scale of EVD epidemic Mano River States. Heymann (2014) also highlighted the challenges associated with containing the infection when it spread to the urban area in the context of existing poor health systems. Folayan and Haire (2016) on the other hand, highlighted how to political, historical and social context of the Mano River States impacted on the EVD health response in the states.

*The antecedents health system dysfunction*: The years of civil wars coincided with the implementation of "structural adjustment programs" in Liberia in 1980, Guinea in 1985, and Sierra Leone in 1992 (Mkandawire and Soludo 1998). The long-term effects of high debt, unfavorable fiscal policies, and the outbreak of civil war embedded in dictatorship, made it nearly impossible to build clinical infrastructure as well as train (and retain) competent medical expertise to address local needs (Reno 1996; Jones 1998; Campbell and Clapp 1995). Structural adjustment programs privatized Guinea, Sierra Leone and Liberia's health care systems, mandated significantly reduced federal spending on health care systems, and introduced user fees. There was also the retrenchment of thousands of health care workers. These measures compounded the poor state of the health systems resulting in dilapidated health care facilities and poor access to health care for the large impoverished populations (Turshen 1999). Public health surveillance systems, epidemic outbreak monitoring, and health communication networks were already broken down prior to the EVD epidemic (Abramowitz 2014). These breakdowns were associated with increases in infectious disease incidence and disease related deaths (Gustafson et al. 2007; Heymann et al. 2015). Only a few dozen physicians were practicing at the time of the epidemic (Sieff 2014). The Mano River States rank low on the human development index; an index largely reflecting the health care status of counties (UNDP 2013).

*The political system and social dysfunction*: As demonstrated by anthropologists, these histories intersect with societal norms and practices that also overlap with political and governance structures. Of note are the long-term activities of outsiders including human extraction(slavery); donors and their relationship to experimental medicine (Bah 2015), transnational raw material extraction and associated corruption scandals that have created longstanding reservations and distrust of both government and outsiders (Bah 2015; Ferme 2001; Shaw 2002).

Throughout the postcolonial era, varying forms of governance also exacerbated distrust. For example, Guinea pursued a post-independence national unity agenda that negatively impacted the inhabitants of the Forest Region where there was high EVD infection rates. These included subordinating their political rights as well as banning social practices, some of which continued in secrecy, such as burials and healing paradigms (McGovern 2012). This marginalization extended into current national politics where EVD was perceived across the entirety of forest communities as getting conflated with other politicized issues.

Nowhere was this more apparent than when members of an EVD sensitization team showed up in the Sous-Prefecture of Womey on September 10, 2014. The delegation included highly distrusted ruling political party members whose EVD sensitization presentation got confused with election campaigning. Community members found it disturbing that they could only discuss EVD and not other grievances they had. Moreover, the delegation's timing coincided with an indigenous initiation ceremony for which some Christian members of the delegation were known to hold in great disdain. After a series of several events that day, the heightened anxiety and distrust resulted in violence and several members of the EVD delegation were killed (Wilkinson and Fairhead 2017). The politicization of EVD throughout the Mano River States resulted in various articulations of resistance to EVD education and treatment.

*Isolation*: Isolation of individuals who have infectious diseases that have the potential to cause public health epidemics is an ethical duty of public health importance. Isolation is effective when early detection of suspected and probable cases is feasible, and where rapid implementation of isolation and prompt administration of other infection control tools occurs (Cetron et al. 2004). While isolation as a public health strategy for containing the spread of EVD is an important public health measure, the associated curtailment the liberty of infected individuals to free movement during the isolation period when they could transmit infection comes with a government's duty for reciprocity. This implies that isolated individuals need to be assured access to adequate health care, food, clothing and means of communication with families and friends (Gostin et al. 2003). When such care is not forthcoming or when it is inadequate, it can be argued that the individual who is legally required to report for isolation does not have a moral obligation to do so. During the EVD epidemic in the Mano River States, patients could not be guaranteed access to adequate health care. Health care institutions themselves became a focal point for EVD spread as in previous epidemics (Heymann 2014; Folayan and Haire 2016).

*Quarantine*: Similar challenges regarding adequate care for individuals also apply to communities that were quarantined. Quarantine is a measure that restricts movement of individuals exposed to contagious diseases for the purpose of observing if they develop the disease. It is a public health measure designed to prevent spread of contagious diseases by reducing the number of disease-exposed individuals people came in contact with. It is effective when used in conjunction with isolation of detected cases, practice of infection control in hospitals and other facilities, community-wide temperature screening, and the monitoring of travelers and response at national borders (Cetron et al. 2004).

While appropriate quarantine is a broadly accepted public health measure, it is expected that those quarantined should not suffer unfair economic penalties in addition to a variety of other negative political and social consequences (Rothstein et al. 2003; Cetron and Landwirth 2005). Importantly, adequate care needs to be provided for affected individuals (Singer et al. 2003) and the curtailment of liberties must be balanced by care for the individuals who acquiesce to these strictures. In the countries worst affected by EVD, the deplorable conditions of crowded, unhygienic EVD treatment centres where the risk of infection is even higher, made people wanted to stay away (Effiong 2014). Escape from quarantine is however deemed a criminal offence punishable by the law in countries like Liberia that inherited laws from the US (Justia US Law 2015), in Sierra Leone that inherited laws from Britain (the Quarantine Act) and in Guinea that inherited laws from France.

Quarantine practices may also require that the movements of whole communities– movement within communities and movement between communities –and not just exposed individuals be restricted as a community containment measure (Folayan et al. 2016). Its maximum duration would be one incubation period. For EVD, this would be 21 days (World Health Organisation 2016). In August 2014, the border region of Guinea, Liberia and Sierra Leone was subject to a 'cordon sanitaire' – an unpassable barrier – for the purpose of confining EVD to a specific geographic area (McNeil 2014). Unfortunately, 'cordon sanitaire' has not been an effective measure for preventing EVD either in the past or in epidemic that happened in Liberia, Sierra Leone and Guinea. Heymann (2014) described how this measured failed in the democratic Republic of Congo in 1995 and how it failed in Liberia in the current epidemic. Bah (2015) narrated how communities in the Guinea showed no respect the call for quarantine. The potential effectiveness of mounted roadblocks to limit movement across borders were undermined by the inefficiency of the process, corruption and the ingenuity of citizens in sabotaging the restrictive orders (Heymann 2014; Bah 2015).

## 17.3 Criminalization of Reckless EVD Transmission

The magnitude of the outbreak in the Mano River States meant that there was a huge strain on both the material and human resources available for decent and humane standards of care within health facilities. Given the poor quality of the health infrastructure in these countries (Jones 1998), the long history of silo-ed or privatized health services (International Crisis Group 2015), longstanding conflicts and even wars waged over colonial public health campaigns that continue today (Wilkinson and Fairhead 2017; Fairhead 2016), the poor standard of care for patients with EVD early in the epidemic (Richter and Farmer 2014), and the high level of stigma associated with EVD infection (Karamouzian and Hategekimana 2015), patients with EVD had legitimate reasons to avoid quarantine and isolation. Unfortunately, prior to the epidemic, citizens had had limited access to the public health care system due to a number of reasons one of which was limited financial capacity to pay for health care services (Wilkinson and Fairhead 2017). This same factor and other factors such as well the lack of reserve resources to survive quarantine, lack of child care and the poor access to safe transport made access to the public health facilities a challenge (Wilkinson and Fairhead 2017).

We consider that upholding criminal sanctions for those in the Mano River States who avoided isolation or quarantine ignores the principle of reciprocity – that people who subject themselves to isolation or quarantine by reporting exposure or symptoms must be assured of a reasonable standard of care (Upshur et al. 2007). Also, that the failure of the government to take a communitarian approach to respond to the public health needs of affected people by negotiating acceptable substitutes for quarantine and isolations in distrusted and unused public health facilities was negligence on the part of the government and an action that delayed prompt control of the epidemic in the worst affected countries.

### 17.3.1 Criminalisation of Evasion of Isolation and Quarantine

Quarantine and isolation are evidence-based actions that prevent harm and protect public health in line with Mill's oft-quoted harm principle: the avoidance of harm justifies the restriction of liberty (Mills 2003). The decision to isolate, or quarantine should be based on public health necessity, and brings with it an obligation to provide adequate food, shelter, clothing and medical care for those whose liberty is constrained by such measures. Certainly, isolation and quarantine appear to be appropriate public health measures for EVD management. But the state's right to exercise this power was undermined in the Mano River States because the public health system to support isolation and quarantine was not in place. Therefore those who were to bear the burden to protect the public's health could not be adequately protected.

Imposing a 'cordon sanitaire' late in the epidemic had limited positive public health effects, given that the virus had already spread beyond the cordoned area (World Health Organisation 2014b). Moreover, there is no evidence to support the effectiveness of community enclosure as this had had very limited success in past EVD epidemics (Heymann 2014; Bah 2015). Further, if the state cannot ensure citizen health protections (and other rights) when imposing quarantine or isolation, it does not have the right to impose laws that criminalise isolation or quarantine avoidance.

### 17.3.2 Criminalising Wilful EVD Transmission

With evolving evidence that EVD can be transmitted through sexual intercourse (Mate et al. 2015), a new perspective on wilful or reckless transmission of EVD infection is possible and people may be legally required to disclose their history of EVD infection to their sex partners as required with HIV infection. The imposition of laws that would criminalize wilful EVD transmission is possible in West African countries that inherited the British legal systems: general offenses relating to the deliberate or reckless infection of a person with a serious disease existed in criminal law, supplemented by common law cases (Groves 2007). We have seen this happen in the case of HIV in countries that inherited the British legal systems: Canada and Australia added new laws to their public health acts, which were either HIV specific or generalized to transmissible diseases such as HIV. Similar HIV-specific legislation broadly criminalising HIV exposure or transmission has already been passed in African countries like Burundi, Djibouti, Kenya, Madagascar, Mozambique and Tanzania. Similar laws are being proposed and/or being debated in other African countries such as Malawi, Uganda, Mauritius and Nigeria (NAM aidsmap 2016).

Criminalization of infectious disease transmission is arguably justifiable when there is evidence to substantiate the accused individual had intentionally committed the action to bring about infection; this may be especially germane in instances where the individual could have exercised forms of influence to prevent the transmission (Flanigan 2014). The argument for criminalisation is premised on the concept that while all parties should be aware of protecting themselves and reducing their own risks of acquiring contagious infections, especially in an epidemic like that of EVD, a person exposed to the infection is in possession of extra facts germane to the situation, which might alter the other party's conduct. If non-disclosure of EVD exposure is counted as a moral wrong, then criminalization and punishment for what may be considered a moral wrong may therefore be deemed justified.

This argument is based upon Western juridical norms and do not account for multiple complexities found in the Ebola outbreak in the Mano River States. For example, patients and/or their ill loved ones may not have access to finances that enables them to present at treatment centres. These include the lack of reserve resources to survive quarantine. The lack of childcare and the absence of safe transport are also reasons that one may have difficulty securing a proper diagnosis (Wilkinson and Fairhead 2017). Moreover, this argument does not consider the consequences of disclosing EVD exposure – mandatory isolation in a facility where if the person was not infected in the first place, she or he is likely to become so.

While the principle of retributive justice may provide justification for criminalization of wilful EVD transmission, advocates against the criminalization of unintentional transmission of HIV infection have demonstrated the relative ineffectiveness of criminal prohibitions and advocated the repeal of such laws (Chalmers 2013). Criminalization and punishment are designed to serve as deterrents to prevent the repetition of antisocial actions. Thus imprisonment is supplemented with rehabilitation programs. Reckless transmission of a virus like EVD is likely to be the result of impulsive acts of desperate people operating within panicked and crisis situations. Thus it is not clear how criminalization would act as a deterrent, other than to discourage people from seeking diagnosis and care. Imposing criminal sanctions for non-compliance with public health authorities may therefore do nothing more practical or pragmatic than send a message of acceptable norms of responsibility and behaviour (Gurnham 2013).

Furthermore, it may be counterintuitive, to place the onus of responsibility for keeping others EVD-free upon those who are infected. Members of society, including health care workers, may interpret the sanction as protective, and may underestimate risks on the assumption that others are taking precautionary measures. Also, the similarity of EVD symptoms with those of common illnesses like flu and malaria and the 21 day incubation period could mitigate efforts to criminalize EVD transmission, based on the 'blameless moral and factual ignorance argument,' which Flanigan articulated in the context of HIV (Mate et al. 2015). Further, criminalizing the conduct of the mortally ill is both futile and paradoxically may add to the kind of stigma that prevents people with EVD symptoms from attending diagnosis and care facilities. We argue that criminalization for non-disclosure of EVD risk status does not pass the test of expediency and is not a fit subject for the operation of law since a legal penalty is not safely applicable in this situation (Jorge, no date).

## 17.4 Trust and Its Implication for Instituting Isolation and Quarantine

The shortcomings in the state of the health care delivery system in the countries that constitute the Ebola Zone constitute what Paul Farmer would describe as a manifestation of structural violence, injustice so extreme and far-reaching that evading care in such facilities would not be unreasonable (Farmer 1996). Yet trust is required especially when isolation and quarantine efforts are necessary in the response to the EVD epidemic (Thomas 2014). Lack of patient trust was associated with reduced utilization of health care service by people with EVD (Musa et al. 2009) and unwillingness to seek out treatment (Elbagir 2014). This contrasts with the 1976 Ebola outbreak in Zaire, where trust of health care workers played a key role in the containment of the EVD outbreak (Breman and Johnson 2014). It also contrasts with the Nigerian experience with Ebola where building trust with contact tracers as well as social workers and medical psychiatrists was a high priority of the government's Emergency Operation Center and a primary reason why the outbreak was so well contained.

The lack of trust, coupled with fear of discrimination, and the potential for stigma by mandatory quarantine and isolation could lead some residents to escape affected areas, as was observed in past epidemics (Tognotti 2013). While the use of isolation and quarantine is an effective public health measure to contain epidemics, vigilant attention needs to be paid to its practice to avoid causing prejudice and intolerance (Tognotti 2013). Efforts also needs to be instituted to gain public trust through regular, transparent, and comprehensive communications that balance the risks and benefits of public health interventions using lessons gained from the past (Tognotti 2013). The implementation of isolation and quarantine should be free from both legal and social forms of coercion (Olveria, Unknown).

### *17.4.1 Liberty to Seek Alternative Care and to Decide on Place for Hospice Care*

Historical distrust of public health authorities in some parts of the Mano River States are directly linked to the governance structures of colonialism, which created local conflicts that continue into the present era (Anoko, no date), in addition to the more recent histories of civil conflict and economic policies such as structural adjustment. Moreover, the World Bank-induced break down of existing health systems have also contributed to eroded trust in public health (Harman 2014). These have implications for public health institutions and use of alternative health systems and structures (Breman and Johnson 2014). While patients have a *prima facie* right to decide what kind of care they want or do not want, the freedom to make such choices is trumped by the need to maximise public safety during an epidemic.

However in submitting to a significant constraint on liberty, affected people maintain the basic rights to food, shelter and medical care.

Individuals however have a right to choose the place to die and how to die (The Choice in End of Life Care Programme Board 2015). Seeking care at designated EVD treatment centres will require individuals to be isolated from family, friends and loved ones though this may not always be the case. For example, in the 2014 Nigeria EVD outbreak, patients and their families received daily psychosocial support from social workers and clinical psychologists. Also, highly protected facilities were created that enabled families and friends to meet with their loved ones in EVD isolation wards (Mohammed et al. 2015). Patients were also able to use electronic devices to communicate (Ada, Nigerian Ebola survivor, personal communication).

Where isolation and quarantine practices may not be able to provide the required standards of care for those whose right to liberty might be infringed on due to a commitment for public health safety of the majority, considerations need to be given to the right of patients to choice preferred alternative health care. For a highly fatal disease like EVD, consideration also needs to be given to the right of choice of place to die even when dealing with infectious diseases. There is currently very little public discussions about these rights and how to address these rights for a highly infectious and fatal disease like EVD where there is need to handle safely the infected and the dead. Safe handling is possible as demonstrated in the EVD epidemic in the Mano River States: many infected individuals were managed successfully at home when the treatment centres were full (Bah 2015) and by traditional healer (Nurhussein 2016). The use of alternative care comes with as many challenges as does the use of poorly equipped public health systems. However, for societies where the respect for rights is increasingly becoming topic in the day to day lives of individuals, we think discussions on these rights and how to ensure rights are respected even during highly fatal infectious disease outbreaks in resource limited setting with challenges as observed in the Mano River States, should commence now.

### 17.4.2 Strengthening the Health Care System

Strengthening existing health systems in the countries as well as the larger subcontinental regions affected by EVD is one approach that should be given the highest priority in the global response to EVD. In addition, international support is required to strengthen the capacity of trusted alternative health care systems in the region to contribute to processes of care, containment and infection control. Treatment facilities for EVD or any other diseases need to be transformed into places that offer some chance of treatment, recovery, and psychosocial support rather than places to die isolated from loved ones and the community (Chertow et al. 2014). Support should include educating and coordinating with alternative caregivers on case management, referral protocols, case reporting, and providing them with EVD support kits including protective gowns, gloves and masks, as well as soap, chlorine and a sprayer, along with instructions on the use and safe disposal of materials (UNICEF 2014). Furthermore, it is important to support government efforts to provide public health education to community members on how to effectively contain the epidemic, strengthen its public health care service delivery systems, and rebuild trust (Wolz 2014). Although the EVD outbreaks have been put under control, systems and structures that were built to contain the EVD outbreak need to be provided the resources to continue providing needed emergency health care services for the country.

### 17.4.3 Motivation to Access Care

In communities like those in the Mano River States, where there is public mistrust for the public health care system, or where there are barriers to health care access in public health facilities due to concerns about cost, transportation, care for family members left behind, and the lack of reserved resources, government can put in place incentives to motivate people to access care – isolation and quarantine - in the equipped medical centres set up to manage EVD. The government should ensure however, that the facilities are adequately equipped to provide EVD care and support. There are a number of programmes that have tried to increase patient access to health care via multiple incentives, including financial incentives (Lorincz et al. 2013). Using incentives to motivate citizens to access quality health care for the purpose of curtailing a rapidly evolving epidemic may be considered apt and may also facilitate prompt responses. This may help to curb delay arising from distrust in public health facilities. The duty to disclose health status during an epidemic for the purpose of making decisions for patient quarantine or isolation places a reciprocal responsibility on the health system to provide adequate care for the medical needs of those patients.

## 17.5 Conclusions

The lessons learnt from the EVD outbreak should not be limited to improved understanding of biological and biomedical issues: the lessons about the human lives and how social, economic and political issues affects personal responses to the epidemic are equally crucial in designing and implementing emergency responses. These issues equally play a role in decisions made about the design and implementation of isolation and quarantine programmes during infectious disease epidemics. Criminalization of EVD transmission or its non-disclosure in the Mano River States and in places with the Mano River States situation would be counterproductive to critical community-building efforts and the public health response.

Criminalization is highly likely to increase the already serious stigma related to EVD, and the consequences of this for people diagnosed with EVD may include rejection, isolation and the possibility of being killed (Davtyan et al. 2014).

Criminalization has the potential to actually increase public health risk by serving as a disincentive for patients to seek early treatment. Thus, we advocate that rather than criminalization, efforts should be made to promote community mobilization and build a supportive environment that encourages disclosure and deters against reckless transmission of EVD to others.

We do acknowledge that beyond the law, there may be 'social criminalisation' of EVD infection suffered in the form of stigma, discrimination and ostracization by community members. This was reported in multiple publications on the subject matter with its impact on low willingness to present for isolations and quarantine by affected persons. This form of sanction for being EVD infected and the oppression that is associated with the 'social criminalisation' process may have worse implications for those who become legally criminalised for EVD related offences – evasion of isolation, quarantine.

Finally, as a proactive public health response for infectious diseases with high fatality, public education needs to be provided for all citizens in countries likely to be worst affected by the epidemic, on how to make home management of people with EVD safe while making efforts to transfer and isolate individuals in healthcare centres. Global and local support for affected nations should continue to promote case isolation in collaboration with other trusted local health care providers in a context where the standard of care provided can offer some real chance of survival.

## References


Abramowitz, S.A. (2014). *How the Liberian Health Sector Became a Vector for Ebola*. *Fieldsights–Hotspots, Cultural Anthropology Online*. http://www.culanth.org/fieldsights/598-how-theliberian-health-sector-became-a-vector-for-ebola. Accessed 1 Jan 2016.

Anoko, J. (No date). *Communication with rebellious communities during an outbreak of Ebola Virus Disease in Guinea: an anthropological approach*. http://www.ebola-anthropology.net/wp-content/uploads/2014/12/Communicationduring-an-outbreak-of-Ebola-Virus-Disease-with-rebellious-communities-in-Guinea.pdf

Bah, C. A. M. (2015). *The Ebola outbreak in West Africa: Corporate gangsters, multinationals and rogue politicians*. Philadelphia: Africanist Press.

Boozary, A. S., Farmer, P. E., & Jha, A. K. (2014). The Ebola outbreak, fragile health systems, and quality as a cure. *Journal of the America Medical Association, 312*(18), 1859–1860.

Breman, J. G., & Johnson, K. M. (2014). Ebola then and now. *New England Journal of Medicine, 371*(18), 1663–1666.

Campbell, B., & Clapp, J. (1995). Guinea's economic performance under structural adjustment: Importance of mining and agriculture. *The Journal of Modern African Studies, 33*(3), 425–449.

Centre for Disease Control and Prevention. 2015. *2014 Ebola outbreak in West Africa – Case Counts*. 30th December. http://www.cdc.gov/vhf/ebola/outbreaks/2014-west-africa/case-counts.html. Accessed 31 Dec 2015.

Cetron, M., & Landwirth, J. (2005). Public health and ethical considerations in planning for quarantine. *The Yale Journal of Biology and Medicine, 78*, 329–334.

Cetron, M., Maloney, S., Koppaka, R., & Simone, P. (2004). Isolation and quarantine: Containment strategies for SARS 2003. In S. Knobler, A. Mahmoud, S. Lemon, et al. (Eds.), *Learning from SARS: Preparing for the next disease outbreak: Workshop summary*. Washington, DC: Institute of Medicine (US) Forum on Microbial Threats; National Academies Press (US).

Chalmers, J. (2013). Disease transmission, liability and criminal law. In A. M. Viens, J. Coggon, & A. S. Kessel (Eds.), *Criminal law, philosophy and public health practice*. London: Cambridge University Press.

Chertow, D.S., C. Kleine, J. K Edwards, R. Scaini, R. Giuliani and A. Sprecher A. 2014. Ebola virus disease in West Africa — Clinical manifestations and management. New England Journal of Medicine 371(22):2054–2057.

Davtyan, M., Brown, B., & Folayan, M. O. (2014). Addressing Ebola-related stigma: Lessons learned from HIV/AIDS. *Global Health Action, 7*, 26058.

Effiong U. 2014. *On Ebola and the challenges of quarantine*. Available at: http://www.huffington-post.com/utibe-effiong/on-ebola-and-the-challeng_b_6015192.html. Accessed 12 Dec, 2016.

Elbagir, N. (2014). *Ebola: Liberian health care system on the brink of collapse*. Khon 2. October 13. hon2.com/2014/10/13/ebola-liberian-health-care-system-on-the-brink-of-collapse/. Accessed 1 Jan 1, 2016.

Fairhead, J. (2016). Understanding social resistance to Ebola response in the forest region of the Republic of Guinea: an anthropological perspective. *African Studies Review*. http://sro.sussex.ac.uk/60074/

Farmer, P. (1996). Social inequalities and emerging infectious diseases. *Emerging Infectious Diseases, 2*(4), 259–269.

Felix, B. (2014). *Liberia says may prosecute man who flew to U.S. with Ebola*. Reuters. October 2. http://www.reuters.com/article/2014/10/02/us-health-ebola-liberia-idUSKCN0HR25U20141002. Accessed 12 Nov 2014.

Ferme, M. (2001). *The underneath of things: Violence, history, and the everyday in Sierra Leone*. London: University of California Press.

Flanigan, J. (2014). Non-culpable ignorance and HIV criminalisation. *Journal of Medical Ethics, 40*(12), 798–801.

Folayan, M.O., & Haire, B.. (2016). History, culture and social norms: Implications for Ebola drug and vaccine clinical trials in affected region. In: *Ebola's message: Public health and medicine in the 21st century*. Rogers Street in Cambridge, MA: MIT Press, 02142.

Folayan, M. O., Haire, B., & Brandon, B. (2016). Critical role of ethics in clinical management and public health response to the West Africa Ebola epidemic. *Risk Management and Healthcare Policy, 9*, 55–65.

Gostin, L. O., Bayer, R., & Fairchild, A. L. (2003). Ethical and legal challenges posed by severe acute respiratory syndrome: Implications for the control of severe infectious disease threats. *Journal of the American Medical Association, 290*(24), 3229–3237.

Groves, M. (2007). The transmission of HIV and the criminal law. *Criminal LJ, 31*, 137–141.

Gurnham, D. (2013). Criminalising contagion: Ethical, legal and clinical challenges of prosecuting the spread of disease and sexually transmitted infections. *Sexually Transmitted Infections, 89*(4), 274–275.

Gustafson, P., Gomes, V. F., Vieira, C. S., et al. (2007). Tuberculosis mortality during a civil war in Guinea-Bissau. *Journal of the American Medical Association, 286*(2001), 599–603.

Harman, S. (2014). *Ebola and the politics of a global health crisis. E-International Relations*. October 20. http://www.e-ir.info/2014/10/20/ebola-and-the-politics-of-a-global-health-crisis. Accessed 31 Dec 2014.

Heymann, D., L. 2014. Ebola: Lessons from the past. Nature, 514(7522):299–300.

Heymann, D., Chen, L., Takemi, K., et al. (2015). Global health security: The wider lessons from the West African Ebola virus disease epidemic. *Lancet, 385*(9980), 1884–1901.

International Crisis Group. (2015). *The Politics behind the Ebola crisis*. Crisis Group Africa Report N°232, October 28. http://www.crisisgroup.org/~/media/Files/africa/west-africa/232-the-politics-behind-the-ebola-crisis.pdf. Accessed 1 Jan 2016.

Jones, J. M. (1998). Economic adjustment programs under stand-by arrangements with the International Monetary Fund (IMF): Liberia's experience 1980–85. *Liberian Studies Journal, 13*(2), 153–177.

Jorge, M.O. (Unknown). *Harm and offence in Mill's conception of liberty*. Faculty of Law, University of Oxford. Available at: http://www.trinitinture.com/documents/oliveira.pdf. Accessed 12 Dec 2016.
Justia US Law. (2015). *Wyoming Code* (WY Stat § 35-4-105). Available at: http://law.justia.com/codes/wyoming/2015/title-35/chapter-4/article-1/section-35-4-105. Accessed 12 Dec 2016.
Karamouzian, M., & Hategekimana, C. (2015). Ebola treatment and prevention are not the only battles: Understanding Ebola-related fear and stigma. *International Journal of Health Policy and Management, 4*(1), 55–56.
Lorincz, I. S., Lawson, B. C., & Long, J. A. (2013). Provider and patient directed financial incentives to improve care and outcomes for patients with diabetes. *Current Diabetes Report, 13*(2), 188–195.
Mate, S. E., Kugelman, J. R., Nyenswah, T. G., et al. (2015). Molecular evidence of sexual transmission of Ebola virus. *New England Journal of Medicine, 17;373*(25), 2448–2454.
McGovern, M. (2012). Life during wartime: Aspirational kinship and the management of insecurity. *Journal of the Royal Anthropological Institute, 18*(4), 735–752.
McNeil, D.G., Jr. (2014). Using a tactic unseen in a century, countries cordon off Ebola-racked areas. *The New York Times*. Available at: http://www.nytimes.com/2014/08/13/science/using-a-tactic-unseen-in-a-century-countries-cordon-off-ebola-racked-areas.html?_r=0. Retrieved October 4, 2016.
Mill, J. S. (2003). In D. Bromwich & G. Kateb (Eds.), *On liberty* (p. 80). New Haven: Yale University Press.
Mkandawire, T., & Soludo, C. (1998). *Our continent, our future: African; perspectives on structural adjustment*. Dakar: Council for the Development of Social; Science Research in Africa (codesria).
Mohammed, A., Sheikh, T. L., Gidado, S., Abdus-salam, I. A., et al. (2015). Psychiatric treatment of a health care worker after infection with Ebola virus in Lagos, Nigeria. *The American Journal of Psychiatry, 172*(3), 222–224. http://ajp.psychiatryonline.org/doi/pdf/10.1176/appi.ajp.2014.14121576.
Musa, D., Schulz, R., Harris, R., Silverman, M., & Thomas, S. B. (2009). Trust in the health care system and the use of preventive health services by older black and white adults. *Journal of Public Health, 99*(7), 1293–1299.
NAM aidsmap. (2016). *HIV and the criminal law*. East Africa. Available at: http://www.aidsmap.com/law-country/East-Africa/page/1444793/. Accessed 12 Dec 2016.
Nurhussein, M. (2016). Cultural competence in the time of Ebola. In J. Kuriansky (Ed.), *The psychological effects of a deadly epidemic*. Santa Barbara: ABC CLO (Praeger).
O'Hare, B. (2015). Weak health systems and Ebola. *Lancet Global Health, 3*(2), e71–e72.
Reno, W. (1996). Ironies of post-cold war structural adjustment in Sierra Leone. *Review of African Political Economy*, (67), 7–18.
Richter, R. and P. Farmer (2014). *We should be saving majority of Ebola patients*. Stanford Medicine News Centre. Oct 14. https://med.stanford.edu/news/all-news/2014/10/paul-farmer%2D%2Dwe-should-be-saving-majority-of-ebola-patients.html. Accessed 1 Jan 2016.
Rothstein, M. A., Alcalde, M. G., Elster, N. R., Majumder, M. A., Palmer, L. I., & Stone, T. H. (2003). *Quarantine and isolation: Lessons learned from SARS, a report to the Centers for Disease Control and Prevention* (pp. 1–160). Louisville: Institute for Bioethics Health Policy and Law, University of Louisville School of Medicine.
Shaw, R. (2002). *Memories of the slave trade: Ritual and the historical imagination in Sierra Leone*. Chicago: University of Chicago Press.
Sieff, K. (2014). *Liberia already had only a few dozen of its own doctors*. Then came Ebola. Washington Post. Oct 11. http://www.washingtonpost.com/world/africa/liberia-already-had-only-a-few-dozen-of-its-own-doctors-then-came-ebola/2014/10/11/dcf87c5c-50ac-11e4-aa5e-7153e466a02d_story.html. Accessed 20 Dec 2014.
Singer, P. A., Benatar, S. R., Bernstein, M., et al. (2003). Ethics and SARS: Lessons from Toronto. *British Medical Journal, 327*, 1342–1344.

The Choice in End of Life Care Programme Board. (2015). *What's important to me. A review of choice in end of life care*. Available at: https://www.gov.uk/government/uploads/system/uploads/attachment_data/file/407244/CHOICE_REVIEW_FINAL_for_web.pdf. Accessed 12 Dec 2016.

Thomas, K. (2014). *Accountability lab: rebuilding trust during a healthcare crisis*. Ebola Deeply. October 24. http://www.eboladeeply.org/articles/2014/10/6313/accountability-lab-rebuilding-trust-healthcare-crisis/. Accessed 12 Nov 2014.

Tognotti, E. (2013). Lessons from the history of quarantine, from Plague to Influenza A. *Emerging Infectious Diseases, 19*(2), http://www.cdc.gov/eid.

Turshen, M. (1999). *Privatizing health services in Africa*. New Brunswick: Rutgers University Press.

UNDP. (2013). *Human development report. The rise of the South: Human progress in a diverse world*. 2013. UNDP. http://www.undp.org/content/undp/en/home/librarypage/hdr/human-development-report-2013.html.

UNICEF Press Centre. (2014) *First batch of 50,000 household protection kits arrives in Liberia*. http://www.unicef.org/media/media_76030.html. Accessed 30 Dec 2014.

United Nation. (2014). *UN Ebola Crisis Centre: External Situation Report*. October 4. Retrieved from http://www.un.org/ebolaresponse/pdf/Situation_Report-Ebola-04Oct14.pdf. Accessed 30 Dec 2014.

Upshur, R. E. G., Faith, K., Jennifer, L., et al. (2007). Ethics in an epidemic: Ethical considerations in preparedness planning for pandemic influenza. *Health Law Review, 16*(1), 33–39.

Wilkinson, A., & Fairhead, J. (2017). Comparison of social resistance to Ebola response in Sierra Leone and Guinea suggests explanations lie in political configurations not culture. *Critical Public Health, 27*(1), 14–27. https://doi.org/10.1080/09581596.2016.1252034.

Wolz, A. (2014). Face to face with Ebola-an emergency care center in Sierra Leone. *New England Journal of Medicine, 371*(12), 1081–1083.

World Health Organization. (2014a). *Field Situation: How to conduct safe and dignified burial of a patient who has died from suspected or confirmed Ebola virus disease*. Available at: http://apps.who.int/iris/bitstream/10665/137379/1/WHO_EVD_GUIDANCE_Burials_14.2_eng.pdf?ua=1. Retrieved 4 Oct 2016.

World Health Organization. (2014b). *Nigeria is now free of Ebola virus transmission*. The "index" case: how it all started. http://www.who.int/mediacentre/news/ebola/20-october-2014/en/index1.html. Accessed 12 Nov 2014.

World Health Organization. (2015). *Ebola response: What needs to happen in 2015*.http://www.who.int/csr/disease/ebola/one-year-report/response-in-2015/en/.Accessed 24 Jan 2016.

World Health Organization. (2016). *Ebola virus disease: Key facts*. Available at: http://www.who.int/mediacentre/factsheets/fs103/en/. Accessed 12 Dec 2016.

# Chapter 18
# Global Emerging Pathogens, Poverty and Vulnerability: An Ethical Analysis

**Mbih Jerome Tosam, J. Radeino Ambe, and Primus Che Chi**

## 18.1 Introduction

Emerging infectious diseases (EIDs) are "*newly identified* or known infectious diseases that have either expanded in geographic range or increased in infection prevalence over the previous two decades" (Liu and Yu 2017, 12). Some examples are the recent Ebola Virus Disease (EVD) in the West African countries of Guinea, Sierra Leone and Liberia, the Middle East Respiratory Syndrome Coronavirus (MERS-CoV) that has had large outbreaks in Saudi Arabia, United Arab Emirates, and the Republic of Korea, and Zika Virus Disease (ZVD) that affected many countries in the Americas and beyond.

Emerging infectious diseases pose serious public health concerns and cause major socio-economic consequences in affected persons and populations. The effects and impact of EIDs on individual and population health may vary from one individual to another and from one society to another. Globally, the distribution of EIDs vary between countries; as well as within each country. A strong health system is critical in effectively combating EIDs through the establishment of strong infection prevention and control programmes. Strong and resilient health systems

M. J. Tosam (✉)
Department of Philosophy, University of Bamenda, Bamenda, Cameroon

Cameroon Bioethics Initiative, Yaounde, Cameroon

J. R. Ambe
Department of Public Health, School of Nursing and Health Sciences, Capella University, Minneapolis, MN, USA

The Global Emerging Pathogens Treatment Initiative, Lagos, Nigeria

P. C. Chi
Cameroon Bioethics Initiative, Yaounde, Cameroon

KEMRI-Wellcome Trust Research Programme, Kilifi, Kenya



G. B. Tangwa et al. (eds.), *Socio-cultural Dimensions of Emerging Infectious Diseases in Africa*, https://doi.org/10.1007/978-3-030-17474-3_18

better tackle these diseases and prevent them from assuming epidemic and pandemic levels.

Socio-economic, cultural and environmental conditions play a fundamental role in the emergence, spread and control/management of EIDs. In poor communities, a large part of the population live in overcrowded and squalid conditions. In these communities, mostly in the major cities of developing countries, there is a lack of clean drinking water, poor hygiene and sanitation. This environment creates opportunities for waterborne diseases and different forms of pollution. It is in the slums of the main cities of developing countries that most EIDs begin and spread and it is also in such areas of the cities that the greatest number of deaths are usually recorded. Infectious diseases like Ebola, HIV, TB, usually spread easily and widely from poor communities in emerging cities and through health workers who serve such communities. Hence, poverty creates a favourable condition for the spread of infectious diseases and makes it difficult for affected people to get adequate access to prevention and care (WHO 2012a, b). The journal of *Infectious Disease of Poverty was* launched in 2012 with the principal aim of fostering "*interdisciplinary and transdisciplinary research that explicitly highlights the intersection of poverty and other ecological factors with disease*" (Xia et al. 2013).

In this chapter, we critically examine the socio-economic and environmental factors that influence the emergence and spread of EIDs and discuss the ethical issues that arise from the global response and management of EIDs.

## 18.2 Trends and Distribution

Globally, the trend in the outbreak of EIDs has been increasing. Jones et al. (2009) analysed the trend of EIDs events from 1940 to 2000, identifying a total of 335 EID events. They found that during this period, the number of EID events ranged from just over 20 between 1940 and 1950 to close to 80 events between 1990 and 2000, with a peak of close to 100 events between 1980 and 1990 as shown on Fig. 18.1. This peak was associated with the HIV/AIDS pandemic.

This increasing trend in EID mirrors the overall global trend in all human infectious diseases. For instance, Smith et al. (2014) found that within a 33-year dataset (1980–2013), 12,102 outbreaks of 215 human infectious diseases were reported, with more than 44 million cases occurring in 219 nations.

Emerging infectious diseases are distributed all over the world, although their rate of emergence and spread varies from one setting to another. Farmer (1996) observed that their emergence and spread appear to be high in areas with huge social inequalities. Additionally, EIDs are more common in areas rich in wildlife and zoonotic pathogens from wildlife while vector-borne pathogens are more concentrated in lower latitudes, such as tropical Africa, Latin America and Asia (Jones et al. 2009). Also, specific EIDs appear to be common within certain geographical regions. For example, EVD has mainly been in sub-Saharan Africa while the ZVD

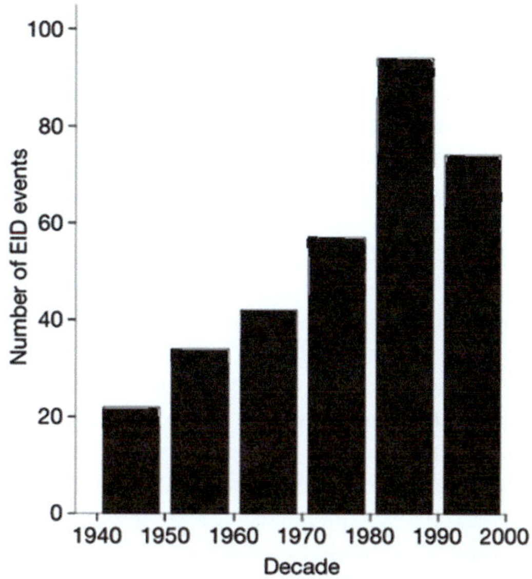


**Fig. 18.1** Distribution of EID events from 1940 to 2000. (Adapted from Jones et al. 2009)

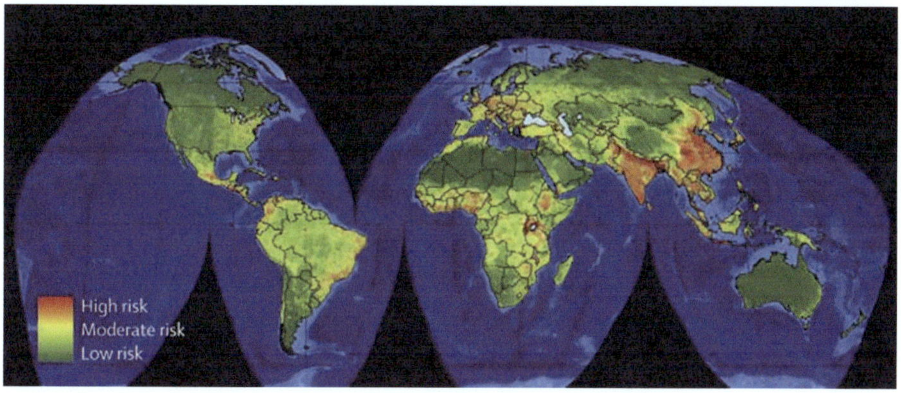


**Fig. 18.2** Global distribution of risk of EIDs originating from wildlife. (Source: Morse et al. 2012)

has been largely limited to the Americas, situations which might be associated with the geographical location of the vectors that spread the disease. Different authors have developed global maps highlighting the areas where EIDs have originated or are most likely to originate. These areas have been described as EID 'hotpots'. One of those maps has been developed by Morse and colleagues, and illustrates the risk of emergence of infectious diseases originating from wildlife as shown in Fig. 18.2 below (Morse et al. 2012).

## 18.3 Factors Affecting the Emergence of Infectious Diseases

The emergence of these diseases is driven by socio-economic, environmental and ecological factors (Jones et al. 2009). The major factors include ecological changes (including those due to economic development and land use), human demographics, behaviour, international travel and commerce, technology and industry, microbial adaptation and change, and breakdown in public health or control measures (Morse 2004). Examples of specific factors affecting infectious disease emergence is shown on Table 18.1. There is a direct correlation between poverty and the emergence of infectious diseases which can be seen through different factors. For instance, the ecological footprint left by humankind is evident by the direct impact on the land, air and water of a specific area or region, used to sustain the depletion of natural resources for an individual or a community.

Among the EIDs of zoonotic origin that make up more than 60% of all EIDs, evidence suggests that between 1940 and 2005 their emergence was largely attributed to changes in land use (18%), human susceptibility to infection (17%), intensification of agricultural practices (13%), and changes in the food industry (13%) (Keesing et al. 2010). A combination of 'other' factors (international travel and commerce, changes in human demographics and behaviour, changes in the medical industry, climate and weather, breakdown of public health measures, and unspecified causes) accounted for 26% of the drivers. Figure 18.3 shows the global percentage of emergence events caused by each driver (a) and the countries in which the emergence events took place, and the drivers of emergence (b) from 1940 to 2005 (Keesing et al. 2010).

This study found that a decrease in the diversity ecosystem that is associated with changes in land use, changes in agricultural and other food production practices such as wildlife hunting, which has led to increasing contacts between humans and other animals has facilitated the emergence of infectious diseases of zoonotic origins (Keesing et al. 2010).

## 18.4 Poverty and the Emergence of Pathogens

There is a close nexus between poverty and infectious diseases. Poverty has provoked a wave of rural urban migration of people in search of new opportunities, which has led to population explosion in the major cities of most developing countries. The result of this has been the growth of slums and expanding cities with "new opportunities for infectious diseases to flourish and spread" (Eisenstein 2016). The concentration of people in squalid conditions leads to waterborne diseases and different forms of pollution. Also, the magnitude and pace of the spread of infectious diseases is usually influenced by overcrowding in tandem with poor hygiene and

**Table 18.1** Factors associated with the emergence of infectious diseases and their relationship with poverty[a]

| Factors | Examples of specific factors | Relationship to poverty |
|---|---|---|
| Ecological changes (including those due to economic development and land use) | Agriculture, dams, changes in water ecosystems, deforestation/reforestation, flood/drought, famine, climate change | Due to poverty, humans may move into new areas (eg. In search of food or shelter - forest clearing for agriculture, wildlife hunting) where there is a higher likelihood for infection. For example forest clearing and wildlife hunting exposes humans more to wildlife that may serve as reservoirs for these infections |
| Human demographics, behaviour | Societal events: population migration (movement from rural areas to cities), war or civil conflict, economic impoverishment, urban decay, factors in human behaviour such as the commercial sex trade, intravenous drug use, outdoor recreation, use of childcare facilities and other high-density settings | Growing urbanisation or conflicts, may force humans, especially the poor into behaviours (risky sexual habits) that may increase the likelihood of mergence and spread of infectious diseases. |
| International travel and commerce | Worldwide movement of goods and people, air travel | Increasing international travels to major international cities may increase the cost of living and force poorer individuals to areas where there is increased contact with EID vectors or engage in risky behaviours that may lead to infectious disease emergence/re-emergence |
| Technology and industry | Food production and processing: globalisation of food supplies, changes in food processing and packaging | Poverty may cause poorer people to sell their organs which may decrease their immune-competence and enhance the re-emergence of infectious disease |
| | Health care: new medical devices, organ or tissue transplantation, drugs causing immunosuppression, widespread use of antibiotics | |
| Microbial adaptation and change | Microbial evolution, response to selection in the environment | Poorer people are more likely to be engage in self-prescription of antibiotics due to the cost associated with seeing a qualified health professional. Such practices might increase the re-emergence of EIDs associated with antibiotics resistance. |

(continued)

**Table 18.1** (continued)

| Factors | Examples of specific factors | Relationship to poverty |
|---|---|---|
| Breakdown in public health or control measures | Curtailment or reduction in disease prevention programmes; lack of or inadequate sanitation and vector control measures | A cutback in public spending on disease and prevention programmes may be more severe in rural areas where the poorer and often less assertive people live compared to major urban centres where the high economic class lives. |

[a]Adapted from Morse (2004)

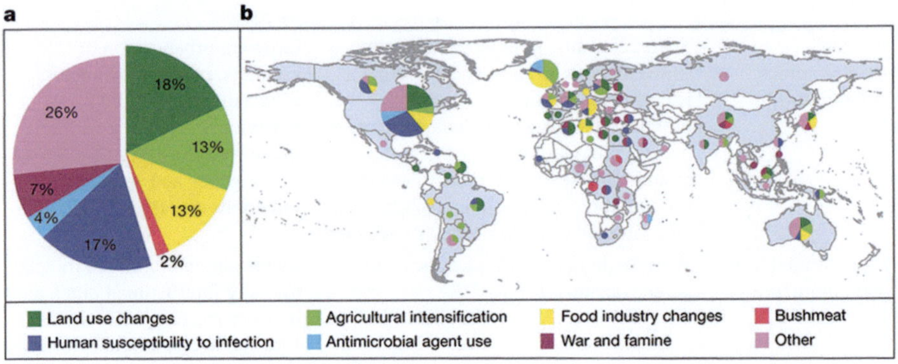


**Fig. 18.3** Drivers and locations of emergence events for zoonotic infectious diseases in humans from 1940 to 2005. (Source: Keesing et al. 2010)

sanitation. For example, it is reported that the recent Ebola outbreak in West Africa spread widely and rapidly in densely populated and highly mobile, urban slums in cities like Monrovia and Conakry (Eisenstein 2016). It was particularly among poor people in the slums, who lacked basic hygiene and sanitation infrastructure in the cities, that there was a serious outbreak. The UN-Habitat estimates that 863 million people- one-third of the developing world's urban population live in slums. Most slums do not have access to safe and clean drinking water and where there exist, it is usually easily open to contamination. These conditions are favourable for the spread of diseases such as cholera, a bacterial diarrhoea and typhoid infections which are transmitted through food and water. For instance, cholera outbreaks were almost an annual occurrence in the northern part of Cameroon during the past 10 years. What accounts for this is extreme water shortage and climate variability, poor sanitation, poor drainage systems with no toilet facilities, in some areas, so that during the rainy season, water carries all human and animal waste into the main sources of water for household use. In some parts of this region, humans and animals depend on the same source of water (Nfor 2014). This exposes the people to waterborne and food related diseases like cholera and typhoid.

Moreover, the “urban poor” usually travel far and wide in search of work, greatly increasing the areas that could be affected by the virus and making contact tracing very difficult (Eisenstein 2016). In slums, there are small ponds, abandoned vehicles, tyres and plastic waste which serve as ideal habitat for the insects that spread dengue and yellow fever as well as malaria. Improvement in living conditions-less crowding, fewer animals and higher quality homes and education may help reduce the possibility of people contracting and spreading infectious diseases.

### *18.4.1 Deforestation, Global Warming and Climate Change*

In addition to the aforementioned factors, high burden of disease, fragile health systems and socio-economic disparity aids in the proliferation of disease vectors and increases vulnerability which can be seen in the patterns of global warming on the African continent. The earth has an ecological system that is comprised of biospheres that are interconnected and rely on each other. Once that is interrupted, for instance, with migration, this disrupts the balance of the biospheres and adds to the burden of this disruption and environmental decay (Abayomi and Cowan 2014). Other factors are increased temperatures, rising sea levels, and increased air pollution. These adverse climatic conditions cause food and waterborne diseases as well as regular ruthless natural disasters (Tosam and Mbih 2015).

Moreover, circumstantial evidence shows that deforestation may have played a role in the West African Ebola Epidemic of 2014/2015. The index case for the West African Ebola Virus Disease Outbreak, lived in a district known as Maliandou, in a village called Guéckédou, in Guinea- Conakry (Marí Saéz 2014). This area is known as the Forest Region, however only approximately 20% of the trees are still standing. The area has lost most of the vegetation due to the mining of iron ore, bauxite, gold and aluminium (Marí Saéz 2014). Wild animals have lost their ecosystems and many use the roofs of thatched huts to nest, living in closer proximity to the villagers. The few remaining trees, are colonized by bats and other animals. It is thought that the insectivorous bats in the hollowed-out tree, in the yard of the index case, may have been the reservoir for the Ebola Virus, Zaire strain (EBOV). Research shows that this particular species (*Mops condylurus*) are able to survive infection by EBOV (Marí Saéz 2014). Amongst the first twelve EVD cases, none were hunters and the index case, was a toddler which led epidemiologists to believe that domestic spaces were in danger for the spread of the disease. Clearly, close living proximity between the bats and the people of the village provides circumstantial evidence of the mode of transmission of this disease, given the issues with deforestation (Borchert et al. 2015).

## 18.5 Ethical Implications in the Context of Poverty

While EIDs have contributed to exacerbating global health inequalities, inequalities in socio-economic conditions globally have arguably also contributed to the emergence and re-emergence of infectious diseases. As has been demonstrated in the earlier sections, developing regions (mostly low and middle-income countries) and impoverished communities and people tend to bear the brunt of EIDs and it negative impacts. Considering the prevailing situation, it would be expected that any efforts in managing the emergence and re-emergence of infectious disease would place more attention and resources in addressing the root causes, especially in developing and low-resource countries. Additionally, one will expect that countries and regions with relatively lower capacity to detect these diseases should receive more attention as the pace with which disease outbreaks are recognized is critical for establishing effective control efforts (Kluberg et al. 2016). However, existing evidence suggests that global resources devoted to countering the emergence of infectious diseases are poorly allocated, with the majority of the scientific and surveillance effort focused on countries from where the next important EID is least likely to originate (Jones et al. 2009). This raises serious ethical issues as it would be expected that for a more effective global response to the prevention and control of EIDs, more resources should be channeled to regions and countries with the greatest risk of experiencing the emergence of these diseases.

Due to our shared elements of vulnerability, there is an urgent need for international cooperative endeavours to promote and preserve health since EIDs know no geographical and economic borders. In the past, vulnerability to EIDs and other health challenges was defined by geographic location and economic factors, but because of the high level of international interactions and movement of persons and goods across borders, this is no longer the case. And since those in affluent countries benefited from the accident of geography and climate as well as efficient health infrastructures which protects them from many threats to EIDs, it is difficult for many to identify with vulnerable people in poor countries. On the contrary, poor people, as a result of their geographical location (mostly in tropical regions) with harsh climatic and economic situations, weak and inefficient health infrastructures; lack access to the health goods needed to prevent them from EIDs (West-Oram and Bux 2016, 1). However, because of globalization and climate change, the tides are changing and vulnerability is being redefined. Today, protection or exposure to EIDs and other tropical diseases is no longer determined by geographical location or economic situation; "all persons are increasingly united in their vulnerability to emerging threats" (West-Oram and Bux 2016, 1). There is need for global cooperation and solidarity between the affluent and poor nations. This can only be effective if both parties identify with each other and acknowledge their shared vulnerability. For example, with the ease in international air travels, an EID in sub-Saharan Africa (sSA) or Asia can reach Europe or the USA within a couple of hours.

The recent EVD and Zika virus pandemics have firmly revealed the extent of global vulnerability and response to EIDs. While EVD-infected expatriate health personnel were flown to their countries for treatment, local EVD-infected health personnel were not accorded such treatment. This attitude was motivated by the failure to recognize the similarity between citizens in rich and poor countries which emerging health threats has exposed us to in our increasingly interconnected interdependent world. It further reflects the discrepancy that existed in international health in the past which does not longer hold today. This calls for a paradigm shift from the charity-based approach to a solidaristic one (West-Oram and Bux 2016, 7). An approach that acknowledges our global interdependence and shared vulnerability to global health threats such as EIDs; and recognizes that if a neighbour's home is on fire, efforts must be made by all to put off the fire, otherwise it may spread and consume more homes (including ours) that may even be further away from the initial home on fire! In fact, the WHO has proposed solidarity as one of the key ethical principles in the management of infectious disease outbreaks globally (WHO 2016). This principle justifies engagement in collective action in the face of common threats such as EIDs, while supporting efforts to overcome inequalities that undermine the well-being of minorities and groups suffering from discrimination. One potential application of this principle globally is the provision of financial, technical, and scientific assistance by high income and developed countries to low-income and impoverished countries to boost their capacities to prevent and manage ongoing and future EIDs. This is in fact one of the obligations of governments and the international community in the WHO 'Guidance for managing ethical issues in infectious disease outbreaks' (WHO 2016).

Therefore, ensuring support for low resource and poorer countries in the prevention and management of EIDs through global solidarity, global health will also be enhanced by reducing the risk of EIDs spreading to other countries. This can be achieved through strengthening LMICs' capacities to adopt and effectively implement the International Health Regulations, a legally binding instrument of international law that aims among others to assist countries to work together to save lives and livelihoods endangered by the international spread of diseases and other health risks.

It is expected that affluent countries have a moral responsibility to support or sponsor research for neglected tropical diseases as well as emerging infectious diseases, and the countries and regions most affected need to take the lead in responding to and in contributing resources to support affected persons, not only as a duty, but on the basis of rational self-interest. Moreover, solidarity does not require that only the rich should identify with the poor; it involves identifying with all persons be they rich or poor. For example, during EVD outbreak in West Africa in 2013–2016, most African countries and the African Union were sluggish in taking the lead in the fight against the disease (Metz 2017). By the time Western countries had pledged 1 billion US dollars, African countries had barely managed to raise $700.000.Cuba, alone, had sent more than 400 health workers whilst the AU had just started deploying only 100 medical personnel (Metz 2017). Developing countries are usually ill-prepared to monitor, prevent and manage the outbreak of these diseases.

## 18.6 Conclusion

In this chapter, we have shown that there is an inextricable link between socio-economic, cultural and environmental conditions and the emergence or re-emergence of EIDs. EIDs have contributed in exacerbating global health inequalities as most areas where EIDs are common are also areas that experience lack of access to basic life-saving and preventive medicines. For any fight against these diseases to be successful, mechanisms must be put in place to redress these determinants as well as bring together the intellectual, financial and health resources of the world for all, especially people from low and middle-income countries where the local capacity to appropriately manage EIDs is relatively weak. This is because in our interconnected and interdependent world, no individual, group or nation is insulated from the threats of EIDs. It is important that rich countries play a fundamental role in dedicating resources and increasing funding for research in capacity-building and drugs for EIDs in developing countries, not only because their own populations are also vulnerable to EIDs, but also for the sake of global solidarity. Also, the countries where EIDs are more likely to occur and those whose capacity to effectively manage EIDs is weak, must also play a leading role in addressing the socio-economic, cultural and environmental conditions which facilitate the emergence and spread of infectious diseases.

## References


Abayomi, A., & Cowan, M. N. (2014). The HIV/AIDS epidemic in South Africa: Convergence with tuberculosis, socioecological vulnerability, and climate change patterns. *South African Medical Journal, 104*(8), 583.

Borchert, M., Saez, A. M., & Kratz, T. (2015). A closer look at the Ebola outbreak in West Africa. *Future Virology, 10*(5), 483–490.

Eisenstein, M. (2016). Disease: Poverty and pathogens. *Nature, 531*(7594), S61–S63. https://doi.org/10.1038/531S61a.

Farmer, P. (1996). Social inequalities and emerging infectious diseases. *Emerging Infectious Diseases, 2*(4), 259.

Jones, K. E., Patel, N. G., Levy, M. A., Storeygard, A., Balk, D., et al. (2009). Global trends in emerging infectious diseases. *Nature, 451*(7181), 990–993.

Keesing, F., Belden, L. K., Daszak, P., Dobson, A., Harvell, C. D., et al. (2010). Impacts of biodiversity on the emergence and transmission of infectious diseases. *Nature, 468*(7324), 647–652.

Kluberg, S. A., Mekaru, S. R., McIver, D. J., Madoff, L. C., Crawley, A. W., Smolinski, M. S., & Brownstein, J. S. (2016). Global capacity for emerging infectious disease detection, 1996–2014. *Emerging Infectious Diseases, 22*(10).

Liu, Y. & Yu, X. (2017). Identification and diagnosis of newly emerging pathogens. *Infectious Diseases and Translational Medicine; 3*(1), 12–16.

Metz, T. (2017). How to deal with neglected tropical diseases in the light of an African Ethic. *Developing World Bioethics*. (Forthcoming).

Morse, S. (2004). Factors and determinants of disease emergence. *Revue scientifique et technique-Office international des epizooties, 23*(2), 443–452.

Morse, S. S., Mazet, J. A., Woolhouse, M., Parrish, C. R., Carroll, D., et al. (2012). Prediction and prevention of the next pandemic zoonosis. *The Lancet, 380*(9857), 1956–1965.
Nfor, M. K. (2014). *Recurrent cholera outbreak in Far-North Cameroon highlights development gaps*. Inter Press Service News Agency. 2http://www.ipsnews.net/2014/08/recurrent-cholera-outbreak-in-far-north-cameroon-highlights-development-gap
Saéz, A. M., Weiss, S., Nowak, K., Lapeyre, V., Zimmermann, F. et al. (2014). Investigating the zoonotic origin of the West African Ebola epidemic. *EMBO Molecular Medicine*, e201404792.
Smith, K. F., Goldberg, M., Rosenthal, S., Carlson, L., Chen, J., Chen, C., & Ramachandran, S. (2014). Global rise in human infectious disease outbreaks. *Journal of the Royal Society Interface, 11*(101), 20140950.
Tosam, M. J., & Mbih, R. A. (2015). Climate change, health, and sustainable development in Africa. *Environment, Development and Sustainability, 17*(4), 787–800.
West-Oram, P. G., & Buyx, A. (2016). Global health solidarity. *Public Health Ethics, 6*(1), 13.
WHO. (2016). *Guidance for managing ethical issues in infectious disease outbreaks*. Geneva: World Health Organization; 2016.
WHO. (2012a). *Social determinants of health: Social exclusion*. 2012. http://www.who.int/social_determinants/themes/socialexclusion/en/
WHO. (2012b). *The global report for research on infectious diseases of poverty*. Geneva: World Health Organization; 2012.
Xia, S., Allotey, P., Reidpath, D. D., Yang, P., Sheng, H. F., et al. (2013). Combating infectious diseases of poverty: A year on. *Infectious Diseases of Poverty, 2*(1), 27.

# Chapter 19
# Why Justice is Good for Healthcare in Africa: Towards an Ethical framework

Samuel J. Ujewe

## 19.1 Introduction

Countries in Sub-Saharan Africa have at least three things in common: cultural heritage, high burden of disease, and low financial commitment to healthcare (Ujewe 2016). The high burden of disease in the region is marked by a persistence of deadly infectious disease epidemics. Such outbreaks are often accompanied by aggressive involvement of donor agencies from the global north. The epidemics tend to present opportunities for the international community to showcase its capacity for good will towards African people. In contrast, this chapter asks questions of justice relating to healthcare issues around Africa. It explores the lack, and need thereof, of an ethical framework of justice to guide health system reforms and intervention strategies in Africa. Acknowledging that Africa is geographically vast and culturally diverse, the chapter focuses on Nigeria as a key microcosm that reflects the broader African picture. A few countries, like South Africa, have better established health systems than Nigeria, but most other countries are worse off. Nigeria is the most populated country in Africa, as well as an economic-index leader in the continent (Focus Economics 2017). An outlook of Nigeria's healthcare would give some insight into that of the broader continent.

In this chapter, "Africa(n)" refers to countries south of the Sahara Desert. The reason being that North African countries (north of the Sahara Desert) have a shared Arab heritage that makes them more culturally aligned to the Arab world, given the historical Arab domination of the region (Abun-Nasr et al. 2016). Also, generally speaking, countries in North Africa are in better economic standing when compared to most in Sub-Saharan Africa. Countries in Sub-Saharan Africa, although variously colonised by Western countries, do not witness the kind of cultural transformation

S. J. Ujewe (✉)
Canadian Institute for Genomics and Society, Toronto, ON, Canada

Global Emerging Pathogens Treatment Consortium, Lagos, Nigeria



G. B. Tangwa et al. (eds.), *Socio-cultural Dimensions of Emerging Infectious Diseases in Africa*, https://doi.org/10.1007/978-3-030-17474-3_19

experienced in North Africa. They have largely maintained their traditional cultural roots, as evident in contemporary social practices. More importantly, the region is widely recognised to have a shared cultural heritage; which is what I mean by "African". This is not to suggest that there are no valuable ethical references from North Africa. Rather, the shared cultural trends in Sub-Saharan Africa make it possible to abstract shared ethical values or principles, which is not the case with North Africa.

In traditional African societies, healthcare was considered a community affair. For instance, a traditional healer had unrestricted access to farmlands or other properties where herbal remedies for particular diseases were to be found (Tangwa 2010). Since much of the African context remains largely communitarian, one would expect that such traditional ideals are carried forward into contemporary healthcare practice. Yet, the continent remains infamous for persistent poor population health, especially when compared to Europe or North America. Also, African health systems are marked by poor infrastructure and limited capacity to manage deadly epidemics, as was evident in the Ebola epidemic in West Africa, between 2013 and 2015 (Moon et al. 2015).

While these facts raise questions of healthcare justice, bioethics in Africa mostly focuses on research ethics (e.g. ethical questions arising in clinical trials). Relevant debates tend to revolve around questions of autonomy and informed consent. Furthermore, global bioethics has largely avoided questions of health inequalities in Africa. In Nigeria, various efforts in healthcare reform do not appear to give priority to ethics-informed measures in reviewing the system and analysing health policies (Ujewe 2016). This appears to be the common trend in other African health systems. Sparse attempts have been made in some countries to include an ethical approach –*Accountability for Reasonableness (AFR)* – to inform health policy and reform (Maluka et al. 2010a, b, 2011a, b; Maluka 2011).

However, these have overlooked the significance of Africa's unique social, cultural and ethical contexts. This chapter aims to establish the place of justice in the bioethical discourse on and outlook of health and healthcare in Africa. It anticipates a specific African ethical approach of justice in the distribution of and access to healthcare, and envisions an ethical framework towards just reforms in African health systems.

## 19.2 Africa's Unfair Share of the Global Burden of Disease

To put it positively, a broad view of the healthcare situation in sub-Saharan African countries presents the population as largely resilient. Exploring the broader context of health and healthcare in Africa would require an entirely different and extended project, which is beyond the scope of this chapter. It would suffice therefore to briefly outline some key aspects for the purpose of clarity. For our consideration, it is worthwhile to explore Africa's share of the global burden of disease, as well as the health systems' incapacity to manage these burdens.

The sub-Saharan Africa region bears a disproportionate weight of the global burden of infectious disease, despite its population largely living below the global poverty benchmark. According to *The World Health Statistics 2017:*

> At the end of 2015, an estimated 36.7 million people were living with HIV. The WHO African Region remains the most severely affected, with 4.4% of adults aged 15–49 years living with HIV… There were an estimated 429 000 malaria deaths globally, with the heaviest burden borne by the WHO African Region – where an estimated 92% of all deaths occurred – and by children under 5 years of age, who accounted for more than 70% of all deaths… there were an estimated 10.4 million new TB cases and 1.4 million TB deaths, with an additional 0.4 million deaths resulting from TB among HIV-positive people… fatality rate …varied widely – from under 5% in some countries to more than 20% in most countries in the WHO African Region. (World Health Organisation 2017, 30)

Compounding the problem of infectious diseases is the high rate of maternal and newborn mortality in the region, as compared to other regions in the world:

> The global under-five mortality rate in 2015 was 43 per 1000 live births, while the neonatal mortality rate was 19 per 1000 live births – representing declines of 44% and 37% respectively compared to the rates in 2000. Newborn deaths represented half or more of all deaths among children under 5 years of age in all WHO regions in 2015 with the exception of the WHO African Region where one third of under-five deaths occurred after the first month of life (Figure 2.1). The WHO African Region also had the highest under-five mortality rate (81.3 per 1000 live births) that year – almost double the global rate. (World Health Organisation 2017, 30)

In terms of performance and health outcomes, *The Global Burden of Disease Study 2016,* does not include any of the mainland sub-Saharan African countries in the top 100 (Fullman et al. 2017). Summarily:

> Although their relative burdens have declined, communicable, newborn, nutritional, and maternal causes such as diarrheal diseases, lower respiratory infections, and protein-energy malnutrition remained the top drivers of health loss in most sub-Saharan African countries, especially in lower-income countries like Niger and Sierra Leone. (Fullman et al. 2017)

Recent data show that in 2015, infectious diseases cumulatively make the major contributions to mortality on Sub-Saharan Africa:

Group I conditions accounted for 5.2 million of deaths (56.4%), down from 5.7 million deaths in 2010 (61.4%). Notable causes of death in this category were:

- lower respiratory tract infections (one million),
- HIV/AIDS (760,000),
- diarrhoeal diseases (643,000),
- tuberculosis (434,000) and
- malaria (403,000).

Non-communicable, or group II accounted for 3.1 million deaths (33.5% of all deaths), rising from 29.4% in 2010. The major killers in this category were:

- stroke (451,000 deaths),
- ischaemic heart disease at 441,000, and
- cirrhosis of the liver with 174,095 deaths. (World Health Organisation 2017; Africa Check 2017)

One does not have to look too far to see how these figures come to life amongst Africa's populations. In 2017, Madagascar, an African island country in the South Indian Ocean, managed to take control of a three-month Plague outbreak that ravaged its population only upon international intervention (Bichell 2017). According to the World Health Organisation (WHO 2017), as at November 2017, 1618 cases were reported and 72 deaths were clinically confirmed as pneumonic plague. Following the epidemic, nine countries and overseas territories in the Africa region were identified as priority for plague preparedness given their visible trade and travel links with Madagascar. In 2016, there was a yellow fever outbreak in the Central Africa region, mostly affecting Angola and the Democratic Republic of Congo, with more than 6000 combined suspected cases and over 400 deaths reported (WHO 2016b). Although yellow fever threatened global populations previously, it has been eliminated in most parts of the world since a vaccine was invented in the 1930s. Yet, the outbreak in Central Africa saw the world struggle to rally enough vaccine doses for the affected countries, as many pharmaceutical companies have pulled out of production due to low profitability of the vaccine (McNeil and Donald 2016).

Finally, between 2014 and 2016, the largest and most devastating outbreak of the Ebola virus took hold of six countries in West Africa, and was declared an international public health emergency by the WHO. The epidemic killed five times more than all other known outbreaks in history, with a total of 28,616 cases and 11,310 deaths as of June 2016 (WHO 2016a). Despite the virus being identified four decades earlier, no urgent effort had been made towards vaccine development, until the 2016 outbreak. Lack of profitability for pharmaceutical companies was blamed as the key limiting factor. The Ebola vaccine developed post the West African epidemic thankfully found use in the 2018 outbreak in the DR Congo (World Health Organisation 2018).

The list of prevailing deadly infectious diseases and epidemics are inexhaustible, as new deadly pathogens continue to emerge. Coupled with the deadly diseases, there are several others that impact on the lives of the populations, commonly referred to as "neglected tropical diseases" (Feasey et al. 2009). These are diseases that, while not deadly, significantly decrease the productive capacities of its victims, and have been classed as diseases of the poor:

> …these diseases predominate in the tropics, but their predilection for hot places results principally from the fact that poverty is found in the greatest concentration in the remote rural communities, urban slums and displaced populations near to the equator… All low-income countries are affected by at least five… simultaneously, and many individuals who live in those countries are concurrently infected by more than one pathogen… infections are at least in part attributable to inadequate access to safe water, sanitation and appropriate housing. (Feasey et al. 2009, *180*).

Most sub-Saharan African countries have these characteristics, and as such provide breading grounds for these diseases. Their persistence means that already disadvantaged populations are being pushed further towards greater health disadvantage, and their productive capacities are greatly diminished.

## 19.3 African Health Systems' Incapacity

The prevalence of deadly infectious diseases and neglected tropical diseases is worsened by the limited capacities of African health systems to control or manage them. In Nigeria, for instance, despite consolidated approaches employed in the health system, access to quality services remains significantly low or non-existent for much of the population (Ujewe 2016). This is despite the country's endowment with vast resources, which if harnessed could make needed healthcare services available and accessible to all. Among other things, primary healthcare in the country is yet to be consolidated, with its development marred by inadequate facilities, personnel and services. As would be the case, if not worse, in several other African countries, the quality of care provided in many public healthcare facilities in Nigeria is sub-optimal (Bonilla-Chacin et al. 2010; Akuki 2015). This means that patients are often compelled to seek healthcare in private facilities that require huge out-of-pocket financial commitment, as most people do not have health insurance.

While various kinds of health insurance schemes exist in many African countries, only those with the financial capacity can afford medical aid cover. To cite an example, Nigeria's National Health Insurance Scheme only covers those in active public service, leaving those in private or self-employment, let alone the unemployed, to entirely self-fund their own cover under the scheme. For non-public employees, or self-employed, the lowest annual premium is N15,000, approximately US$50, per person (National Health Insurance Scheme 2015). While this cost appears to be considerably low, it is unaffordable to many in the Nigerian context. The national minimum wage remains N18,000, approximately US$50, per month; and negotiations are underway for a proposed increment to N56,000 (US$155) per month (Inyang 2017). At the current rate, the insurance scheme is not affordable to many citizens, especially in the light of the undesirably high rate of unemployment in the country. To show the ineffectiveness of the insurance scheme, only about 3% of the population has enrolled on all of its program since its inception in 2005 (Arin and Hongoro 2013).

Compare the situation with South Africa, which arguably has the leading health infrastructure in sub-Saharan Africa, and one finds little to no encouraging news. Public healthcare facilities are accessible to all citizens; yet, adequate health services are mostly only available in private healthcare facilities (Young 2016; Patel 2017). Private health facilities are expensive, and are only affordable to those who can buy private insurance. The lowest monthly premium for the most basic medical aid plan is R1,100, approximately US$80, for the principal member (Writer 2017), with some discounted rates offered for adult and child dependants. The current national minimum wage for cashiers, for instance, is R3,395.47 per month (Mywage.co.za and WageIndicator.org 2017). This means that in a family of four, where the couple both earn minimum wages, they cannot afford medical aid, and hence cannot access healthcare services offered in the private sector.

Given the persistence of deadly infectious diseases and NTDS, and the fact that all citizens are at risk of being infected with at least one of these diseases at any given period, the question comes down to who can afford treatment or full course of vaccinations when it matters. In Nigeria, South Africa, as with most countries in the region, one can argue that epidemics are largely a function of the lack of or inadequate capacity of the health systems, which results in undue healthcare disadvantage to poorer population groups. The Ebola epidemic, which caused great havoc in Liberia, Sierra Leone, and Guinea, was brought under control in Nigeria within a very short period (WHO 2014). Nigeria's Ministry of Health deservedly received praises from around the world for its efforts at halting the epidemic. The virus was brought into the country through its foremost international airport by a high profile personnel, who arrived the country for a regional conference (Adekunle 2014). Hence, one can also attribute a luck-factor to Nigeria's early success: an important personality, arriving through the foremost and most secure airport in the country means that it was easier to detect the virus and to isolate the carrier. Suppose, he was a local merchant, and entered Nigeria through the land border at Seme (the south-western border town of Nigeria with Benin Republic), which is notoriously porous, chaotic and highly populated, one can only imagine what the story of Ebola in Nigeria would have been.

## 19.4 A Question of Healthcare Justice

The considerations above raise questions of justice in healthcare for African populations. In part, one can argue that Nigeria's ability to avoid the Ebola catastrophe, as suffered by Liberia, Sierra Leone, and Guinea, was largely because of its higher economic prosperity, a more functional health system and luck. As a result, Nigeria's population was spared the devastation that was suffered in Liberia, for instance, which had not fully recovered from the long-term effects of civil war. The lack of capacity in Guinea to detect the virus for several months was a key factor that led to its spread into Liberia and Sierra Leone (Moon et al. 2015). This phase underscored the issue of inadequate investment in healthcare infrastructure, despite the government's formal commitment to do so. Also, there is a question around the slow international support, despite awareness that these low-income countries had no capacity to control the epidemic. Failures of the relevant governments to adequately invest in healthcare represent a healthcare injustice to their populations. Likewise, the international community's slow operational response raises a question of healthcare justice from a global perspective.

Like many other epidemics in Africa, Ebola variously attracted sympathies from around the world, and the international support offered appeared to be largely motivated by a sense of beneficence. The principle – *the end justifies the means* – appears to be the key consideration guiding various decisions taken and strategies adopted during the epidemic, given the speed with which they were executed. Nevertheless, viewing support for a disadvantaged population's health predicament from a beneficence perspective places them at a greater disadvantage, as they cannot adequately negotiate the terms of such help. By allowing a beneficence outlook to inform international action in the time of Ebola, affected countries were relegated to the bane of total surrender of their health systems. They were saliently expected to accept whatever measures, strategies or support that were offered, even if they may wish to disagree. And whatever was offered would be considered ethically acceptable, if a potentially favourable outcome was anticipated. Power differential between the suffering population and sponsoring agencies was thus normalised – with the typical subjects being affected African populations.

However, where the situation is viewed in terms of justice, approaches suggested or employed would reflect the inherent wishes of the populations for their own health and wellbeing. Prioritising the ideals of justice in healthcare intervention would present the power relations differently. It is established that the WHO and the international community took several months following initial warnings to react to the West African Ebola epidemic (Kelland 2015); and that it was only taken seriously when individual health workers from Western countries became infected (Kerridge and Gilbert 2014). Thus, underpinning the slow response is the outlook of beneficence with which the situation was initially viewed. Other countries saw their contribution towards ending the epidemic as a supererogatory gesture – i.e. going beyond the requirements of the duty to do good – despite being aware that the affected countries had no adequate capacity to address the problem. A quick response was thus stalled by the underpinnings of beneficence.

If justice for the affected population was the priority consideration from the initial alerts on the Ebola epidemic, a swift response may have been motivated, and the scale massively curtailed. Response to epidemics in Africa needs to be underpinned by considerations of justice; not a beneficence outlook. In the light of justice, affected populations would be viewed as partners or equal stakeholders in the pursuit of the global health initiative; not simply as beneficiaries or subjects. Where partnership underpins the process, key decisions like skipping several trial stages of an unproven vaccine for advance trial in humans would be undertaken differently. Viewing African health problems from a justice perspective would raise the consciousness that the benefits are not only for African people, but also for people in other parts of the world. If health epidemics on the continent are viewed as uniquely African problems – as was the case in the early stages of the West African Ebola epidemic – the nature of obligation for the rest of world to respond would remain that of beneficence. This would engender a slow international response, and escalate the epidemic to a global scale, affecting all populations – as was potentially the case with the Ebola epidemic. However, where justice for the health and wellbeing of affected African populations is prioritised, a swift response would be motivated, the epidemic curtailed sooner, and populations in other parts of the world would be safe.

### *19.4.1 The Preoccupation of African Bioethics*

While imminent questions of healthcare justice abound for the continent, health research ethics is presently the most developed aspect of bioethical considerations in/for Africa. The trend is pronounced in the existing literature, as mostly developed by scholars of African origin. For instance, (Ezeome and Simon 2010) evaluate the ethical implications of the infamous research trial by the pharmaceutical corporation Pfizer, in Nigeria. In establishing the ethical flaws of Pfizer's trial, they employ the international guidelines for conducting research in low and middle-income countries. They make no recourse to how substantive African ethical values should inform these guidelines, despite the uniqueness of the context. Similar routes have been taken by others, as seen in exploratory discourses on: informed consent practices in Nigeria (Ezeome and Marshall 2009); the promotion of health research integrity in Africa (Kombe et al. 2014); and ethics and researcher identity (Simon and Mosavel 2011).

Although health research ethics remains a significant concern in Africa, we must also broaden our focus to include considerations of justice for the populations' health and wellbeing. Moreover, if significant issues in health research, like informed consent, are to be specifically relevant in African contexts, research participants would require guaranteed access to basic health services or resources, as justice demands. We cannot, for instance, talk about patient autonomy when patients do not have access to the most basic treatments; nor is the discourse on informed consent compelling where participants do not have access to basic health services and/or needed treatments. Likewise, it is difficult to talk about informed consent in health research or medical trials when participants have desperate health status, as was the case with the numerous trials conducted during the Ebola epidemic in West Africa. Their desperate health situations already make them vulnerable; they are likely to 'give consent' out of desperation for a remedy.

Thus, it is imperative to first seek and address considerations of justice in Africa's populations' health. When this is established, only then can we better engage with other relevant ethical considerations. The relevant pathway should seek to abstract from specific African ethical values in addressing Africa-specific issues in healthcare or health research. It should be an appropriate representation of *African bioethics in an African frame*. Since the reality and effects of healthcare inequality rages on in contemporary Africa, we are obliged to provide relevant solutions. The answers can still be found in the ethical imperatives underlying African traditional healthcare approaches. We must however, abstract from these imperatives to make the effects of justice real for population health.

A specific African ethical approach to justice in healthcare or health promotion is yet to be established, as African bioethics endeavours appear to focus exclusively on the clinical and medical research fields. This reflects the enormous challenge facing population health in Africa, especially regarding the broad range of ethical considerations needed to consolidate the various health systems. What exists in current literature could serve as a platform towards further research on broader issues, especially those relating to justice in population health. As Tangwa (2016) notes, there is a vast area of research in African bioethics which still lies fallow, including ethical considerations in: disease and treatment, poverty and disease, medical practice, healthcare and professionalism, among others. As a possible way forward, Azetsop (2011) suggests integrating elements of solidarity, especially those of mutuality and interdependence, in considering effective strategies for health promotion in Africa.

## 19.5 Towards an African Ethical Framework of Justice for Africa's Healthcare

To effectively address the varied questions of justice arising in healthcare around the continent, it is crucial to develop a framework of healthcare justice that would guide relevant approaches in population health. Norman Daniels provides a viable framework which has been developed over three decades. His ethical approach has been applied to healthcare reforms in the United States, and adopted in a WHO health improvement program for Africa. Attempts have also been made to adapt it towards health care reforms in low and middle-income countries (Daniels et al. 2000, 2005; Daniels 1985, 2007; World Health Organization 2004). In Daniels' view, we need to focus on justice in promoting effectiveness in populations health: "justice obliges us to pursue fairness in the promotion of health, but policy needs the guidance of ethics in determining what this means"(Daniels 2006, 23). He develops a theory of justice for health, against which one can evaluate or measure fairness in health outcomes. Daniels theory of just health is guided by three basic explanations (Daniels 2007):

1. Health is of special moral importance because it contributes to the range of opportunities open to us;
2. Health is produced not just by having access to medicine and treatment, but also by accumulated social experience of life conditions; and
3. We can only meet health care needs fairly under limited resource availability through a fair deliberative process.

Against this background, Daniels develops the framework of *Accountability for Reasonableness* (AFR), which he offers as an ethical tool to legitimise policy processes, as well as guide effective and just healthcare reforms. The framework requires health policy reforms to be guided by a fair process:

> Key elements of fair process will involve transparency about grounds for decisions; appeals to rationales that all can accept as relevant to meeting health needs fairly; and procedures for revising decisions in light of challenges to them…Fair process must also be empirically feasible (Daniels 2000).

Being the most established ethical approach of justice in healthcare (Segall 2010), Daniels' framework requires close consideration towards improving populations health in African settings. However, the AFR framework faces two key challenges regarding its applicability in African settings, which are mainly contextual and conceptual limitations: (1) the framework was originally formulated for health reforms in the United States, the context of which is significantly different from those in Africa; and (2) the AFR framework is substantiated by a strictly Western approach to justice, as encapsulated in John Rawls' idea of *fair equality of opportunity* (Ujewe 2016).

In contrast, healthcare reforms in African contexts should be guided or informed by a framework of justice that appreciates the nature of African healthcare contexts, and the interwoven socio-cultural dynamics. Without discounting the value of Daniels' approach, it is crucial that local socio-ethical contexts be taken seriously in formulating a justice framework for African health system reforms. Rather than simply import the AFR framework into Nigeria's health system, for instance, considerations must be given to specific socio-cultural dimensions that were not anticipated in Daniels' original formulation.

The relevant ethical framework towards just reforms in African health system must take the shape of the socio-ethical context. Insisting on universalising one ethical model for just healthcare reforms across the board would perpetuate the dominance of one moral worldview against several others in different parts of the world. Such approach simply extends the current trend in global bioethics, where specific societies' ethical ideals are taken as universal principles. This minimises the significance of the varied social, cultural and contextual factors, like social relationships and interactions that shape moral precepts, attitudes and behaviour:

> [It] …disparages the social and cultural differences that exist within and between societies, negates the importance of recognising and respecting otherness and the many ways of being in the world, and rather ironically mask what is particularist about bioethical thought by attributing universalism to some of the Western and specifically American culture patterns with which it is imprinted (Fox and Swazey 2010, 278).

At the same time, it may not be helpful to completely abandon the significant benefits or lessons we could draw from innovative approaches like the AFR framework, for an entirely new or opposing framework. If we insist on a strictly "African" ethical approach, without recourse to some universal principles in the current framework, we may forego some features that effective reforms in African health systems may need. The way forward is to pursue an even-handed approach healthcare justice in African settings. This should also account for the varied social and cultural conditions, as well as universal phenomena:

> There can be no culturally and psychologically perspective ethics without taking account of the diversity of moral lives, but there can be no ethics at all without universals, allowing a means of trying to stand aside from particulars to make meaningful ethical assessments (Callahan 2000, 38).

The viable ethical framework towards healthcare justice in African settings must consider both the African modes of moral explanations and relevant universal dynamics. While not discounting relevant universalist perspectives, such as those informing the AFR framework, it must be underpinned by specific African principles of justice, such as the principle of restoration (Ujewe 2016).

## 19.6 Conclusion

The health and wellbeing of populations in Sub-Saharan Africa seeks more than a beneficence outlook for the kind of support it desires. What is mostly contributed towards healthcare aid to the region by affluent countries is largely viewed as supererogatory. This implies that at best, Africans should be thankful for every drop of support they get. Additionally, African governments have been largely unable to mobilize the needed resources to revamp population health, thereby sustaining the disadvantage chain for most citizens. A viable way forward for effective health system reforms must incorporate a justice framework that is informed by African principles. In the foregoing, I have explored the underlying ethical dynamic guiding approaches to health epidemics in Africa. I refer to the beneficence model reflected in recent response strategies as a limiting factor that is detrimental to Africa's population health. Healthcare resources invested in Africa's populations by both African governments and the global community will be more effective if motivated and directed by an outlook of justices. This chapter has thus aimed to motivate the development of a justice approach to healthcare in Africa. The approach to justice in healthcare would be particularly beneficial in responding to and managing epidemics around the continent.

## References

Abun-Nasr, J. M., Warmington, B. H., & Brett, M.. (2016). 'North Africa'. *Encyclopædia Britannica*. Encyclopædia Britannica, inc. https://www.britannica.com/place/North-Africa.

Adekunle. (2014). How Ebola disease got to Nigeria. *Vanguard News* (blog). 22 October 2014. https://www.vanguardngr.com/2014/10/ebola-disease-got-nigeria/.

Africa Check. (2017). *FACTSHEET: Africa's leading causes of death*. Africa Check. 4 August 2017. https://africacheck.org/factsheets/factsheet-africas-leading-causes-death/.

Akuki, A. (2015). Salvaging Nigeria's health care challenges. *Independent Nigeria* (blog). 20 January 2015. https://independent.ng/salvaging-nigerias-health-care-challenges/.

Arin, D., & Hongoro, C. (2013). *Scaling up national health insurance in Nigeria: Learning from case studies of India, Colombia, and Thailand*. Washington, DC: Futures Group Health Policy Project.

Azetsop, J. (2011). New directions in African bioethics: Ways of including public health concerns in the bioethics agenda. *Developing World Bioethics, 11*(1), 4–15.

Bichell, R. E. (2017). *How Madagascar took control of its plague outbreak*. NPR.Org. 19 November 2017. https://www.npr.org/sections/goatsandsoda/2017/11/19/564821692/how-madagascar-took-control-of-its-bubonic-plague-outbreak.

Bonilla-Chacin, M. E., Okigbo, A., Malife, N., Sherburne-Benz, L., & Ruhl, O. (2010). *Improving primary health care delivery in Nigeria: Evidence from four states*. Washington, DC: World Bank.

Callahan, D. (2000). Universalism & particularism: Fighting to a draw. *Hastings Center Report, 30*(1), 37–44.

Daniels, N. (1985). *Just health care*. Cambridge: Cambridge University Press.

Daniels. (2000). Accountability for reasonableness: Establishing a fair process for priority setting is easier than agreeing on principles. *BMJ: British Medical Journal, 321*(7272), 1300.

Daniels. (2006). Toward ethical review of health system transformations. *American Journal of Public Health, 96*(3), 447–451.

Daniels. (2007). *Just health: Meeting health needs fairly*. Cambridge: Cambridge University Press.

Daniels, N., Bryant, J., Castano, R. A., Dantes, O. G., Khan, K. S., & Pannarunothai, S. (2000). Benchmarks of fairness for health care reform: A policy tool for developing countries. *Bulletin of the World Health Organization, 78*(6), 740–750.

Daniels, N., Flores, W., Pannarunothai, S., Ndumbe, P. N., Bryant, J. H., Ngulube, T. J., & Wang, Y. (2005). An evidence-based approach to benchmarking the fairness of health-sector reform in developing countries. *Bulletin of the World Health Organization, 83*(7), 534–540.

Ezeome, E. R., & Marshall, P. A. (2009). Informed consent practices in Nigeria. *Developing World Bioethics, 9*(3), 138–148.

Ezeome, E. R., & Simon, C. (2010). Ethical problems in conducting research in acute epidemics: The Pfizer meningitis study in Nigeria as an illustration. *Developing World Bioethics, 10*(1), 1–10.

Feasey, N., Wansbrough-Jones, M., Mabey, D. C. W., & Solomon, A. W. (2009). Neglected tropical diseases. *British Medical Bulletin, 93*(1), 179–200.

Focus Economics. (2017). 'Nigeria Economic Outlook'. *Focus Economics: Economic Forecasts from the Wolrd's Leading Economists*, 14 November 2017. https://www.focus-economics.com/countries/nigeria.

Fox, R. C., & Swazey, J. P. (2010). Guest editorial: Ignoring the social and cultural context of bioethics is unacceptable. *Cambridge Quarterly of Healthcare Ethics, 19*(3), 278–281.

Fullman, N., Barber, R. M., Abajobir, A. A., Abate, K. H., Abbafati, C., Abbas, K. M., Abd-Allah, F., Abdulkader, R. S., Abdulle, A. M., & Abera, S. F. (2017). Measuring progress and projecting attainment on the basis of past trends of the health-related sustainable development goals in 188 countries: An analysis from the global burden of disease study 2016. *The Lancet, 390*(10100), 1423–1459.

Inyang, I. (2017). Labour Kicks, Says Reps N30,000 Minimum Wage Not Good Enough. *Daily Post Nigeria* (blog). 15 October 2017. http://dailypost.ng/2017/10/15/labour-kicks-says-reps-n30000-minimum-wage-not-good-enough/.

Kelland, K. (2015). Two new trials of Ebola vaccines begin in Europe and Africa. *Reuters*, 15 July 2015. https://www.reuters.com/article/us-health-ebola-vaccines/two-new-trials-of-ebola-vaccines-begin-in-europe-and-africa-idUSKCN0PP1BH20150715.

Kerridge, I., & Gilbert, L.. (2014). Epidemic ethics: Four lessons from the current ebola outbreak. *The Conversation*, 24 August 2014. http://theconversation.com/epidemic-ethics-four-lessons-from-the-current-ebola-outbreak-30534.

Kombe, F., Anunobi, E. N., Tshifugula, N. P., Wassenaar, D., Njadingwe, D., Mwalukore, S., Chinyama, J., Randrianasolo, B., Akindeh, P., & Dlamini, P. S. (2014). Promoting research integrity in Africa: An African voice of concern on research misconduct and the way forward. *Developing World Bioethics, 14*(3), 158–166.

Maluka, S. O. (2011). Strengthening fairness, transparency and accountability in health care priority setting at district level in Tanzania. *Global Health Action, 4*(1), 7829.

Maluka, S., Kamuzora, P., Sebastián, M. S., Byskov, J., Ndawi, B., & Hurtig, A.-K. (2010a). Improving district level health planning and priority setting in Tanzania through Implementing accountability for reasonableness framework: Perceptions of stakeholders. *BMC Health Services Research, 10*(1), 322.

Maluka, S., Kamuzora, P., Sebastiån, M. S., Byskov, J., Olsen, Ø. E., Shayo, E., Ndawi, B., & Hurtig, A.-K. (2010b). Decentralized health care priority-setting in Tanzania: Evaluating against the accountability for reasonableness framework. *Social Science & Medicine, 71*(4), 751–759.

Maluka, S., Kamuzora, P., Sebastián, M. S., Byskov, J., Ndawi, B., Olsen, Ø. E., & Hurtig, A.-K. (2011a). Implementing accountability for reasonableness framework at district level in Tanzania: A realist evaluation. *Implementation Science, 6*(1), 11.

Maluka, S. O., Hurtig, A.-K., Sebastián, M. S., Shayo, E., Byskov, J., & Kamuzora, P. (2011b). Decentralization and health care prioritization process in Tanzania: From national rhetoric to local reality. *The International Journal of Health Planning and Management, 26*(2), e102–e120.

McNeil, Jr., & Donald, G. (2016). Yellow fever epidemic in Africa shows gaps in vaccine pipeline. *The New York Times*, 5 December 2016, sec. Health. https://www.nytimes.com/2016/12/05/health/yellow-fever-africa-vaccine.html.

Moon, S., Sridhar, D., Pate, M. A., Jha, A. K., Clinton, C., Delaunay, S., Edwin, V., Fallah, M., Fidler, D. P., & Garrett, L. (2015). Will Ebola change the game? Ten essential reforms before the next pandemic. The report of the Harvard-LSHTM independent panel on the global response to Ebola. *The Lancet, 386*(10009), 2204–2221.

Mywage.co.za, and WageIndicator.org. (2017). *Minimum Wage, Minimum Wages South Africa – Mywage.Co.Za*. 2017. https://mywage.co.za/main/salary/minimum-wages.

National Health Insurance Scheme. (2015). *Nigeria national health insurance scheme: Operational guidelines, October 2015*. Abuja: National Health Insurance Scheme. https://www.google.ca/search?rlz=1C1CHBF_enCA761CA762&biw=1013&bih=945&ei=FaI6Wv6lN8G7jwSDj6_4CA&q=Nigeria+National+Health+Insurance+Scheme%3A+Operational+Guidelines&oq=Nigeria+National+Health+Insurance+Scheme%3A+Operational+Guidelines&gs_l=psy-ab.3...752709.757066.0.757858.9.9.0.0.0.0.280.880.0j3j2.5.0....0...1c.1.64.psy-ab..4.2.430...0j0i13k1.0.Wu2X3UyNhgM.

Patel, A. D. (2017). A World of difference between private and public healthcare in South Africa - Google Search. *The Daily Vox*, 8 March 2017. https://www.google.ca/search?rlz=1C1CHBF_enCA761CA762&biw=1013&bih=945&ei=Wac6WosFovYjwTenYiYDQ&q=a+world+of+difference+between+private+and+public+healthcare+in+south+africa&oq=a+world+of+difference+between+private+and+public+healthcare+in+south+africa&gs_l=psyab.3...200473.222941.0.223430.81.64.3.12.12.0.353.8205.6j34j8j2.50.0....0...1c.1.64.psyab..16.49.5509...0j0i67k1j0i131k1j0i10k1j0i22i30k1j33i22i29i30k1j0i13i30k1j33i21k1j33i160k1.0.e-bf_oo-y-o.

Segall, S. (2010). Is Health (Really) special? Health policy between rawlsian and luck egalitarian justice. *Journal of Applied Philosophy, 27*(4), 344–358.

Simon, C., & Mosavel, M. (2011). Getting personal: Ethics and identity in global health research. *Developing World Bioethics, 11*(2), 82–92.

Tangwa, G. B. (2010). *Elements of African Bioethics in a Western Frame*. African Books Collective.

Tangwa, G. B. (2016). Leaders in ethics education: Godfrey B. Tangwa. *International Journal of Ethics Education, 1*(1), 91–105.

Ujewe, S. J. (2016). *Just health care in Nigeria–The foundations for an African ethical framework*. Preston: University of Central Lancashire. Clok.uclan.ac.uk.

WHO. (2014). *WHO declares end of Ebola outbreak in Nigeria*. WHO. 20 October 2014. http://www.who.int/mediacentre/news/statements/2014/nigeria-ends-ebola/en/.

WHO. (2016a). *Ebola Virus Disease: Situation Report*.

WHO. (2016b). *WHO | Yellow fever situation report*. WHO. 15 July 2016. http://www.who.int/emergencies/yellow-fever/situation-reports/15-july-2016/en/.

WHO. (2017). *WHO | Plague – Madagascar*. WHO. 15 November 2017. http://www.who.int/csr/don/15-november-2017-plague-madagascar/en/.

WHO. (2018). *Ebola virus disease – Democratic republic of the Congo*. WHO. 23 May 2018. http://www.who.int/csr/don/23-may-2018-ebola-drc/en/.

World Health Organisation. (2017). *World health statistics 2017: Monitoring health for the SDGs*. Geneva: World Health Organization.

World Health Organization. (2004). *Guidance on ethics and equitable access to HIV treatment and care*. Geneva: WHO.

Writer, S. (2017). South Africa's cheapest Medical aid schemes and hospital plans in 2017. *BusinessTech*, 4 May 2017. https://businesstech.co.za/news/lifestyle/173415/south-africas-cheapest-medical-aid-schemes-and-hospital-plans-in-2017/.

Young, M. (2016). *Private vs. Public Healthcare in South Africa*. Western Michigan University. Honors thesis. Paper 2741. https://scholarworks.wmich.edu/cgi/viewcontent.cgi?referer=https://scholar.google.co.za/&httpsredir=1&article=3752&context=honors_theses. Accessed June 2019.

# Part V
# Narratives from the Field: The Ebola Virus Disease Experience

# Chapter 20
# Beyond Mere Statistics: Case Studies from the Field During the Ebola Epidemic in West Africa

**J. Radeino Ambe, Nchangwi Syntia Munung, and Godfrey B. Tangwa**

## 20.1 Introduction

Significant progress has been made in reducing the burden of disease globally. Life expectancy has increased in many regions of the world. In sub-Saharan Africa, for example, life expectancy has generally increased in most African countries and there has been an overall decline in the prevalence of communicable diseases in the last 10 years. Despite the decline in global disease burden and an increase in life expectancy across most regions of the world, sub–Saharan Africa (sSA) still bears the highest disease burden. For example, of the 36.7 million people living with HIV/AIDS globally, about 25.6 million are in sub-Saharan Africa (WHO 2017a, b). The African region has a disproportionate amount of malaria cases. In 2015, 90% of malaria cases worldwide, occurred in Africa (WHO 2016b). Currently there is a threat with multidrug resistant tuberculosis in many countries in sub-Saharan Africa. The region is also witnessing a sharp rise in non-communicable diseases such as hypertension, diabetes, stroke, depression and obesity, (Naghavi and Forouzanfar 2013).

J. R. Ambe (✉)
Department of Public Health, School of Nursing and Health Sciences, Capella University, Minneapolis, MN, USA

The Global Emerging Pathogens Treatment Initiative, Lagos, Nigeria
e-mail: jambe@capellauniversity.edu

N. S. Munung
Department of Medicine, University of Cape Town, Cape Town, South Africa

Global Emerging Pathogen Treatment Consortium (GET) Consortium, Lagos, Nigeria

G. B. Tangwa
Department of Philosophy, University of Yaounde 1, Yaounde, Cameroon

Cameroon Bioethics Initiative (CAMBIN), Yaounde, Cameroon

Global Emerging Pathogen Treatment Consortium (GET) Consortium, Lagos, Nigeria

 
G. B. Tangwa et al. (eds.), *Socio-cultural Dimensions of Emerging Infectious Diseases in Africa*, https://doi.org/10.1007/978-3-030-17474-3_20

Management and control of these health conditions have been challenged by a high level of poverty and poor health systems in many African countries. The combination of abject poverty, poor health systems and lack of basic infrastructure, in many areas, enables an environment where epidemics can easily thrive and spread. This results in loss of life and further complicates an already distressed socio-economic system. While statistics on the global and national burden of disease are important in setting public health priorities and in resource allocation, it may easily be forgotten that there is also a human face to each statistic presented during an epidemic. Each statistical number is someone's mother, father, son, daughter, uncle, aunt, cousin or grandchild, belonging to a particular socio-cultural community and milieu, country and region. The health needs of any community, be it during an epidemic or in normal times, cannot be addressed without taking into consideration their existential situation and conditions, their beliefs and understanding, especially of disease and wellness, their social and cultural practices and daily habits. Several issues overarch statistics no matter how diligently collected and accurate they are.

The importance of a holistic approach to address disease burden, besides the focus on statistics, can best be illustrated in the case of epidemics. In this chapter we focus on the "human face" of the Ebola epidemic in sSA using real people and cases from the 2014 Ebola outbreak in West Africa.

The Ebola outbreak started in December 2013 and lasted until June 2016; when all three countries (Sierra Leone, Liberia and Guinea- Conakry) were declared "Ebola-free". An end to the transmission was declared in March of 2016 when emergency measures were lifted by the World Health Organization, at a meeting in Geneva, Switzerland. (WHO 2016a).

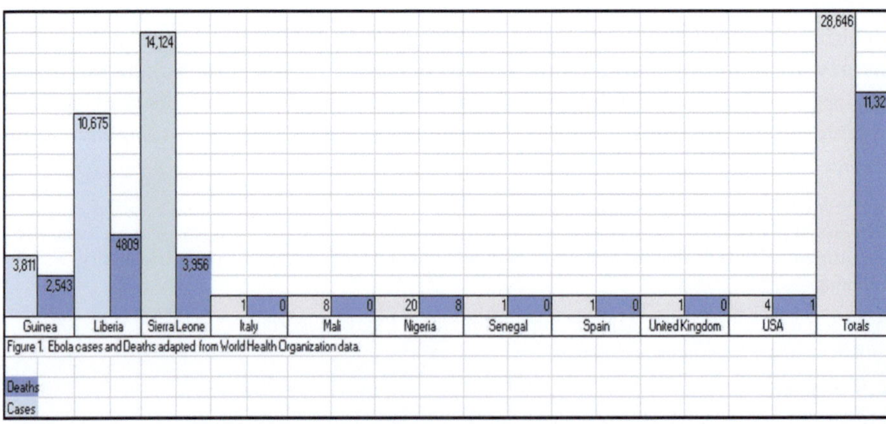

Figure 1. Ebola cases and Deaths adapted from World Health Organization data.

These cases involve multi-faceted ethical dilemmas and it is hoped that issues relating to the abuse of individual rights and/or lack of respect for the dignity of affected persons that occurred as part of actions to control the epidemic are sufficiently highlighted in this chapter for future reference. These instances are drawn upon as a means of reflection in an effort to learn from the situation and to provide guidance should similar situations arise during a future outbreak.

Treating those who have been afflicted by a disease during an epidemic, appropriately with empathy and sympathy, is central to the success of any epidemic control programme. The abuse of individual rights and lack of respect for their dignity are some of the factors that perpetuate mistrust between people, governments and researchers. However, while there have been numerous epidemics in a number of African countries, with anecdotal reports of actions which could be considered abuses of individual rights and/or lack of respect for the dignity of affected persons, there has been no systematic documentation of such abuses. These case studies present information and illuminate the concerns around these issues and the need for development and/or application of guidelines to address these issues in future epidemics.

## 20.2 CASE 1: Patient Zero, Emile Ouamouno

The first person to contract a disease during an epidemic, is known as the *index case* and is given the epidemiological name of "Patient Zero". It is befitting to start the Case Studies for this chapter, with the index case, as reported in research conducted by Health Officials, in Guinea, Conakry, by the World Health Organization (WHO) and the German institution known as the Robert Koch Institute (RKI). The 2014 Ebola epidemic started in Maliandou, a village in Guéckédou District of Guinea-Conakry with only 31 households (Marí Saéz et al. 2015), Guéckédou is close to the borders of Liberia and Sierra Leone in southeastern Guinea. A laterite road leads to the village which sits on top of a hill. This area is known as the Forest Region although approximately 80% of the forest has been obliterated due to mining of gold, aluminium, iron and bauxite. Guinea holds the largest reserves of iron ore with high iron content in the southern mountains of Simandou. (The Economist 2014). Much of the mining is done by foreign investors and exploiters who do not give so much of an afterthought to the ecology; the replanting of trees and/or vegetation, much less the environmental impact or the ecology. It is owing to this deforestation that wild animals have lost their habitats and are brought closer in proximity to humans, sometimes even substituting treetops for rafters under the thatched roofs of huts.

Patient Zero, Emile Ouamouno, a toddler between 18 and 24 months old, lived in Maliandou with his parents and three sisters. His immediate older sister, Philomene, was 3 years old. His grandparents also lived in the family compound. Maliandou has become known as ground zero from which Ebola Virus Diseasespread across the "red" or "hot zone". This zone is shaped like a triangle. Maliandou is close to where three national borders converge. The countries of Guinea- Conakry, Sierra Leone and Liberia had all had years of wars and unrest; were impoverished and had no proper public health system to assist those who did not have the means to pay for healthcare services.

Emile would play with his sister and other children outside, under the tree in the backyard. This hollowed out tree was home to a colony of insectivorous bats *(Mops condylurus)* which are thought to have been a reservoir for the Ebola Virus. (Callaway 2016). Early discussion and research shows that this bat species, is able to survive infection induced by experiments, which shows their hardiness and inability to succumb to the Ebola Virus (Marí Saéz 2015). Emile's father, Etienne Ouamouno, stated that his children usually danced and played outside with a ball (Ghoulipour 2014).

Although there are conflicting dates, it is clear that, in the month of December 2014, Emile got ill with a high fever accompanied by vomiting and the passing out of dark stool mixed with blood. Within two days, Emile, an active toddler, who loved to play outside, was declared dead (WHO 2015). Within a week, following his death, his younger sister, Philomene, also died, after presenting the same symptoms – black stool, vomiting and fever. Shortly after that, their pregnant mother presented with exactly the same symptoms. Emile's grandmother also died shortly after that. At this point, the health officials thought the deaths were from cholera. They later declared it was Lassa fever, before realizing it was Ebola Virus Disease (EVD).

When the zoonotic origins of the West African Ebola Epidemic was investigated using interviews, surveys, and laboratory analyses of samples taken from bats and the environment, there was no evidence of outbreak of the disease in wildlife. This led to the conclusion that this was not a case of the ingestion of bush meat, although it cannot be concluded that the fruit bat is not a reservoir for EVD. (Callaway 2016). In the case of the West African outbreak and from prevailing research, it is more likely that Emile became infected by playing around insectivorous bats in the hollowed out tree. There is much debate but little proof that the outbreak started from bat reservoirs and some argue that as common as bats are in West Africa, if bats are reservoirs, there should have been more than just this one major outbreak (Callaway 2016). Research and the arguments on this issue are still inconclusive.

In conclusion, little Emile Ouamouno, a toddler likely to have been between 18 to 24 months of age, was the index case of the West African Ebola epidemic. Emile's sister, mother and grandmother died within a month of his death, triggering a trail of deadly infections and deaths across three countries in the affected zones of Guinea, Liberia and Sierra Leone. There is no conclusive evidence on how Emile got infected with Ebola Virus Disease. It is unlikely that he was out hunting bush meat, since he was a toddler. His exposure to bush meat would have been minimal. Despite the presence of insectivorous bats in the hollowed out tree behind their house, there were no large colonies of fruit bats in the area.. Thus this index case was traced to a toddler who would not, in all likelihood, have hunted or handled bush meat.

## 20.3 CASE 2: Reverend Brother Patrick Nshamdze

The second case study is on Patrick Nshamdze, a Cameroon-born missionary of the Hospitaller Order of Saint John of God. One of the very first people of the Nso' ethnic tribe of the Northwest region of Cameroon to join this religious order, he had dedicatedly been serving for 23 years and spent the last years of his life in Monrovia, Liberia, working as director for the Saint John of God Catholic Hospital (Osei-Owosu 2014), Monrovia. The Hospitaller Order of St. John of God was founded in Spain and is an International Roman Catholic health care organization with over 50 hospitals around the world.

Though serving as director of the hospital, Bro Patrick, as he was fondly called, found himself assisting the clinical staff during the recent Ebola outbreak. This was partly driven by the ever increasing number of patients that were coming into the SJGH and the shortage of staff in the hospital, particularly as many workers tended to stay at home due to the fear of getting ill from the deadly disease. On 08th July 2014, in the course of assisting a patient who had been brought in by a high ranking Liberian official, bleeding and convulsing, Bro Patrick probably contracted the Ebola virus disease (EVD). A few days after this incident, Brother Patrick felt ill and complained of severe headache. He also felt heartbroken when he learnt that the patient he had recently helped had died of EVD.

Although Bro Patrick had had direct contact with this patient, he felt he could continue with his duties at the hospital and ordered that all staff who had been in contact with the patient (12 out of 28 nurses at the hospital) undergo a 21 day observation period (Osei-Wusu 2014). An initial test on July 18th, by the Liberian Ministry of Health's Ebola testing centre, indicated that Bro Patrick was negative for EVD. However, after 2 weeks of being sick, he tested positive for EVD on July 29th. Bro. Patrick finally succumbed to the deadly virus on the second of August 2014 at the age of 52 (SJCH 2014).

News of his death was received with absolute consternation and disbelief in Cameroon, especially in his native village of Shiy and the entire Nso' clan. In a community where the burial ritual is very important, everyone was waiting for the corpse of Bro Nshamdze to be convinced of his death, but the corpse never arrived. Worth noting are the medical tests that were carried out on Bro Patrick. Before the second EVD test results that turned positive, a test at the St. John of God Hospital, following the negative first EVD results, had shown that he could be suffering from Brucellosis. Despite treatment, his health deteriorated and plans were made to evacuate him to Ghana for treatment. For this, a hard copy confirmation from the Ministry of Health of Liberia that he was EVD negative was needed. The testing centre reported that the test result was no longer in their system and that a new test would be required. The results of the new test showed that Bro Patrick was positive for EVD. Following this, it was agreed that that Bro. Patrick would be treated at the SJGH but, a few days later, the Ministry of Health insisted that he be transferred to one of the Ebola treatment centres. This was done in the evening of the 31st of July (Osei-Owusu 2014). Bro Patrick died 2 days later at ELWA Hospital.

The SJGH was shut down on the first of August, as an increasing number of persons who had been caring for Bro Patrick also succumbed to the EVD disease. Following the sad situation, the religious order consulted with the Spanish government and decided to evacuate all the religious personnel at the SJGH to Spain. However, when the military jet that was sent for the purpose arrived, it turned out that only personnel of Spanish nationality were to be evacuated (Richardson 2014).

When the Order received news of the death of Bro Patrick, they requested to know the precise burial arrangements and the possibility of some loved ones attending the burial. Anecdotal information has it that the Catholic authorities in Liberia had also requested that his remains be buried differently so that the church, friends and relatives could have the opportunity to pay homage to a man who had, for 27 years, given his life unreservedly for the service of humankind. However, none of this happened and he was buried in Johnsonville, Monrovia, in one of the mass graves of victims of the EVD. News of Bro Patrick's death spread like wild fire in Monrovia and beyond. Newspapers in Monrovia carried the story alongside his picture and the pictures of some of the people who had been in direct contact with him. This caused a lot of panic. The honorific distinction of Grand Commander in the order of the star of Africa, was later conferred upon Bro Patrick by the president of the Republic Liberia, Madam Ellen Johnson Sirleaf, in consideration of his contributions to the cause of humanity, especially the people of Liberia.

## 20.4 CASE 3: Fatu Kekula

Fatu Kekula, a 22 year old, nursing student lived in Kakata, Liberia, with her father, Moses, her mother, Victoria, her older sister, Vivian, and cousin, Alfred. On July 27th, Moses had a spike in his blood pressure and Fatu took him to the Kakata Hospital. He was admitted to the hospital due to his elevated blood pressure and placed on the newly vacated bed of a patient. When he was admitted, it was not known that the patient died from EVD. Moses, contracted EVD and within a short time had a fever, was vomiting and having diarrhea (Dixon et al. 2014). Unfortunately, several nurses from Kakata Hospital, where Moses was admitted, died from EVD and Kakata Hospital was shut down.

Fatu took her father to the capital city of Monrovia, which was over an hour's drive away, in an effort to see if she could get him admitted in an Ebola Treatment Unit (ETU) or any hospital or clinic; however, there were no beds available. They got turned away again and again from one hospital to another. Upon returning to Kakata, Fatu took her father to another hospital but there was very little they could do for him. Fatu prayed about it and since she had no choice, she took him home to the rest of the family in an effort to take care of him by herself. She prepared a space in an unfinished part of the building for him as an isolation unit. It was soon clear that the other family members had what ailed her father, the dreaded Ebola Virus Disease that many were succumbing to. Doctors in the hospital where she was receiving her training soon heard and called her on phone urging her to stay away from her sick family members. But Fatu would not abandon her family. She knew she was their last hope and could not just sit and watch them die without any care. In order to protect herself, Fatu bought plastic bags, face masks, rubber boots, a raincoat and bleach. She prayed and felt confident that her prayers would be heard. Then she set aside fear and wore the mantle of faith and determination. She received phone assistance on protective gear use from her family doctor and devised a makeshift protective equipment from trash bags. She put trash bags over her socks, put on rain boots and then more trash bags. She used stockings to cover her head then tied a trash bag, like a scarf on her head, covering the stocking. She also used trash bags as gloves. To cover her clothes, she wore a raincoat which she could easily disinfect with chlorine bleach solution. Fatu did this several times a day so as to be able to care for her sick family. Unfortunately, her cousin, 14 year old Alfred, succumbed to the disease but the rest of the family recovered. (Dixon et al. 2014).

After the outbreak was brought under control, Fatu Kekula went on to study nursing at Emory University in Atlanta, United States. Coincidentally Emory was also treating four Ebola patients at the same time.

## 20.5 CASE 4: Sarh Conteh (Anonymized)

At the time of the 2014 West Africa Ebola outbreak, Sarh Conteh, a young man in his mid- 20's, was working as a doctor's assistant at the Medvale Hospital in Monrovia, Liberia. Sarh was very fond of one of his colleagues, Sia, a young nurse, in her late 20s who worked many long shifts with him. Sia was a dedicated and caring nurse who often went out of her way to help patients and their caregivers. Sia took ill and Sarh remained by her side, nursing her, feeding her and cleaning up after. He hardly left her side. Sarh cared for Sia until she died, approximately 2 weeks into his caring for her. Looking back, Sarh realized that Sia was one of the very first people he knew to have come down with EVD.

A few days afterwards, one of the doctors in the hospital who had treated Sia tested positivefor EVD and was taken to the Sunydale Ebola Treatment Unit (ETU), about five kilometers away from Medvale Hospital where he worked. A few days after, another nurse, Kumba, in the same hospital took ill but eventually survived the infection. Sadly, the doctor died about a week after admission to the Sunydale ETU.

Sarh became terrified as it dawned on him that he had worked closely with all the sick people taken to Medvale Hospital. It appeared that no one who had been admitted at the Sunydale ETU ever came out alive. Sarh does not remember when he was tested for EVD, but he woke up in the Sunydale ETU on June 28, 2014, to see two persons dressed in Personal Protective Equipment (PPE) bending over him and peering down at him. It seemed all so surreal and his thoughts were of certain death. As time went by, Sarh lost all hope and became depressed. Moreover, while Sarh was at the Sunydale Hospital, his death was falsely announced.

Another nurse from Medvale, Findah, joined Sarh at the Sunydale ETU. Upon hearing she was diagnosed with EVD, Findah became hysterical. She attacked Sarh the moment she saw him, raining blows on him and accusing him of having infected her with Ebola. Both of them, however, were fortunate to survive the infection, although she has remained "emotionally distressed" even after her recovery.

Sarh was declared Ebola free and discharged from the Sunydale ETU on the 16th of July, 2014. Sarh's eyes smarted as he tried to adjust to the bright sunlight. He emerged confused and realized, as he tried to make his way back home that people who recognized him fled in apparent terror. Some people mistook him for a ghost and others for someone still infected with Ebola. He was lucky, however, because his family received him home with open arms. He was later to hear of others who were shunned by their own families. His mother cooked for him and cared for him.

Despite the support he received from family, the nights were difficult times for Sahr. He struggled to sleep and every time he closed his eyes he was transported back to the Sunydale ETU. Sarh started doubting whether he was really alive or dead. For several days he was unable to sleep and had pains all over his body.

One day, a team of health researchers came to ask Sarh to donate his blood for research purposes. They explained that, as a survivor of EVD, he was immune to developing a new infection and that his blood might act like a "medicine" for those suffering from EVD. Following the encounter with the health researchers, Sarh started regaining composure and his thoughts started fixating on how he could help his country and those still suffering from EVD infection. His morale lifted and he started to derive meaning from all he had been through.

## 20.6 Conclusion

According to the Centers for Disease Control, 11,325 people died from EVD; a total of 28,652 cases had been recorded out of which only 15,261 were confirmed in a laboratory (CDC, n.d.). The Ebola epidemic raised a plethora of dilemmas and ethical issues concerning human rights, access to care, and inequality. Moral dilemmas, heroism, failings and unanswered questions are evident through the case studies presented in this chapter. They provide but a small glimpse through a handful of real lives, in situ and context, at the time of the epidemic. It is a quite different view from that of those who were mainly concerned with preventing the epidemic from crossing borders and becoming a pandemic; those mainly concerned with containing the epidemic and preventing its future recurrence; those concerned with testing a possible cure or vaccine and worrying about risk-benefit ratios and informed consent; and those excited about the commercial possibilities and prospect of catapulting a molecule previously tested in rats and primates for other purposes into a knockout cure for the epidemic disease.

Unfortunately, by virtue of their birth, thousands of people live in areas of high mortality and morbidity from many tropical diseases. There is an inverse relationship between disease, mortality, morbidity and education, income level and access to healthcare. (Gapminder, n.d.). Four indicators for measuring the health of a community or group of people have been identified as: how long a person lives, the quality of the years during which the person is active, the number of deaths in that population and, finally, how theenvironment and society accommodate persons withdisabilities, physical, mental or cognitive (Holtz 2017). All these indicators are lower in sub-Saharan Africa. There is an ethical obligation to provide improvement to African health systems in an effort to reduce the socio-economic injustice and unfairness suffered by many. People are counted as mere statistics when documenting public health epidemiological or situation reports, as was seen during the Ebola epidemic, by institutions such as the Center for Disease Control (CDC) and the World Health Organization (WHO); however, in reality, each statistic was a person with loved onesbelonging to a family, clan, tribe, nation or region.

## 20.7 Questions for Ethical consideration:

1. What are the key ethical challenges posed in the cases and how could they best be addressed?
2. In an epidemic situation, such as the 2014 Ebola outbreak, what ethical considerations should be taken into account when recruiting survivors into a clinical study?
3. Who should be responsible for the needs of patients during an outbreak?
4. To what extent is the health system in place appropriate for the actual context it is supposed to be serving?

**Note**
One of the anonymized case studies presented in this chapter was first presented, in substance, at the Global Forum on Bioethics in Research (GFBR), November 2015, in Annecy, France. The meeting theme, "Emerging epidemic infections and experimental medical treatments" drew attendees from across the globe. During Session 1: Trust and Community Engagement, the anonymized case study, Bonglam Kromah, Physician's Assistant: using convalescent blood from Ebola survivors, was presented. We hereby acknowledge the sponsorship of the GFBR which made this possible. The meeting report may be of interest to the readers of this chapter and the link can be found in the reference section of this chapter (GFBR 2015).

## References

Anonymous, Crying foul in guinea; mining and corruption. (2014). *The Economist 413*(8916), 78.

Callaway, E. (2016). Ebola hunters go after viral hideout. *Nature, 529*(7585), 138–139. https://library.capella.edu/login?url=http://search.proquest.com.library.capella.edu/docview/1757965618?accountid=27965.

Citation (posthumus). Retrieved from https://www.barmherzige-brueder.at/dl/pKqmJKJLlMNnJqx4KJK/Posthume_Ehrungen.pdf. Accessed 17 Dec 2017.

Dixon, M. G., Schafer, I. J., & Centers for Disease Control and Prevention (CDC). (2014). Ebola viral disease outbreak — West Africa, 2014. *Morbidity and Mortality Weekly Report, 63*(25), 548–551.

GapMinder Tools. n.d.. Retrieved from http://www.gapminder.org/tools/#_

GFBR. (2015). *Meeting report for annecy.* http://www.gfbr.global/past-meetings/10th-forum-annecy-france-3-4-november-2015/

Gholipour, B. 2014. Ebola patient zero: How outbreak started from single child. *Live Science.*

Holtz, C. (2017). *Global health care: Issues and policies* (3rd ed.). Burlington: Jones & Bartlett Learning. ISBN: 9781284070668.

Marí Saéz, A., Weiss, S., Nowak, K., Lapeyre, V., Zimmermann, F., Düx, A., . . . Leendertz, F. H. (2015). Investigating the zoonotic origin of the west african ebola epidemic. EMBO Molecular Medicine, 7(1), 17–23. doi:https://doi.org/10.15252/emmm.201404792.

Naghavi, M., & Forouzanfar, M. H. (2013). Burden of non-communicable diseases in sub-saharan africa in 1990 and 2010: Global burden of diseases, injuries, and risk factors study 2010. *The Lancet, 381*(S2), S95–S95. https://doi.org/10.1016/S0140-6736(13)61349-5.

Osei-Owusu, E. (2014). *The Ebola crisis in St. Joseph catholic hospital, Liberia -As witnessed.* Retrieved from http://www.myjoyonline.com/opinion/2014/October-2nd/the-ebola-crisis-in-st-joseph-catholic-hospital-liberia-as-witnessed.php

Richardson, V. (2014). *Spanish priest infected with Ebola to be treated with experimental drug*. Washington Times. http://www.washingtontimes.com/news/2014/aug/10/spanish-priest-infected-ebola-be-treated-experimen/.

St. Joseph's Catholic Hospital. SJCH. (2014). *Br. Patrick Nshamdze, our Hospital Director, dies at 52*. http://www.sjcatholichospital.com/2014/08/03/br-patrick-nshamdze-our-hospital-director-dies-at-52/. Accessed 12 Dec 2017.

World Health Organization. (2015). *Origins of the 2014 Ebola epidemic*. http://www.who.int/csr/disease/ebola/one-year-report/virus-origin/en/

World Health Organization. (2016a). *Statement on the 9th meeting of the IHR emergency committee regarding the Ebola outbreak in west Africa*. African Press Organisation. Database of Press Releases Related to Africa.

World Health Organization. (2016b). *Malaria fact sheet*. http://www.who.int/mediacentre/factsheets/fs094/en/

World Health Organization. (2017a). *HIV/AIDS Fact Sheet*. http://www.who.int/mediacentre/factsheets/fs360/en/

World Health Organization. (2017b). *Tuberculosis Fact Sheet*. http://www.who.int/tb/en/

# Chapter 21
# Lagos the Mega-City: A Report on How the Metropolis Handled an Outbreak of the Ebola Epidemic

**Jide Idris and Adesina Fagbenro**

## 21.1 Context

Lagos State is a mega-city with an estimated population of 16–21 million people.[1] In the last ten years, the megacity has made tremendous progress in terms of: sustained rapid economic growth, improved infrastructure and services, and a significant reduction in crime rates. This has provided an enabling environment for millions of Lagos state inhabitants to find their way out of poverty. Lagos State Government has also made great strides in its quest to: increase value for money in public spending; improve the business climate in Lagos; maintain fiscal sustainability; and properly monitor and manage financial and health risks.

[1] The State attained megacity status in early 2000 with a population of above 10,000,000 people.

J. Idris (✉)
Commissioner for Health, Lagos, Lagos State, Nigeria

A. Fagbenro
Mothergold, Lagos, Nigeria



G. B. Tangwa et al. (eds.), *Socio-cultural Dimensions of Emerging Infectious Diseases in Africa*, https://doi.org/10.1007/978-3-030-17474-3_21

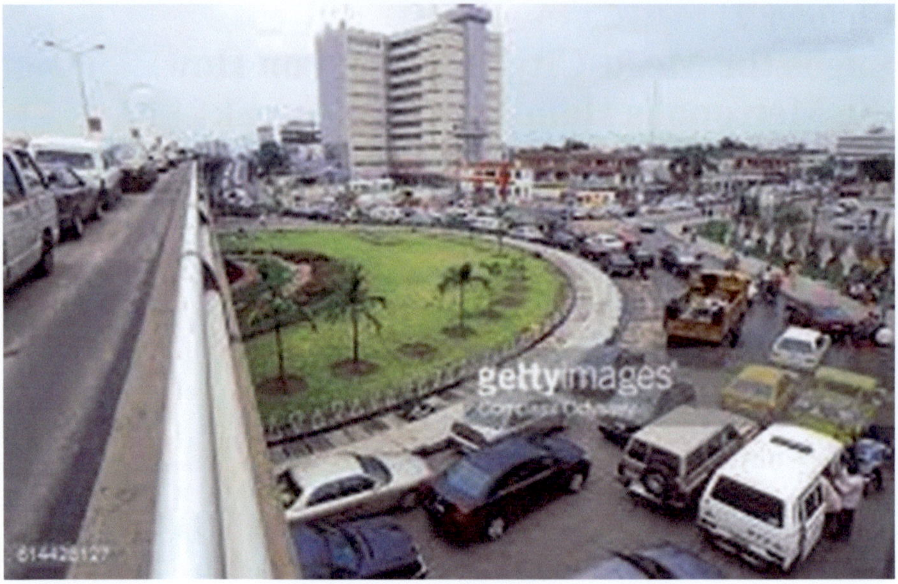


Lagos is the most densely populated state in Nigeria, with over 5% of the national population estimated to reside in its environs (Ayeni 2017; Aliyu and Amadu 2017). Ironically, it is the smallest state in terms of land mass. The state has an area of 356,861 hectares of which 75,755 hectares are wetlands. Metropolitan Lagos, an area covering 37% of the land area of Lagos State, is home to over 85% of the state's population making it densely populated. The United Nations estimates that at its present growth rate, the state of Lagos may, in the near future be one of the top most populous mega-cities in the world joining, Tokyo in Japan and Bombay in India (UN 2016). Poverty levels in Lagos remain at about 48–50%. While access to health and education is quite high, poverty remains a huge challenge especially with rapid population migration into Lagos from other Nigerian states especially in the North and East.

## 21.2 Implications of Transportation, Security, Commerce, Housing, Environment, Healthcare/Safety

To make Lagos an economic hub and attraction that is liveable for all, a strong health dimension comes to significance as the liveability of a city, town or any community for that matter will require an efficient and effective health care delivery service and system. For Lagos to be liveable for all its inhabitants, Government authorities, as well as the local population would have to create and maintain an enabling environment that allows Lagosians to meet their maximum human capability. Above all, it would need to establish a health service delivery system that is accessible, qualitative, affordable and diverse. This process can best be fascilitated by using innovative public health approaches and the use of technology. It would also have to revisit its existing public health services and infrastructure to meet the growing health needs of populations in the megacity. The Lagos state government, in collaboration with the federal government is already making major investments in health and it is hoped that these investments, both human and infrastructural would would prepare Lagos state public health authorities to quickly manage a disease outbreak. However, at this stage, the state is directing much of its efforts towards preventive measures, especially after its experience with Ebola in 2014. To achieve these goals, Lagos state has adopted a number of policies aimed at improving overall population health.

Current policy direction includes environmental infrastructure such as the much needed drainage and sewage systems. Others are policies on waste management, green areas, the reduction of pollution, slum reclamation, multimodal-transportationl system, Lagos bus rapid transit system, traffic law, Security-trust fund, disaster management, low-cost housing, health care, Safety-infrastructure, public health financing, health promotion and disease prevention.

### 21.2.1 *Incident Management Approach: Existing Institutional Structures, Mechanisms and Capacity Plan*

The following are established mechanisms to ensure there is an effective health incident management plan which will mitigate risks to safety:

- Rapid Response Teams
- Lagos State Emergency Management Agency (backed by law)
- Functional and effective Emergency Preparedness and Response Committees in all the tiers of health care delivery.
- Infectious Disease Hospital i.e. Mainland Hospital, Yaba (MHY)
- Lagos State Ambulance Service (LASAMBUS) – was very useful in transporting suspects who took ill from their homes to EVD isolation/referral center
- Public Health Law
- Coroner's Law/crematorium
- Sanitation Law
- State Environmental Health Monitoring Unit
- Integrated Disease Surveillance and Response (IDSR) system at both the State and Local Government levels for routine surveillance and notification, with this platform taken advantage of in tracing of contacts
- Lagos State Waste Management Authority
- Experience garnered in tackling previous emergencies and epidemics e.g. cholera, SARS, bomb blast, DANA air crash, etc.

## 21.3 Ebola Virus Disease Outbreak: Pre-outbreak General Measures

The following measures have been taken for pre-outbreak readiness: the development of Fact Sheets which contain advocacy on the preventive/protective measures from more general and immediate information such as: frequent hand washing, avoidance of contact with infected people, professional handling of corpses.

Advocacy has continued after the 2014 outbreak and significant investments have gone into rapidly institutionalizing emerging infection-control procedures such as: establishing standard operating policies / procedures on the use of Personal Protective Equipment (PPE); the activation of collaboration protocols with the Federal Ministry of Health's Port Health Services in the screening of persons coming into the Lagos via air, sea and land borders. The Lagos state health authorities have designated the Infectious Disease Hospital, Yaba (MHY) as the referral center for any suspected/confirmed cases of any emerging infectious disease, including Ebola and Lassa fever. Also, the Lagos state government has mandate all public health facilities to create an isolation ward for suspected cases of Ebola and Lassa fever, and to provide healthcare workers with a buffer stock of PPEs and body bags.

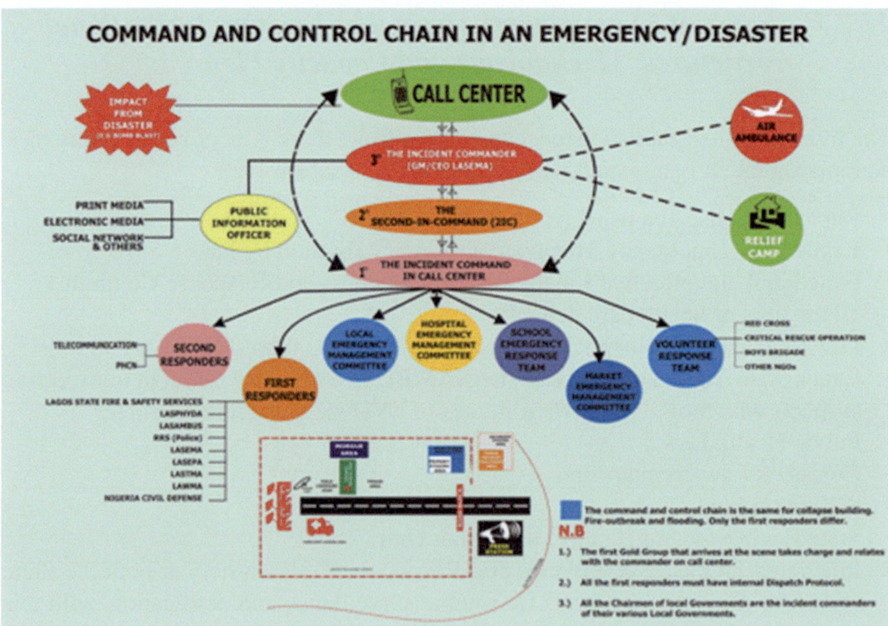

## 21.4 Lessons from Nigeria: Foundations of a Successful Emergency Response

Nigeria's experience in putting a stop to the spread of the deadly EVD virus has clearly been a learning experience. As a result here are some points which sum up what was learned; teamwork, fear is a good motivator, the need for expert technical leadership and technical assistance, incentives for health workers, the need for operational efficiencies and the importance of data and information sharing (Fig. 21.1).

### *21.4.1 Response Teams*

The following response teams are crucial for a successful public health emergency: Epidemiology/Surveillance (to include all points of entry to the country), case management/infection prevention & control. Other important infrastructural elements are; laboratories, appropriate management and coordination leadership teams.

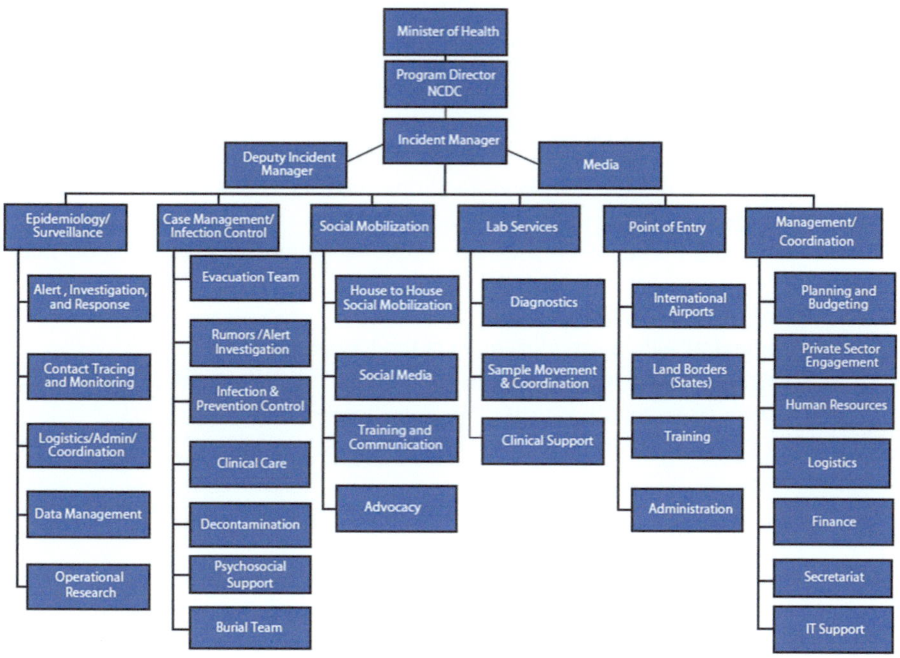


**Fig. 21.1** Diagram showing different stakeholders and processes required for effective response to outbreaks. (Source: WHO Facts Sheet: Ebola Virus Disease. http://www.who.int/news-room/fact-sheets/detail/ebola-virus-disease. Assessed on 19th July, 2018)

#### 21.4.1.1 Post-outbreak Immediate Measures-Response-1

- Epidemiology & Surveillance
- Adoption of the *Incident Management* approach
- Initiation of WHO protocol governing management of the disease
- Constitution of a broad-based multi-agency Rapid Response Treams (RRT)
- Establishment of the Incident Management/Ebola Emergency Operations Center, Core Strategic Planning and Decision-making team and Response Teams
- Development of strategic plan of action.
- Commencement of active and immediate contact tracing regarding primary contacts
- Press conference held to sensitize Lagosians and indeed Nigerians on the arrival of EVD in the state and country
- Same day cremation of the corpse of the index case, following due preparation, decontamination, evacuation
- Decontamination of the affected hospital
- On-the-spot training of all relevant staff (morticians and environmental health workers) on evacuation

#### 21.4.1.2 Post-outbreak Immediate Measures-Response 2

- Laboratory confirmation of cases
- Aggressive tracing of primary *(70)* and secondary/tertiary *(298)* contacts
- Decontamination of affected health facilities and homes of suspected/confirmed cases admitted
- Evacuation and burial of corpses and implementation of a protocol on mass gathering
- Shut down of NNPC Clinic, Lagos.
- Establishment of a Point of entry team at the Lagos airport
- The Screening of persons entering Lagos through the different national borders
- Development of screening instruments

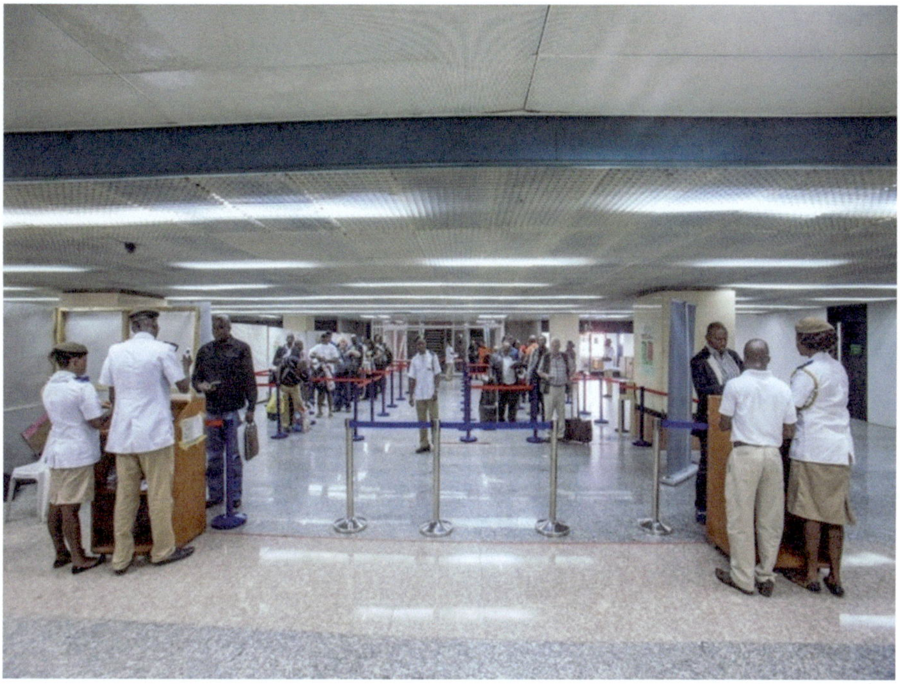

#### 21.4.1.3 Post-outbreak Immediate Measures-Response 3

- Case Management/IPC Team
- Upgrading of MHY as referral/isolation center. 40-bed Male and Female Wards for confirmed cases
- Eight (8_-bed Isolation Ward upgraded to hold suspected cases, backed up by
- Two (2) emergency tents to hold additional 24 suspected cases
- Dedicated 60KVA generator
- Dedicated borehole
- Burn and bury pit for waste management
- 2–5000 liter septic tanks (one each for urine and faeces) – ready for decontamination prior to evacuation
- Activation of the crematorium to cremate corpses of confirmed cases.

#### 21.4.1.4 Post-outbreak Immediate Measures-Response 4

- Case Management/IPC Team (Cont'd)
- Dedicated ambulances for transport cases to referral center
- Dedicated environmental health purpose built vans to transport corpses
- Development of treatment SOPs

- Capacity building of relevant health workers
- Provision of psycho-social support to cases and their families
- Call for volunteers to fill critical human resource gap with same backed with life insurance cover, safe work environment, and daily incentives
- Establishment of additional isolation center outside of MHY to play host to quarantining some suspected cases.

#### 21.4.1.5 Post-outbreak Immediate Measures-Response 5

- Social Mobilization Team
- Initial Mapping – community, stakeholders (including health workers), risk, political, incidence and contact.
- Advocacy to/sensitization of relevant stakeholders (Community Development As, CDCs, market men and women association, traditional and religious leaders, Lagos State Public Servants, Association of Private School Proprietors, NYSC, transport operators, morgue operators, etc.)
- Development of messages in different formats (public service announcements, jingles fan-tapes for motorized campaign and bulk SMS) and in different languages to cater for the different population
- IEC materials (fact sheets, FAQs, and hand-washing)
- Media appearances to allay fears and address concerns which include possible cure, denial i.e. need to report early for treatment, and stigmatization

**Engaging Communities**

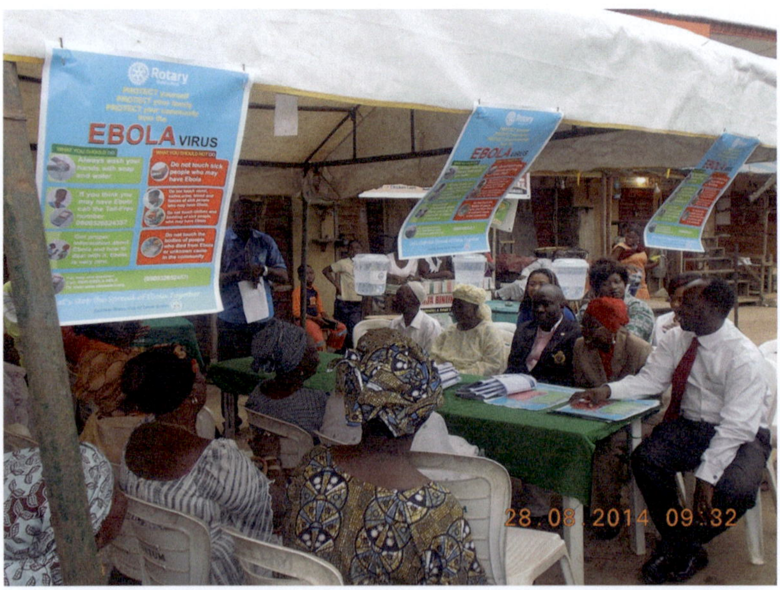

#### 21.4.1.6 Post-outbreak Immediate Measures-Response 5

- Social mobilization Team
- Frequent press briefings on cases of Ebola and respond strategies
- Use of social media platforms communicate information on Ebola. This included the use of services like
- Bulk messages on the prevention to subscribers of two major networks in Nigeria, that is- MTN and Airtel
- The introduction of n Ebola Help Line: **0800 EBOLA HELP (0800 32652 4357)**
- The development of a website that provided up-to data information on Ebola in Nigeria as well as other useful resources on Ebola prevention and management: **www.ebolaalert.org**
- The use of LiveChat messaging platforms:
- Facebook: **fb.com/ww.ebolaalert**
- Twitter: @ebolaalert

Community engagement took the form of grassroots mobilization (house-to-house, motorized campaigns, for example, road shows and engagement of town announcers, collaboration with Nollywood stars and high profile musicians, community dialogue in high risk communities).

### *21.4.2 Role of Traditional Medical Practitioners*

Since 1980, the Lagos State had enacted a law establishing the Traditional Medicine Board[2]. The board was established to regulate the code of conduct and practice of traditional medicine practitioners in Lagos state to accredit, monitor and license all traditional medicine practitioners and traditional clinics/health facilities premises. To this end, and while a great population of Lagosians patronize traditional medicines and health service providers, it was easy to mobilize and partner with persons and establishments that provided alternative medicine and healing. Lagos has an inclusive framework.

---

[2]The Board was established by the administration of Alhaji Lateef Jakande. Then the executive governor in 1980, by law 13th of governor in the Laws of Lagos 1980 caps 103 of 19194

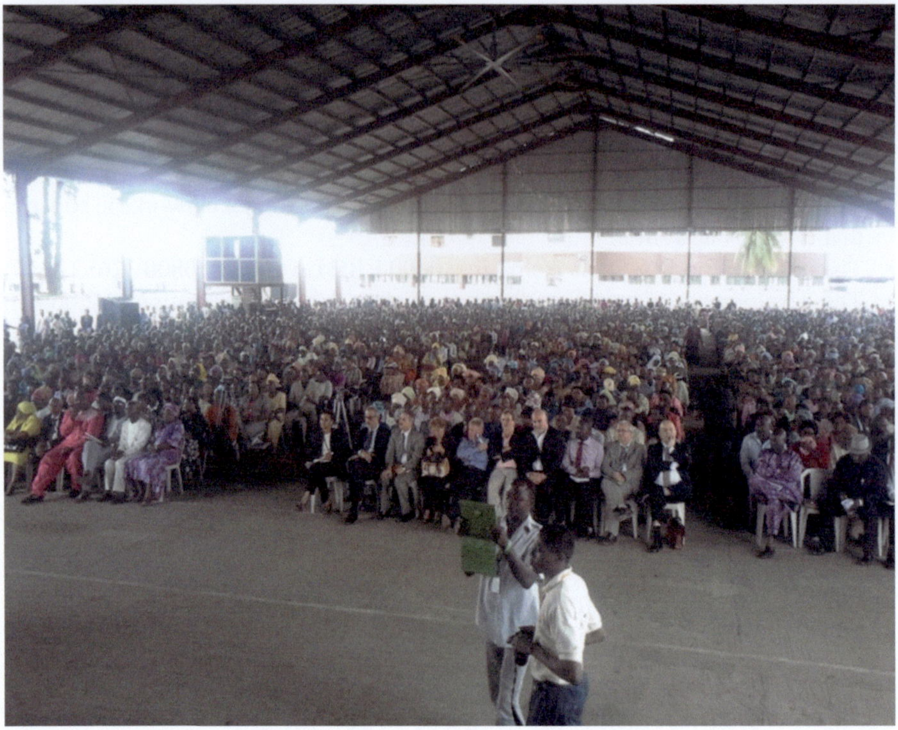

### 21.4.3 Training

Infection prevention and control, inter-personal communication, case management includes the handling of Level III Pandemic Personal Protective Equipment (PPE); emergency crisis communications management; school health officers on preventive measures and referrals; emergency preparedness for port health services staff; the use of hand-held radios for volunteers at primary screening points (Port Health Services) and evacuation and decontamination procedures and training.

### 21.4.4 Capacity Building

Capacity building and strengthening cut across disciplines. In the Sciences this occurred for all staff, clinical and non-clinical including laboratory science, bio-banking and disease surveillance teams In the Public Health. Also, Research and Data Management, Disaster and Emergency response and communications teams received training. Supply logistics in the field of administration and management; in governance, policy development, operational frameworks, regulatory capabilities and legal teams to include that of advocacy and ethics participated in capacity building exercises.

## 21.5 Challenges

At the inception of the outbreak, there was a strike by medical doctors in Nigeria. This led to a delay in securing adequate health care teams (especially doctors, nurses, public health experts) to effectively respond to the Ebola crisis. There was a lot of panic, fear and anxiety amongst health care workers, political leaders and the population, in general. During contact tracing, some people were difficult, evasive and downright hostile. They hid information and others preferred discrete follow-up. Stigmatization of both contacts and cases was a serious issue. Rumors, especially through the social media platforms travelled fast. There was community resistance due to ignorance in the spheres of religion and culture. For instance, in terms of religion, there was the tendency for some who suspected that they might have been contracted Ebola to make the churches or mosques the first port of call, while many traditionalists preferred to visit traditional medicine practitioners. Of course there were the rumors that the use of traditional medical potions had been used to treat persons infected with Ebola in certain communities. Undoubtedly, all these were anecdotes with hardly any evidential basis. If anything, they only made it difficult for public health authorities to contain the spread of the disease.

## 21.6 Key Success Factors

The factors which led to the success of the outbreak were of a diverse nature and could be grouped into: political will, good leadership, teamwork; robust inter-governmental, inter-agency and inter-sectorial collaboration; aggressive contact tracing, monitoring; effective surveillance and contact tracing activities with case management (basic instruction – temperature monitoring etc.); active rumour and alert investigation; aggressive public enlightenment campaign (role of media); availability of SOPs, protocols and other relevant materials from partners that were quickly adapted for use in Nigeria; use of mobile phone technology enabled real-time follow-up of contacts and prompt detection of those with symptoms; data management from the beginning and use of data to monitor response; training and re-training of health workers and support from the private sector mainly non-governmental organizations.

## 21.7 Post Containment

External vigilance remained the watchword during and after the outbreak. During post containment, public engagement activities were used to provide psychosocial support to survivors and affected communities. These public health activities also helped to address issues of stigmatas and created a sense of awareness amongst the population. Increasingly, the public became more alert and willing to report suspected EVD cases in their communities. They also demonstrated knowledge on, and had access to, the proper procedures for reporting suspected cases. Equally all Ports of entry into Lagos, for example airports and national/international borders were equipped with the necessary resources required for early detection and reporting of all suspected cases of Ebola.

Training and continues education of health care workers on management of EIDs were prioritised by the Lagos state government. This was in addition to: building research capacity for EIDs, scaling up of emergency preparedness and response activities at health care facilities; upgrading the infectious disease hospital in Lagos, through the acquisition of an apheresis equipment to examine the use of convalescent serum; as well as an upgrade of the isolation units. The majority of these activities were funded by the international donor agencies such as the Bill and Melinda Gates Foundation.

## 21.8 Key Conclusions for Health Sector Reform and Service Delivery Systems

Following the curbing of the spread of Ebola in Lagos, and Nigeria as a whole, the World Health Organisation made key recommendations that LMICs need to adopt in terms of preparedness for infectious disease outbreaks (WHO 2015). These recommendations centre on leadership, timely intervention; autonomy of policy makers, incentives for health care workers, evidenced based decision making and technical assistance to resource limited countries. The effective management of a case of Ebola in Lagos state is reflected in these recommendations, giving credence to arguments that if African countries were to implement the WHO recommendations, they will stand a good chance to bringing an outbreak under reasonable control. Details of these are provided below:

**Effective Coordination and Leadership** The ability of the Lagos state government to effectively stop the spread of EVD in Lagos was, in a large part, due to strong political and technical leadership. Despite the fact that Lagos is densely populated and that a good proportion of the population stays in slum, coupled with systemic weaknesses in the health system, the Lagos State and indeed the Nigerian government was able to reorganise itself and to effectively respond to the first and subsequent cases of Ebola in Lagos. Firstly, Nigeria had a first-rate virology laboratory that is affiliated to the Lagos State University Teaching Hospital. This unit is equipped with the appropriate infrastructure and resources to diagnose a case of Ebola virus disease. Therefore, there was some level of preparedness. Secondly, once it was confirmed that there was a case of Ebola in Nigeria, the government reacted promptly and quickly allocated funds for an emergency response. This was crucial in planning interventions to curb the spread of the disease.

**Timely Actions** The timely reaction by the Nigerian government to news of a case of Ebola in Nigeria had a spiral effect on planning and management. The Federal government immediately declared that there was a national public health emergency and this led to health facilities taking timely action to prevent the spread and to educate staff members. This shows that early ownership by the government that the health system is in crisis is important where there is the threat of an epidemic. As a result of this, the government, quickly asked that designated Ebola treatment and isolation facilities be set up built in Lagos and Port Harcourt, the tow cites that had reported cases of Ebola. More so, the government quickly set up sensitisation campaigns including: house-to-house health education programs, radio programs in English and local dialects. Much investment also went into contact tracing with the government adopting to use real-time contact tracing and daily contact mapping.

**Meaningful Autonomy** Giving mid-level managers control over their operations circumvents unwieldy bureaucracy that can throttle a rapid response. It allows them to find innovative solutions and can catalyse the efficient decentralization of functions. This is consistent with the findings of performance-based financing interventions which shows that health care results are achieved not by policy makers but by technical cadres at optional levels, particularly when they are granted autonomy.

**Incentives for Health Care Workers** In the wake of an outbreak, the workload on health care workers is further stressed. When the epidemic is one that kills fast, the chances or emotional burn out could lead to an inertia of heath care workers to respond to the increasing workload. Incentives can help motivate health care workers. Such incentives could be monetary or otherwise. However, it must be done such that it is in line with the broader socio-economic, political, cultural, lineage of the country.

**Available Infrastructure** It is important that governments, through their ministries of health, and associated government structures, identify existing assets and resources, infrastructural, human or fiscal that could be easily accessed and used during an outbreak and in curbing a possible outbreak. For example, once it was announced that there was a case of Ebola in Nigeria, the government instructed that available technologies that were in place for use in polio eradication program, be repurposed to support the Ebola response.

**Data Driven Decision Making** It is important that decisions during an outbreak are evidence-based driven. During an infectious disease outbreak, lots of data is generated but is not used to guide decision making. This should not be the case. During an outbreak, it is important that healthcare facilities make information on the epidemic available for use by policy makers. The advantage being that, if information is available and properly generated, it could foster the potential for real-time learning and effective decision making.

**Relevant Technical Assistance** In an outbreak situation, the importance of technical assistance, especially in resource limited settings, cannot be overemphasized. International health agencies and non-governmental organisations such as the WHO, and MSF stand a good chance to support national governments to quickly respond to threats of an outbreak. It is important that such a response be provided in a timely fashion taking into consideration local systems, organizational culture and political dynamics of the affected country. This can be best achieved if these organisations collaborate with local experts and national governments.

## Key Statistics on the Ebola Outbreak in Lagos, Nigeria

| S/N | Cases | | National | Lagos | Rivers |
|---|---|---|---|---|---|
| 1 | Cumulative No. of cases | Confirmed | 19 | 15 | 4 |
| | | Probable | 1 | 1 | 0 |
| | | Suspected | 0 | 0 | 0 |
| 2 | Cumulative No. of deaths (+ index case) | Confirmed | 7 | 5 | 2 |
| | | Probable | 1 | 1 | 0 |
| | | Suspected | 0 | 0 | 0 |
| 3 | Case Fatality Rate – Confirmed + Probable | | 40% | 37.5% | 50% |
| 4 | No. of patients in isolation facility | Confirmed | 0 | 0 | 0 |
| | | Suspected | 0 | 0 | 0 |
| 5 | Date of last discharged case | Confirmed | - | Sept 2 | Sept 7 |
| 6 | Cumulative No. of discharges | Confirmed | 12 | 11 | 1 |
| 7 | Cumulative confirmed cases among health care workers | | 11 | 9 | 2 |
| 8 | Cumulative deaths among health care workers | | 5 | 4 | 1 |
| 9 | Cumulative No. of contacts listed | | 891 | 365 | 526 |
| 10 | Contacts under follow-up as at Oct 8 | | 0 | 0 | 0 |
| 11 | Contacts that have completed 21 days follow-up | | 890 | 365 | 525 |
| 12 | Contacts lost to follow-up | | 1 | 0 | 1 |

Source: Lagos State Ministry of Health. 2014 Joint Ebola Emergency Operations Files. Available on request from the Office of the Commissioner, Lagos State Ministry of Health, Lagos State Secretariat, Alausa, Lagos.

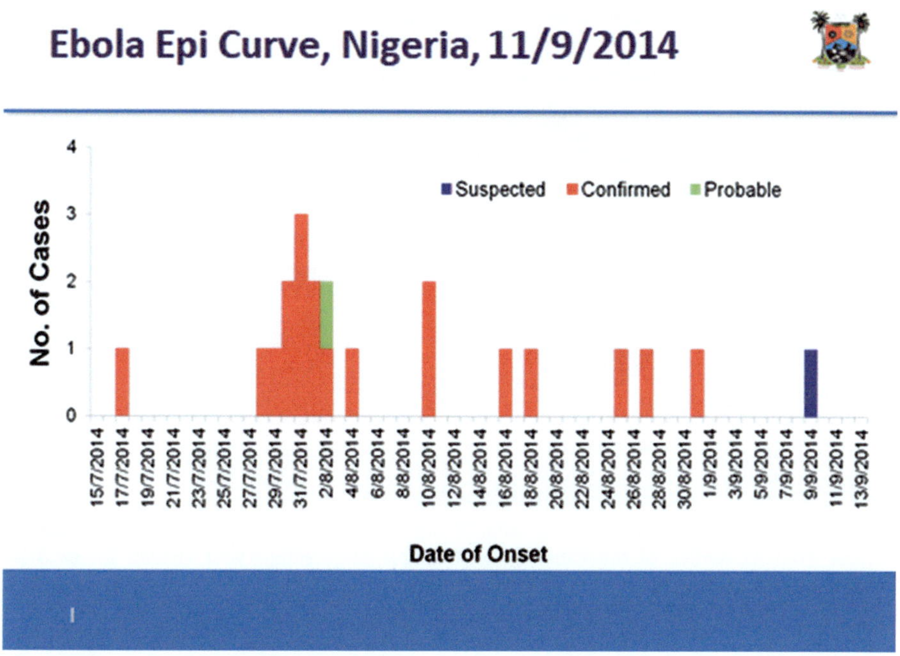
Ebola Epi Curve, Nigeria, 11/9/2014
Suspected
Confirmed
Probable
No. of Cases
0
1
2
3
4
15/7/2014
17/7/2014
19/7/2014
21/7/2014
23/7/2014
25/7/2014
27/7/2014
29/7/2014
31/7/2014
2/8/2014
4/8/2014
6/8/2014
8/8/2014
10/8/2014
12/8/2014
14/8/2014
16/8/2014
18/8/2014
20/8/2014
22/8/2014
24/8/2014
26/8/2014
28/8/2014
30/8/2014
1/9/2014
3/9/2014
5/9/2014
7/9/2014
9/9/2014
11/9/2014
13/9/2014
Date of Onset

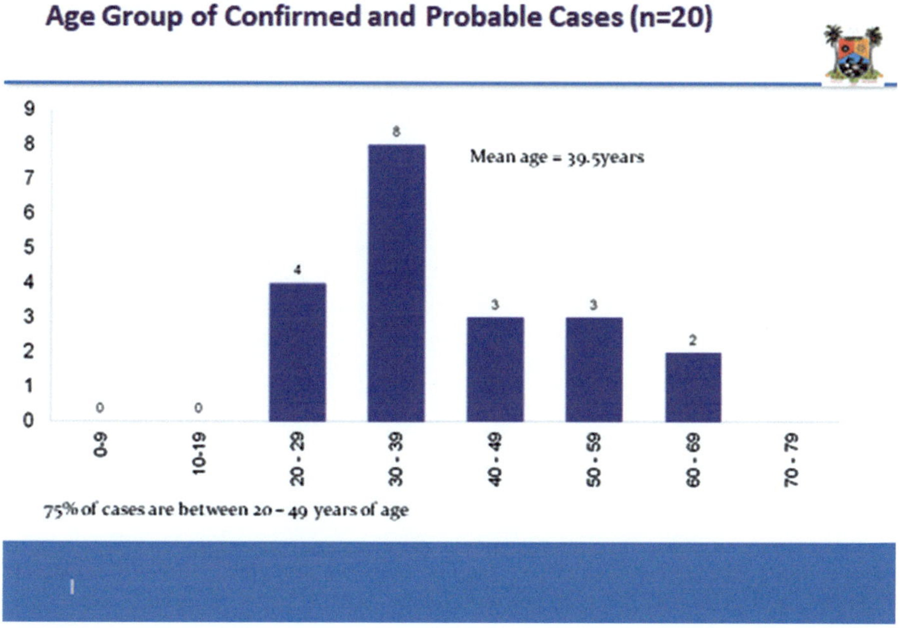
Age Group of Confirmed and Probable Cases (n=20)
Mean age = 39.5years
0
1
2
3
4
5
6
7
8
9
0-9
10-19
20 - 29
30 - 39
40 - 49
50 - 59
60 - 69
70 - 79
75% of cases are between 20 – 49 years of age

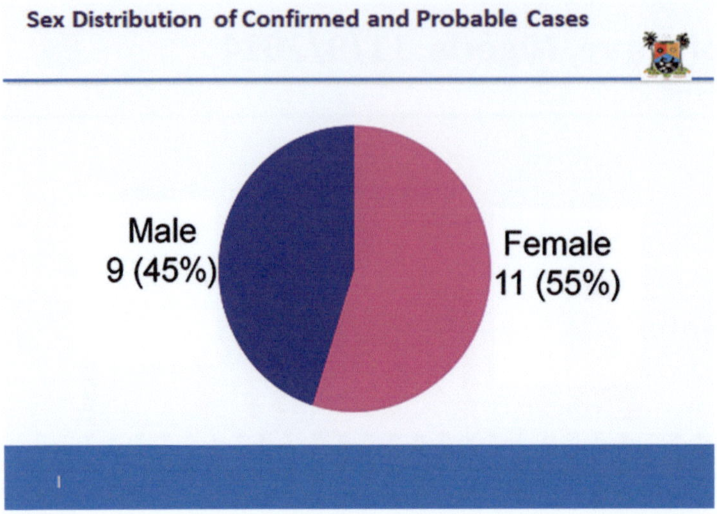


Lagos State Ministry of Health. 2014 Joint Ebola Emergency Operations Files. Available on request from the Office of the Commissioner, Lagos State Ministry of Health, Lagos State Secretariat, Alausa, Lagos.

## Frequency of signs and symptoms

| Symptom* | Frequency | Percent |
|---|---|---|
| Fever | 12 | 85.7% |
| Fatigue | 8 | 57.1% |
| Vomiting | 8 | 57.1% |
| Diarrhea | 8 | 57.1% |
| Anorexia | 7 | 50.0% |
| Headache | 3 | 21.4% |
| JointPain | 3 | 21.4% |
| Conjunctivitis | 2 | 14.3% |
| MusclePain | 2 | 14.3% |
| BleedingNose | 1 | 7.1% |
| BleedingSkin | 1 | 7.1% |
| BleedingUrine | 1 | 7.1% |
| BleedingVagina | 1 | 7.1% |
| Confused | 1 | 7.1% |
| PainEyes | 1 | 7.1% |
| SoreThroat | 1 | 7.1% |

Case presentation in line with case definition currently in use

*For confirmed and probable cases only

Source: Lagos State Ministry of Health. Internal Epidemiology Files: 2014 EVD Outbreak. Available at the office of the Commissioner, Lagos State Ministry of Health, Lagos State Secretariat, Alausa, Lagos.

### Type of contact with source case (n=20)

| Contact Type | Frequency | Percent |
|---|---|---|
| Had direct physical contact with the body | 14 | 70 |
| Touched body fluids | 4 | 20 |
| Touched or shared linens, clothes | 1 | 5 |
| Unknown | 1 | 5 |
| TOTAL | 20 | 100.0 |

Lagos State Ministry of Health. 2014 Joint Ebola Emergency Operations Files. Available on request from the Office of the Commissioner, Lagos State Ministry of Health, Lagos State Secretariat, Alausa, Lagos.

## Some Key Timelines

- Average duration from onset to admission (for discharge patients) = 3 days
- Average duration from onset to admission (for deaths) = 5 days

  Differences were not statistically significant
- Average hospital stay = 10 days (range: 2 – 21 days)
- Average duration of illness (Date of onset to discharge) = 15 days (range: 7 – 25 days)
- Average duration of illness for dead (Date of onset to death) = 11 days (range: 6 – 19 days)

  Differences were not statistically significant

DATA prepared by Dr. Jide Idris Commissioner for Health, Lagos State Nigeria.

*Pictures of persons included in this chapter were taken by the Federal and Lagos State Ministry of health, Nigeria during its public health awareness campaigns against Ebola. Approval to publish pictures is provided by the Commissioner of Health, Lagos State Government.*

## References

Aliyu, A. A., & Amadu, L. (2017). Urbanization, cities, and health: The challenges to Nigeria – A review. *Annals of African Medicine, 16*(4), 149–158.

Ayeni, A. O. (2017). Increasing population, urbanization and climatic factors in Lagos State, Nigeria: The nexus and implications on water demand and supply. *Journal of Global Initiatives: Policy, Pedagogy, Perspective, 11*(2), 6.

UN. (2016). *The world's cities in 2016.* Data Booklet. http://www.un.org/en/development/desa/population/publications/pdf/urbanization/the_worlds_cities_in_2016_data_booklet.pdf. Accessed 26 Oct 2018.

WHO. (2015, January). *Successful Ebola responses in Nigeria, Senegal and Mali. One year into the Ebola epidemic.* http://www.who.int/csr/disease/ebola/one-year-report/nigeria/en/ Accessed 27 Oct 2018.